Canine and Feline Dermatology

Canine and Feline Dermatology

K. P. Baker MA MSc PhD DVD FRCVS
Professor
Faculty of Veterinary Medicine
University College
Ballsbridge
Dublin
S. Ireland

L. R. Thomsett DVD FRCVS
Senior Lecturer
Royal Veterinary College
London

BLACKWELL SCIENTIFIC PUBLICATIONS
OXFORD LONDON EDINBURGH
BOSTON MELBOURNE

Editorial offices:
Osney Mead, Oxford OX2 0EL
25 John Street, London WC1N 2BL
23 Ainslie Place, Edinburgh EH3 6AJ
3 Cambridge Center, Suite 208
Cambridge, Massachusetts 02142, USA
107 Barry Street, Carlton
Victoria 3053, Australia

First published 1990

Set by Setrite Typesetters Ltd, Hong Kong
Printed and bound in Great Britain
by William Clowes Ltd, Beccles and London

DISTRIBUTORS

Marston Book Services Ltd
PO Box 87
Oxford OX2 0DT
(*Orders*: Tel: 0865 791155
Fax: 0865 791927
Telex: 837515)

USA
Year Book Medical Publishers
200 North LaSalle Street
Chicago, Illinois 60601
(*Orders*: Tel: (312) 726–9733)

Canada
The C.V. Mosby Company
5240 Finch Avenue East
Scarborough, Ontario
(*Orders*: Tel: (416) 298–1588)

Australia
Blackwell Scientific Publications
(Australia) Pty Ltd
107 Barry Street
Carlton, Victoria 3053
(*Orders*: Tel: (03) 347–0300)

British Library
Cataloguing in Publication Data

Baker, K. P.
Canine and feline dermatology.
1. Livestock: Dogs. Skin. Diseases 2. Pets: Cats. Skin. Diseases
I. Title II. Thomsett, L. R.
636.7'08965

ISBN 0–632–02092–X

Contents

Preface

For many years both authors have had the privilege of specializing in dermatology, teaching generations of veterinary students and presenting courses on continuing education to veterinary graduates. We hope to pass on the benefits of our experience to a wider audience in this text. It is intended for undergraduates as an aid to clinical diagnosis and therapy, for practitioners, and to all those interested in comparative dermatology. Descriptive matter has been limited as far as possible for clarity to permit the inclusion of as many illustrations as production costs would permit.

The majority of illustrations are by the authors. Credit is given in the text where the illustrations of others have been used. We are most grateful to those who have aided us in this way.

1 / Biology and Physiology of the Skin

The skin is the organ which protects the body from the environment, and its functions are numerous. Whilst most functions are basic to most mammals, special functions may have been developed in some. The basic structure and functions of the skin are shown in Fig. 1.1.

If skin is cut vertically to the surface, three distinct layers are seen, the epidermis, dermis and subcutis. The skin is of variable thickness in different parts of the body, e.g. it is thickest over the dorsal trunk and thinnest on the ventral abdomen. It is elastic and variably moveable, the skin being relatively immobile on the lower limbs yet freely mobile over the lateral trunk.

Most of the body surface is covered by hair which is of variable length but it is absent or sparse in some areas, e.g.

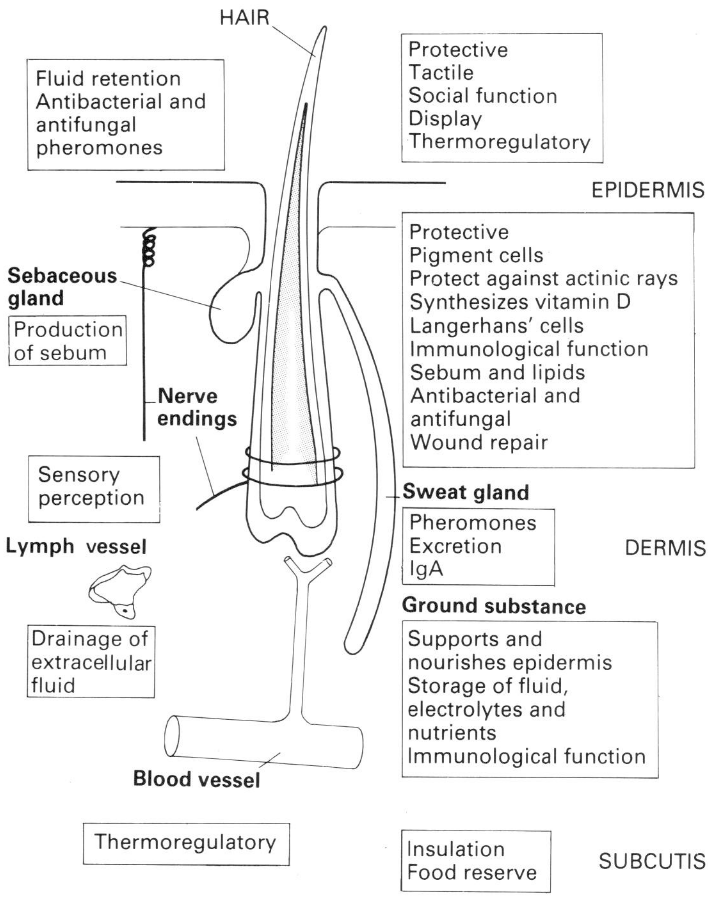

Fig. 1.1. Basic structure and function of the skin.

around the body orifices, the ventral surface of the proximal end of the tail and the inner aspects of the pinna.

Some parts of the body show extreme modification of the skin, e.g. the distal phalanges are modified into claws which have various functions. These specialized areas will be described in detail later.

Close examination of the surface reveals it is not smooth: if the hair covering is clipped off and the skin examined with the light microscope the surface is seen to be irregular with small prominences — these are the tylotrich pads (epidermal papillae) containing mechanoreceptors (Straile, 1960; Brown & Iggo, 1967).

Hairs leave the epidermis at an acute angle and are arranged in groups of compound follicles of two to five, most of them in triads (Fig. 1.2). Each compound follicle will contain a single stout primary (guard) hair, which extends somewhat more deeply into the dermis and subcutis, and several secondary (undercoat) hairs of variable diameter. Hairs of different colour may occupy the same compound follicle. The primary hair of the central follicle in a triad will usually be the stoutest. Compound follicles share a common pilary canal to the openings of the sebaceous ducts into the pilary canal. The flow of the hair follows the tension lines in the skin (Langer's lines).

Examination of the surface of the skin using the scanning electron microscope shows the epidermis to be covered by a very thin lipid sheet which in places is seen to be detached in fine flakes from the underlying surface (Fig. 1.3) revealing

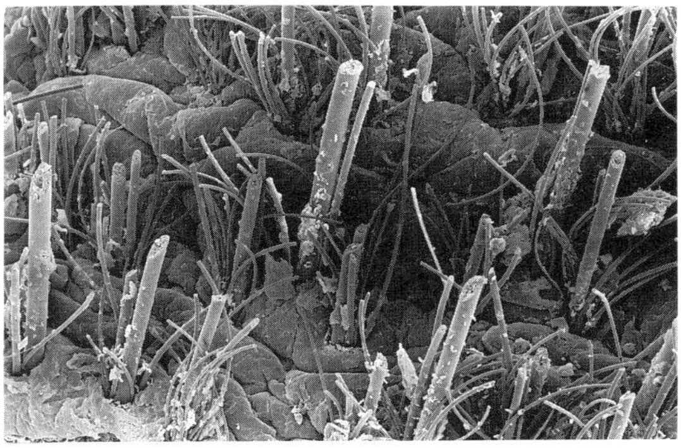

Fig. 1.2. Scanning electron micrograph of the interscapular skin of the dog revealing compound hair follicles.

There is a single, stout primary hair per compound follicle.

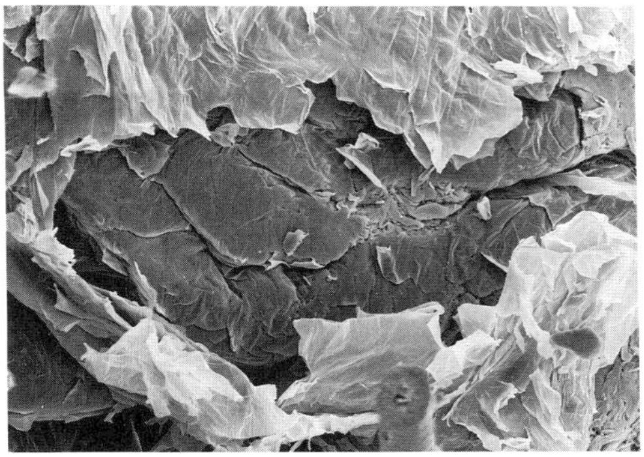

Fig. 1.3. Scanning electron micrograph of the epidermis of the interscapular region of the dog. The surface is covered by a thin lipid sheet which in some places is displaced to reveal individual keratinocytes of the stratum corneum.

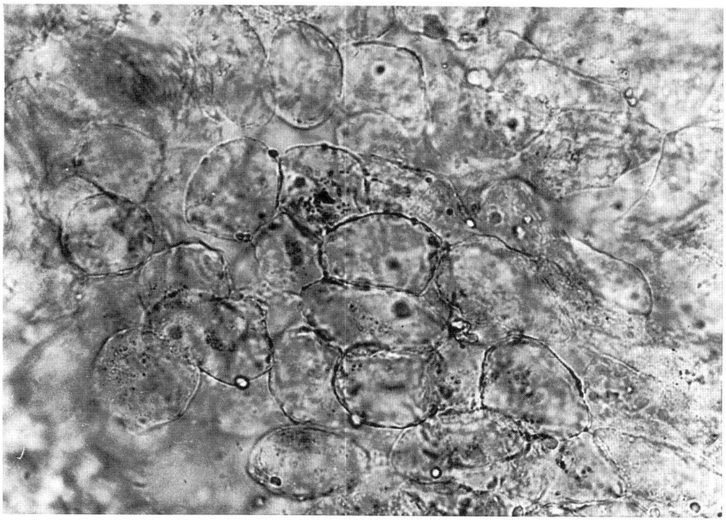

Fig. 1.4. Potassium hydroxide digest of the stratum corneum revealing individual exfoliating keratinocytes.

individual keratinocytes. These are very thin, flattened, keratinized epidermal cells — the final product of the stratum germinativum. Potassium hydroxide digests show them to be hexagonal without nuclear remnants (Fig. 1.4). Exfoliation of normal skin is a continuous process and apparently occurs by small groups of keratinocytes, one cell thick, leaving the surface. In normal animals, the pilary canals are usually patent and not plugged by lipidaceous material and exfoliated keratinocytes.

The epidermis

The epidermis contains a number of cells with different functions and origins whilst the relatively acellular dermis is of dense connective tissue containing vascular and neural networks, with glands and epidermal appendages descending into it. It is separated from the epidermis by the basement membrane. The epidermis of hirsute skin is considerably different in appearance from that of the glabrous, specialized areas like the lips and foot pads. In the former, it is much thinner (approximately 20 μm), and clear division into several layers is not seen (Baker, 1966). Hirsute skin is made up of usually two to three layers of cells upon which rest the compact keratinized cells of the stratum corneum (Fig. 1.5). The cells resting on the basement membrane are cuboidal in shape with large vesicular nuclei and one or two nucleoli; this is the germinal layer. Paraffin processing of this layer often produces some nuclear shrinkage so that the nuclei may appear to be surrounded by a halo. In hirsute skin, it is usually possible to see a further layer of germinal cells which are not yet undergoing keratinization. Some of these cells in dog skin contain brown melanin pigment. The cells in this layer stain less deeply with basophilic stains.

Above the germinal layer is the stratum granulosum layer in which cells undergo rapid keratinization and become flattened as they are subjected to pressure from below and above. In hirsute skin, the thin stratum granulosum merges imperceptibly into the stratum corneum in which individual cell outlines cannot be seen. Paraffin processing results in some separation of the thin stratum corneum giving it a honeycomb appearance. The epidermis of glabrous skin in some regions resembles that of human skin (Fig. 1.6).

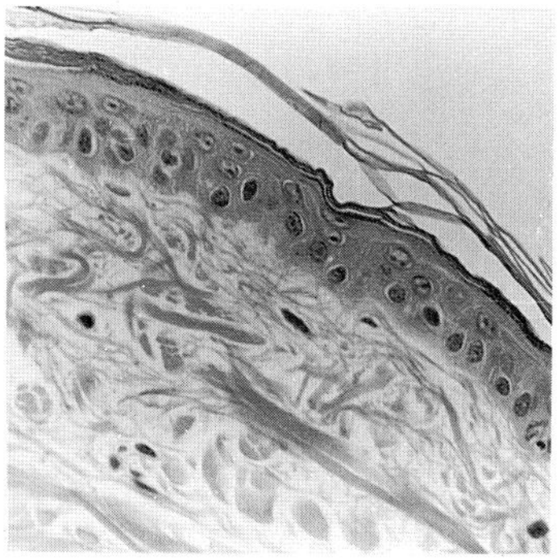

Fig. 1.5. Hirsute epidermis of the cat.

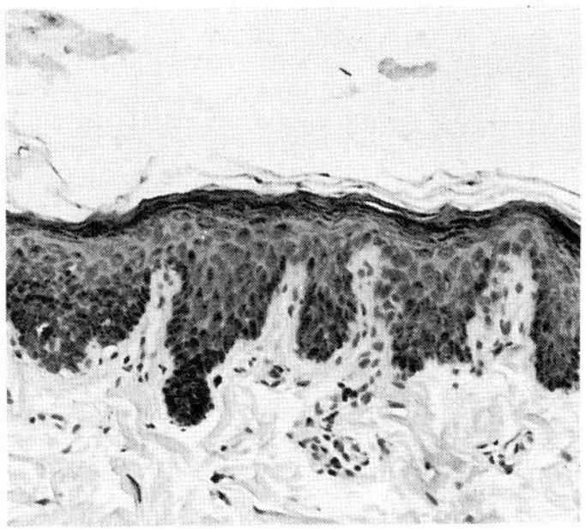

Fig. 1.6. Glabrous epidermis (cat lip). The epidermis is much thicker than the hirsute epidermis (Fig. 1.5).

In the stratum corneum the cells are hexagonal in shape with a regular alternative overlapping between the edges of cells with individual hexagons surrounded by two sets of three hexagons. Desquamation only occurs when a hexagon is not overlapped by its neighbouring six hexagons.

It is estimated that 10% of cells in the stratum basale of human skin undergo mitosis daily. It is calculated that a single keratinocyte enters each column daily as a keratinocyte is desquamated (Allen, 1977). As each keratinocyte moves towards the surface, its shape changes radically from that of a cylinder. It becomes progressively keratinized and flattened indicating a pressure gradient towards the surface. The nucleus becomes flattened, deeply staining and is finally lost. The surface keratinocyte is now a very thin, flattened squame in the stratum corneum, which is composed of soft keratin in contrast to the hard keratin of the hair and claws. In the normal hirsute skin of beagle dogs, the time taken for keratinocytes to pass from the basal layer to the stratum granulosum is estimated to be 22 days (Baker *et al.*, 1973). There is evidence that keratinocytes pass to the surface of the stratum corneum in single-cell stacks (the epidermal proliferation unit); each stack is maintained by vertical migration in the group of 10 basal cells beneath it.

Clear cells of the epidermis

These are the melanocytes, Langerhans' cells and Merkel cells.

MELANOCYTES

When the epidermis is stained with haematoxylin and eosin, about 10% of the cells in the basal layer are revealed to have dark-staining nuclei and clear cytoplasm. These are the melanocytes. Melanocytes are located in the basal layer of the epidermis and in the hair papillae. Bloch's dopa reaction or silver stains reveal them because they contain tyrosine. Melanocytes have numerous dendritic processes and unlike basal cells are not attached to their neighbours by intercellular bridges. The melanocyte is derived from the neural crest, migrating to the epidermis during early embryonic life. Its function is to produce pigment which is passed to the keratinocytes by long, slender cytoplasmic projections. Those in the hair follicles produce melanin during the anagen (active) stage of the hair cycle; during the telogen (resting) stage, activity is not detected.

The hirsute surface epidermis of the cat contains no melanin granules. However, the prepuce, the scrotum, teats and anal sac do contain pigment (Strickland & Calhoun, 1963; Baker, 1974).

The degree of pigmentation of the skin is determined by the activity of the melanocytes and not by increasing numbers: thus, pigmented skin contains the same number of cells as unpigmented skin.

Melanocytes are characterized by containing the enzyme tyrosinase which is essential for the production of melanin within organelles — the melanosomes — which are then passed to the keratinocytes in the stratum germinativum.

Greying of the hair in humans results from reduced production of melanosomes by the melanocytes and is age dependent. However, there is considerable variation in the age when this commences in different breeds of dog. It becomes apparent first around the eyes, mouth and tips of the ear. Subsequently, grey hairs appear scattered throughout the body pelage.

Melanosomes may be passed to histiocytes in the upper dermis in senility (Baker, 1967b) and in some diseases as a result of disease-initiated degeneration of the cells of the basal layer.

The degree of production of melanosomes is under the control of the melanocyte-stimulating hormone produced by the pituitary gland. Ultraviolet light increases production of melanin and this protects the skin from the harmful effects of prolonged exposure to ultraviolet rays.

LANGERHANS' CELLS

These are epidermal dendritic cells and are the first cell type meeting foreign antigens in the skin (Halliday *et al.*, 1986).

These cells also appear as clear cells in the epidermis with shrunken nuclei when stained by haematoxylin and eosin. The Langerhans' cells have dendritic processes like melanocytes but are not derived from the neural crest and are considered to be of mesenchymal origin. They may be located in the basal layer of the epidermis or stratum germinativum and are occasionally found in the normal dermis. Langerhans' cells migrate to the skin via the blood from the bone marrow. When examined by electron microscopy, these cells have a distinctive appearance characterized by a cytoplasmic organelle — the Langerhans' granule — which is shaped like a tennis racket. The cells are found in other stratified epithelia, the spleen, thymus and lymph nodes. Their function is considered to be immunogenic, concerned with the uptake and processing of antigenic substances (Silberberg *et al.*, 1975). Stingl *et al.* (1977) first demonstrated that Langerhans' cells have cell-membrane receptors for certain immunologically important molecules and are capable of presenting antigen to responsive T-cells and are therefore responsible for the immunizing capacity of antigen applied to the skin (Fig. 1.7). Of significant importance is their discovery that this facility can be destroyed by ultraviolet light. Keratinocytes are also apparently important in the epidermal immune system, producing hormone-like molecules which significantly influence T-lymphocytes migrating through the epidermis (Endelson & Fink, 1983). Another immunological dendritic cell in the epidermis — the Grandstein cell — has recently been reported with a tendency to interact with suppressor rather than with helper T-cells.

MERKEL CELLS

Merkel cells were formerly considered to be of neural crest origin but there is now evidence that they are of keratinocytic origin (English, 1974, 1977). They are found in small knobs which are scattered over the corporal epidermis at intervals — the so-called tylotrich pads. A terminal neuraxon derived from a myelinated nerve is associated with the dermal and sometimes the lateral aspects of the Merkel cell. These cells are thought to be part of a unit of a slowly adapting mechanoreceptor (Breathnach, 1980).

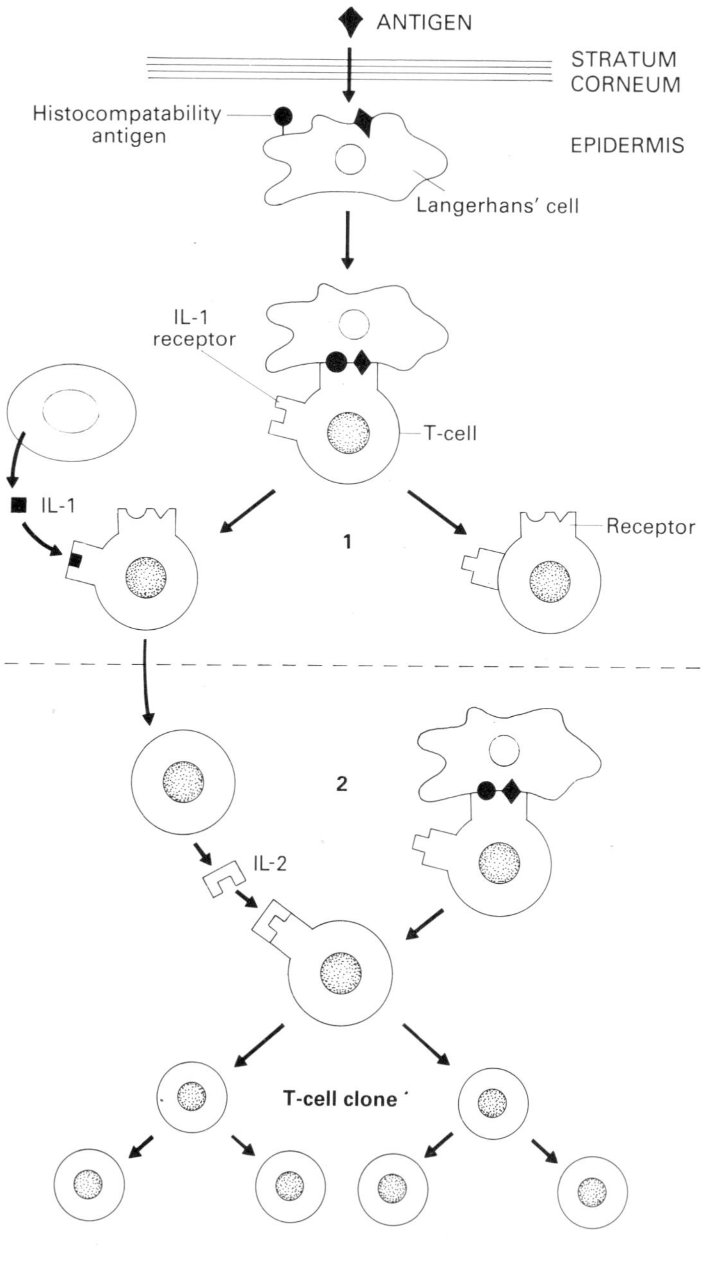

Fig. 1.7. The role of the Langerhans' cell in the immune system of the skin.

The basement membrane

This structure marks the boundary between the dermis and the epidermis and exists also in other organ systems. In hairy skin, it is gently undulating. It has two main functions:

1 Support.

2 Selective filtration.

When stained with eosin, the basement membrane appears homogeneous and is 3–4 μm thick (Lichtenstein, 1979). Staining with *p*-aminosalicylic acid indicates the presence of a glycoprotein. Electron microscope examination reveals the following (Lichtenstein, 1979):

1 Basal-cell plasma membrane with attaching structures — the hemidesmosomes.

2 Lamina lucida (the intermembranous space).

3 Basal lamina (basement membrane of epidermal origin).

4 Sub-basal lamina (fibrous elements consisting of anchoring fibrils).

5 Microfibrils and collagen (produced by dermal fibroblasts) (Briggaman & Wheeler, 1975).

In composition, the basement membrane is 80% protein and 20% carbohydrate. Lichtenstein (1979) states that, experimentally, antibodies produced against whole basement membrane are directed primarily to the non-collagenous peptides of its glycoproteins. The basement membrane may be the site of immunological diseases like systemic lupus erythematosus, and direct immunofluorescence techniques have shown antibody and complement involvement in immune reactions at the junction of the membrane with the dermis.

The basement membrane is a barrier to the migration of tumour cells. However, malignant cells can disrupt it and then pass through it. Liotta *et al.* (1980) report that the metastatic potential of tumour cells correlates with the enzymatic degradation of basement-membrane collagen.

The dermis

The dermis is made up of amorphous ground substances and fibrous proteins — collagen, reticulin and elastin tissues. Hair follicles and glands project into this layer and it also supports the vascular, lymphatic and nervous systems of the skin. In addition, it contains a population of various cells.

The dermis should not be thought of as a uniform layer between the epidermis and subcutis — its boundaries are irregular and they may project for a considerable distance into the subcutis. The distinct division between the papillary and reticular layers of human dermis is not seen in cat and dog skin; however, the collagen fibres in the upper dermis are much finer than those in the lower dermis.

When viewed with the light microscope, collagen is composed of large bundles of fibres. Electron microscopy reveals bundles of microfibrils aligned in parallel with regular cross striations approximately 70 μm apart.

The collagen molecule has an approximate molecular weight of 290 000 and is made up of three polypeptide chains — α-chains — each of which is closely coiled in a triple-helical structure like the coils of a rope. Each chain has approximately 1000 amino acids with glycine representing about 33% of all the amino acids and occupying every third position along each α-chain. The chain of polypeptides is actually a repetitive triplet sequence which may be represented as (*X* — *Y* — Gly)333. Numerous amino acids can occupy the *X* and *Y* position but proline more commonly occupies the *X* position with hydroxyproline occupying the *Y* position. Proline and hydroxyproline constitute about 22% of the amino acid composition of collagen (Uitto, 1979).

Elastic fibres

These require special stains for demonstration. In normal skin, they are comparatively sparsely distributed, much branched, predominantly in the upper dermis and particularly related to the epidermal adnexae. They provide physiological elasticity in the skin. With age, there is marked deterioration. Elastic fibres consist basically of straight polypeptides rich in alanine, valine, glycine and proline. Unlike collagen, glycine is not evenly distributed along the polypeptide chains. As in collagen, about 30% of the amino acid content consists of glycine. Elastic fibres have cross links which hold the polypeptide straight chains in a network (Partridge, 1962; Gray *et al.*, 1973). In cutis laxa there is alteration of the structure with deficiency in cross links.

Ground substance

The collagen and elastic fibres of the dermis are permeated throughout by amorphous material — the ground substance — which is mostly mucopolysaccharide with glycoproteins, various salts and water present in similar proportions to plasma. Hyaluronic acid, dermatan sulphate and chondroitin-6-sulphate are the mucopolysaccharides which particularly constitute ground substance. Heparin derived from the mast cells is also present but its function is not known. Ageing skin has fewer mucopolysaccharides, particularly hyaluronic acid, and has a decreased water content.

The ground substance constitutes only a small fraction of the total dry weight of the skin. It is supportive, acts as a water carrier permitting salt and water movement and cell migration.

Earlier scientists researched widely into the effects of hormones on the ground substance: hyaluronic acid accumulates periodically in the sexual display skin of primates — this can be produced experimentally using oestrogen therapy (Reinits, 1960). Prednisolone therapy decreases the concentration of chondroitin sulphate and there is an increase in hyaluronic acid (Schiller, 1965). The thyroid gland has a profound effect on ground substance, as shown experimentally by hypothyroid rats which develop an increased concentration of hyaluronic acid and a decreased concentration of chondroitin-6-sulphate and dermatan sulphate in their skin (Schiller *et al.*, 1962; Schiller *et al.*, 1963). The dermal mucopolysaccharides are influenced by diabetes mellitus and insulin; synthesis of the mucopolysaccharides is decreased in diabetic subjects.

Free cells in the dermis

Examination of the dermis with conventional light-microscope methods will not differentiate all dermal cells, though mast cells characteristically appear as large oval cells with granular cytoplasm and a round nucleus.

THE MAST CELL

These cells are usually found related to blood vessels. They are oval in shape with a long axis of 10–20 μm. Staining with haematoxylin and eosin does not clearly reveal the granular nature of the cytoplasm which contains numerous granules which stain metachromatically with basic thionine dyes like toluidine blue.

The structure of the granules is complex, each being enclosed within a membrane, and it is not possible to differentiate heparin, histamine or proteases within individual granules as they are enclosed within membranes. The granules are released from the cell without damage to the cytoplasm or cell membrane. Immunoglobulin E has the capacity to bind to mast cells and basophils in a stable manner until activated by an antigen, when a complex series of events indicates release of the granules (degranulation). Several differing stimuli may cause degranulation. Non-immunological stimulants are therapeutic drugs like codeine, thiamine, polymyxin and toxin (e.g. bacterial, snake venom). Reactions between antibodies and antigens on the surfaces of the mast cells are immunological stimulants of degranulation. Direct physical effects — stroking of the skin, the effects of hot water, acetylcholine or acetylcholine activators — can cause degranulation of mast cells that have cholinergic receptors on their plasma membranes. Immunological interactions (more commonly Type I) can cause degranulation. The granules contain a number of mediators with numerous functions, some important in tissue defence. However, if the mast-cell response is not limited, disease may result.

FIBROBLASTS

These are large cells present in the normal dermis in small numbers. They have an oval- or spindle-shaped nucleus which has a distinct nuclear membrane. Their prime function is the production of collagen and collagenase and they are responsible for both production and degradation of collagen. Immature fibroblasts are phagocytic. Fibrocytes, histiocytes and macrophages develop from a common precursor cell.

HISTIOCYTES AND MACROPHAGES

Some texts refer to two different types of cells which are macrophagic and increase in number at inflammation. They are probably varieties of a single cell. This has an indented nucleus, prominent Golgi apparatus, many cytoplasmic vesicles, a few mitochondria and primary lysosomes. It is considered by some authorities that these cells may also differentiate into Langerhans' cells.

Arrectores pilorum muscles

These are composed of smooth-muscle fibres — the muscles which are involuntary. They are attached to the hair follicles and raise the hair by their contraction. They are under adrenergic control and their function is thermoregulatory and also behavioural. At their distal extremity, they are attached to the basement membrane of the epidermis and are inserted on the lower third of the hair follicle where they may be branched to connect adjacent follicles. They are particularly well developed and more numerous along the dorsal midline from the cervical region to the tail. In hypothyroidism the muscles may be hypertrophied and vacuolated.

Cutaneous nerves

The skin contains two functional nerve types: several different receptors convey impulses by somatic sensory nerves, whilst autonomic motor nerves act on glands, the arrectores pilorum muscles and vessels. Motor nerves to apocrine and sebaceous glands have not been demonstrated and only tactile hairs receive motor nerves.

Cauna (1976) has reported two types of free endings in hairy skin: papillary and penicillate. The former are derived from myelinated axons and give a positive cholinesterase reaction. They are possibly concerned with the reception of cold stimuli. In contrast, the latter are derived from non-myelinated fibres and do not show cholinesterase activity: they form an extensive network but their exact sensory function has not been determined. Sensations of itching, temperature difference and pain may be subserved by these terminals; Merkel cells, Meissner corpuscles and Pacinian corpuscles act as mechanoreceptors. There is considerable difference in the population of receptors from region to region.

The autonomic nervous system is apparently sympathetic. Vessels and the arrectores pilorum muscles are supplied by adrenergic and cholinergic fibres, whilst the eccrine glands are innervated by cholinergic fibres. A direct nerve supply to the sebaceous glands and apocrine glands has not been found.

Sensation is conveyed by a dermal network of nerve endings located beneath the epidermis and around hair follicles and by specialized nerve endings. Hirsute skin has many less sensory nerve endings per unit area than glabrous skin. Specialized nerve endings are particularly numerous and developed in specialized areas of the skin — lips, foot pads, integumentary papillae — and are related to the tactile hairs. The integumentary papilla contains a specialized nerve — a touch receptor making contact with local Merkel cells in the epidermis (Mann & Straïle, 1965). The hair follicle network conveys touch reception with specialization in the tactile hairs or sinus hairs prominent on the muzzle, chin and legs. Nilsson (1970) has described four mechanoreceptors in the forelegs of cats.

Itch and pain sensations are the result of activation by stimuli of free nerve endings at the dermo-epidermal junction (Fig. 1.8). In humans, there is variation in the threshold level of stimulation in different regions; however, there are no visual microscopic differences in nerve ending frequency or distribution between such areas; apparently, other non-anatomic factors determine the itch and pain sensitivity in different regions (Greaves, 1987).

The itch-producing mediators are possibly histamine, unidentified peptides with prostaglandins and related compounds having synergistic functions. There is increasing evidence that opioid peptides in the central nervous system

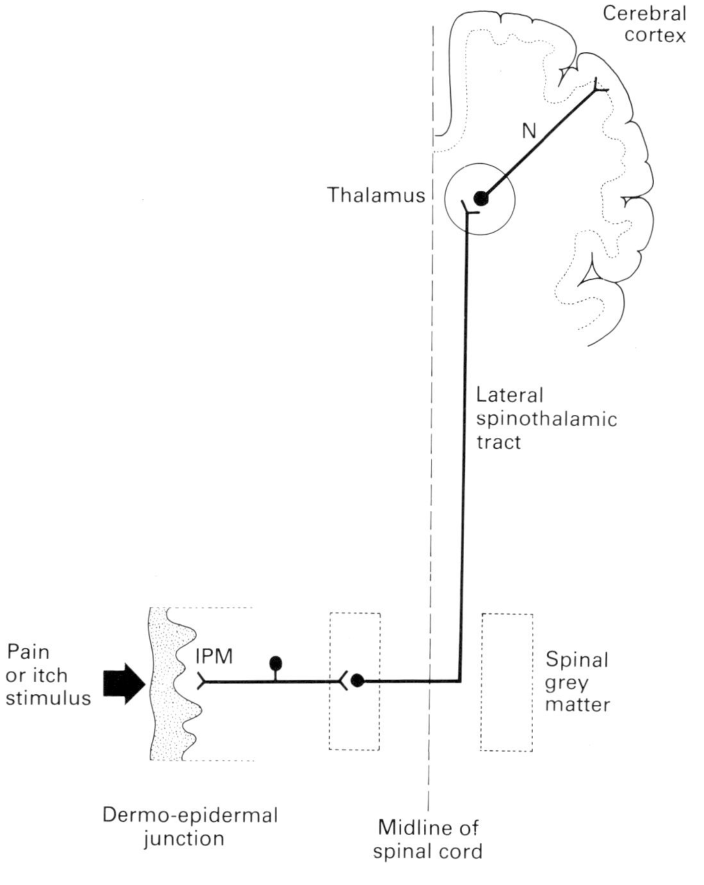

Fig. 1.8. Neural pathways of itching. IPM = itch-promoting mediator, N = tertiary neurons (not yet identified).

have a role in itch perception (Greaves, 1987). The importance of histamine in the medication of pruritus is not known in dogs and cats and antihistamines are of no value. Other mediators are probably more important.

In diseases characterized by pruritus, the production of polypeptide kinins from the activation of proteases resulting from tissue damage may be important in inducing nerve uptake, resulting in pruritus.

The response to itching is scratching — a spinal reflex. Scratching may actually destroy the free endings of the itch receptors at the dermo-epidermal junction since, following scratching, pruritus is relieved for a considerable period.

The lymphatic system

The lymph vessels are extremely thin walled and are rarely discernible in sections of normal skin. They are lined by a single layer of flattened endothelial cells (Fig. 1.9). They begin as blind endings in the upper dermis and form a network with other vessels, becoming larger, valved and thicker walled as they drain towards their collecting vessels. In the deep dermis and subcutis they develop muscular walls providing a one-way draining system for the removal of water, protein and other products including those of immunological reactions. A regular arrangement of the lymph vessels has not been detected, therefore the system, although very extensive, appears to have no definite structure.

The blood vascular system has been extensively studied whilst the lymphatic system, which is probably as extensive, has been comparatively neglected.

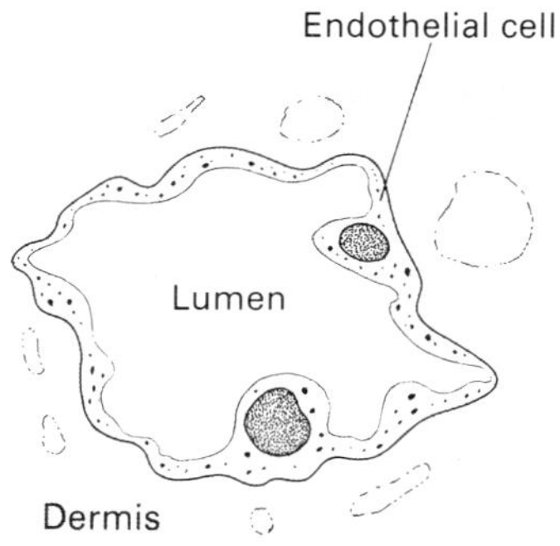

Fig. 1.9. A lymphatic vesselent transversely.

The vascular system

Hughes and Dransfield (1959) list the arteries which supply blood to the skin and report three distinct arterial plexuses arranged in parallel to the surface. Arteriovenous anastomoses occur in the lower layers of the skin. They are:

1 The deeper subcutaneous plexus.
2 The middle or cutaneous plexus.
3 The superficial plexus.

The deep plexus is situated at the junction of the subcutis and dermis. Branches pass to the hair papillae, in which they form capillary loops, to supply the follicles, tubular glands and arrectores pilorum muscles, while others pass directly upwards as radicles to the middle plexus.

The middle plexus also supplies ascending and descending vessels to the hair follicles, tubular glands, arrectores pilorum muscles, and the sebaceous glands. In turn it passes radicles to the superficial plexus. In humans, this plexus is well developed to supply capillary loops of the dermal papillae. In the mainly hirsute skin of the cat and dog, the epidermis is gently undulating without dermal papillae so this plexus is a flattened capillary network. However, in the specialized glabrous areas, like the foot pads, dermal papillae are well developed and this plexus provides numerous ascending capillary loops. The veins, which are somewhat larger than the arteries, are arranged with them; arteriovenous anastomoses are located in the deeper layer of the skin, the pinnae and the tail tip.

The vascular supply has the potential for considerable development and changes, as will be observed in inflammatory changes, wound healing or during the various stages of the hair growth cycles.

The cutaneous blood vessel is composed of three basic elements: the endothelial cell, the pericyle and the basal lamina.

Apocrine sweat glands

Mammalian skin contains two types of sweat glands: apocrine and eccrine. In the former, the secretions usually discharge into a hair follicle; in the latter, they discharge directly onto the surface of the skin. The apocrine glands are distributed evenly throughout the hirsute skin but are absent from specialized areas like the foot pads. They may be aggregated in large numbers in particular areas, e.g. the interdigital spaces and around the anal sacs. Their prime function in the cat and dog is probably to produce pheromones. The apocrine glands of most mammals are active from birth, but in humans activity begins with puberty. Those scattered more or less uniformly throughout the hirsute skin of dogs and cats are probably excretory and thermoregulatory in function, whilst those grouped together are odiferous and concerned with scent marking.

The glands open into the pilary canal at the level of the sebaceous gland duct from which they descend following the follicular axis to terminate in a serpentine manner in the subcutaneous tissue (Fig. 1.10). In the embryo, they arise as buds from the upper third of the simple follicle and then

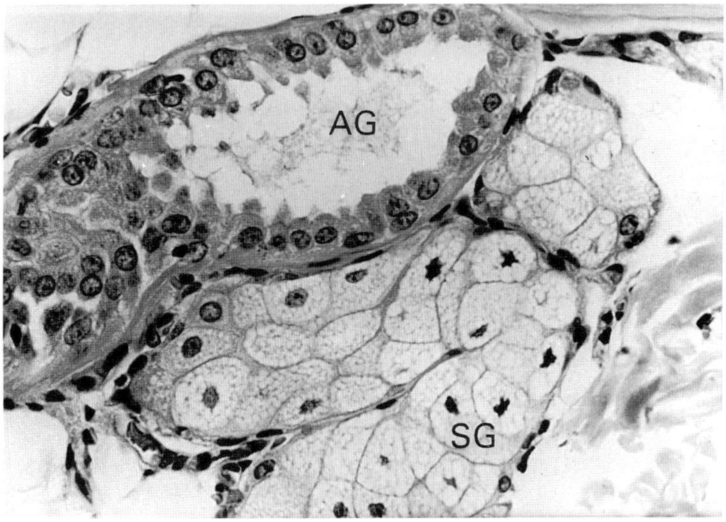

Fig. 1.10. Apocrine and sebaceous glands.

grow down through the dermis (Baker, 1966).

The secretory cell is cuboidal in shape, the nucleus is large and the cytoplasm is somewhat granular. Secretion is apocrine without cell disintegration as in the holocrine secretion of the sebaceous gland cell. The cell is flattened if the gland becomes cystic. The secretory epithelium is continuous throughout the length of the gland. The cells discharge their secretion into the lumen of the gland which is roughly circular in cross section. The secretions are expelled from the gland by the contractions of the myoepithelial cells which surround the secretory cell. They are controlled by the sympathetic adrenergic system. Stimulation of the glands in the Canidae is activated by α-receptors (Allen & Bligh, 1969). There is some variation in the morphology of the gland. In the interdigital spaces and external auditory meatus they are convoluted whilst over the general body surface they are simple serpentine tubes. The mammary glands are large aggregates of apocrine glands.

Eccrine sweat glands

These are located only on the foot pads and are described under that heading (p. 28). Their sweating activity is often clearly demonstrated in foot imprints observed on the examination table when nervous cats and dogs are examined.

Sebaceous glands

Sebaceous glands develop during fetal life as buds from the primordial hair follicle, and are found in all areas of the skin with the exception of the foot pads, muzzle and lips. In some areas, they are not associated with hair, i.e. the external auditory meatus, anus, eyelids (meibomian glands). In the external auditory meatus they are not to be confused with the ceruminous glands — these are apocrine glands.

In hairy skin, the glands tend to be unilobular with several placed around each compound follicle. Each gland opens by a wide duct into the pilary canal. The duct is composed of cells which may be considered to be composed of transitional cells between those cells making up the stratified epithelium of the pilary canal and the lipid-producing cells of the sebaceous gland. Each individual gland is composed of an outer layer of small, deeply staining basophilic cells — the reserve cells. They surround larger cells with foamy cytoplasm (appearing vacuolated in paraffin-processed sections) containing lipid: as these cells enlarge their nucleus is compressed and becomes smaller and finally disappears. The cells rupture to release sebum. Sebaceous glands are therefore holocrine, with the whole cell discharging its contents into the sebaceous duct. Sebaceous glands have no nerve supply and are under hormonal control: experimentally, testosterone produces hypertrophy whilst cortisol and oestrogen cause involution.

The composition of canine and feline sebum awaits detailed study: sebum probably makes up 95% of the skin-surface lipid. Greene *et al*. (1970) consider that in humans, glycerides and free fatty acid make up 57.5% of sebum, wax ester 25%, squalene 12%, cholesterol esters 3% and cholesterol 1.5%.

In good health, sebum flows from the pilary canals over the surface of the skin and hair: the dull coat and hair of unhealthy or poorly nourished animals may be explained as resulting from diminution of the flow. Mixing of apocrine secretion and sebum results in the formation of an emulsion which dries on the surface to form an impermeable seal with antibacterial, antiviral and antifungal properties.

The circumanal glands

A large mass of modified sebaceous glands surrounds the anus of the dog. They are not found in the cat. Their function is not known but they are of considerable importance clinically.

They must be distinguished from the glands associated with the anal sacs. The term 'hepatoid gland' is often used for these glands because cells of the mature gland resemble liver cells. The mature gland is composed of sheets of acini with numerous short, blind ducts present. Developing as buds from the upper third of the hair follicle at birth, the glands increase in size throughout life, and are responsible for the prominence of the anal ring in the older dog (Fig. 1.11). In a middle-aged, normal dog this may extend in an irregular manner around the anus to a distance of 2 cm, and they may be 9 mm thick in normal male dogs and less thick in normal female dogs. They are therefore more extensive in male dogs than in female dogs (Baker, 1967a).

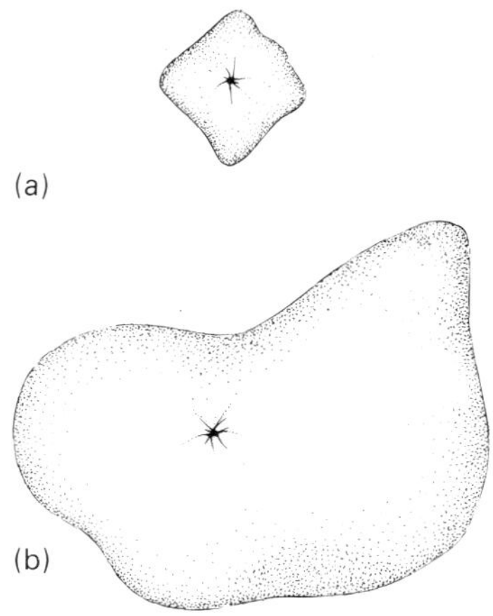

Fig. 1.11. Circumanal glands of the male dog. Relative area of gland at: (a) 7 months, (b) 13 years.

Supracaudal glands

The dorsal surface of the proximal third of the tail of most dogs contains a large oval area (1500 × 750 μm diameter) of extremely well-developed, functional sebaceous glands. It is particularly prominent in some breeds (Labrador retriever, Staffordshire bull terrier). In the cat, they are distributed along the dorsal midline of the tail; individual glands are 1500 μm in length and 750 μm in diameter (Baker, 1974).

The glands are each associated with single, large hairs and they discharge on to the surface. In some older dogs, the area is hairless, prominent and covered with yellow-grey waxy scale: the supracaudal glands are probably influenced by androgen. In male cats they are involved in the disease stud tail, whilst in older dogs they may be the site of seborrhoea.

Hair

The coat contains longer stouter primary hairs (topcoat) and finer shorter hairs (undercoat). However, there is considerable variation between breeds; in some, the undercoat hairs may be longer than the primary hairs. The length of the hair is extremely variable according to the breed as is the number of follicles per cm^2 (range 120–486/cm^2 dorsal thoracic region; Baker, 1966). The hairs are produced in follicles arranged in groups of two to five compound follicles, with three being the most usual. The central follicle in a triad is the largest and usually contains the thickest of the primary hairs. It may be accompanied by several fine secondary hairs. The lateral follicles are smaller and usually contain two finer primary hairs and six to 12 thin secondary hairs. The angles at which the follicles descend into the dermis and subcutis are variable, becoming more oblique in thinner skin.

Hair vortices are prominent in short-haired dogs and are less obvious in those with long-hair. There are two on the nose around the eyes and ears, one on the dorsal cervical region and one on the ventral cervical region. A hair ridge may be present on the lateral neck. Vortices and ridges are seen on the anterior and ventral thorax. A vortex is present on the medial aspect of the forearm, the forelimbs also have a hair ridge on the caudolateral aspect, and there is a vortex over each hip. A hair ridge is usually present in the perineal area of bitches. Both cats and dogs have a vortex over the sciatic tuberosity with a conjoint hair ridge to the anus. Rhodesian ridgebacks have an anteriorly directed ridge of hair along the dorsal midline of the body. Both cats and dogs have tactile hairs provided with sensory nerve plexuses. These tactile or sinus hairs have prominent palpable bases. The stiff eyelashes (cilia) are not sinus hairs. Sinus hairs have well-developed blood sinuses encircling them and are well supplied with sensory branches of the trigeminal nerve. Typically, the sinus hair has a large upper sinus and numerous smaller lower sinuses (Table 1.1).

Hairs consist of a central medulla, cortex and cuticle. The medulla is much wider in guard hairs than secondary hairs

Table 1.1. Distribution and number of sinus hairs

Location	Number of sinus hairs
Dog	
Zygomatic bundle	3
Mental bundle	1–3 lateral to buccal commissures
Cheek bundle	1–3 on each cheek
Medial canthus	4–8 on both sides
Upper lip	4 rows } 30–40 on each side
Lower lip	2 rows } 30–40 on each side
Cat	
2 cheek bundles	—
Above each eye	8–12
Upper lip	4 rows (the whiskers, white other than in black cats)
Carpus	3 dorsal to the carpal pad

(Fig. 1.12). Each hair is a cylinder of impacted keratinized cells and is formed by the intense mitotic activity of the cells of the matrix which surrounds the dermal papilla. They are covered with scales, which are most pronounced in secondary hair where the free edges are slightly raised (imbricated) (Figs 1.12 and 1.13a). The cuticle of the sinus hair is smoother (Fig. 1.13b).

The hair follicle consists of the hair, inner sheath and outer hair sheath. At its lower end, during its active period of growth (the anagen phase), it has a hollow, knob-like expansion containing the hair matrix cells which surrounds the dermal papilla and which is well supplied with blood vessels. The hair matrix cells form the hair and the inner root sheath, whilst the outer root sheath is a downward projection of the epidermis. Hair matrix cells have large vesicular nuclei and deeply basophilic cytoplasm; among them are the dopa-positive melanocytes.

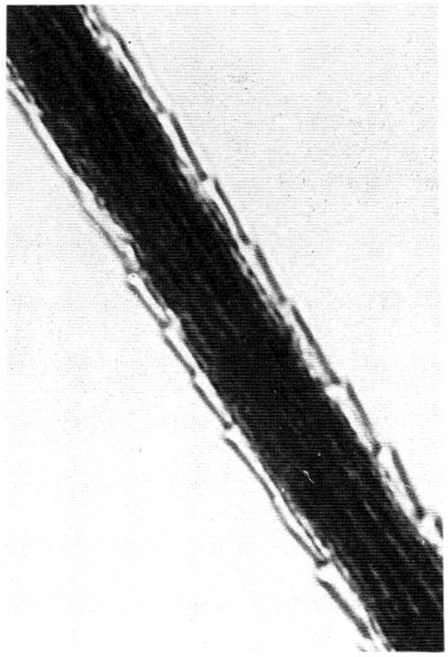

Fig. 1.12. Medulla of secondary hair of cat. Note the prominent cuticular scale.

The bulb (Fig. 1.14)

At the base of the follicle in anagen there is an expanded mass of cells which is invaginated to enclose the dermal papilla. The cells in its lower hemisphere are actively dividing, in the upper hemisphere to the zone of keratinization is the zone of differentiation, although some mitotic activity occurs here as well (Epstein & Maibach, 1964). It is the cells of the matrix that produce the hair medulla, hair cortex, cuticle and the inner root sheath.

The medulla

This is produced by matrix cells at the apex of the dermal papilla. Cells of the cortex project into the medulla, giving a ladder-like appearance, an effect most noticeable in the finer secondary hairs of the cat where the rungs may touch.

The cortex

The main mass of hair is composed of fused keratinized cells.

The hair cuticle

These are the last cells to differentiate from the matrix and they form the outer 'tile'-like covering to the hair, encircling

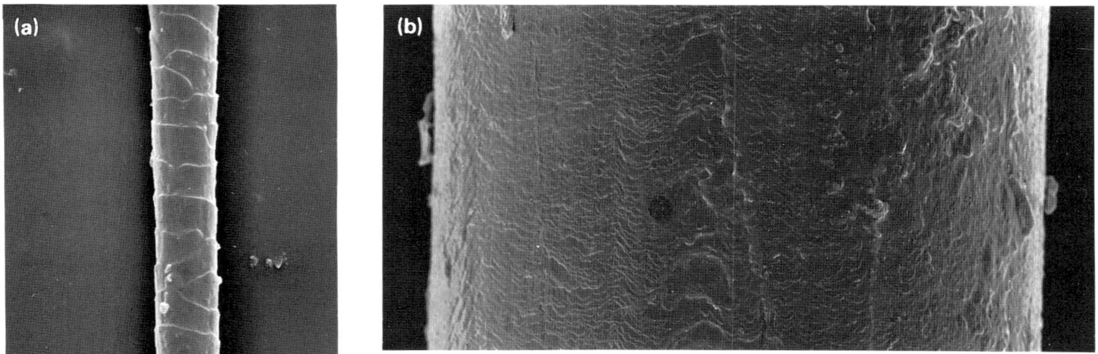

Fig. 1.13. Scanning electron micrographs of: (a) a secondary canine hair, (b) a primary canine hair.

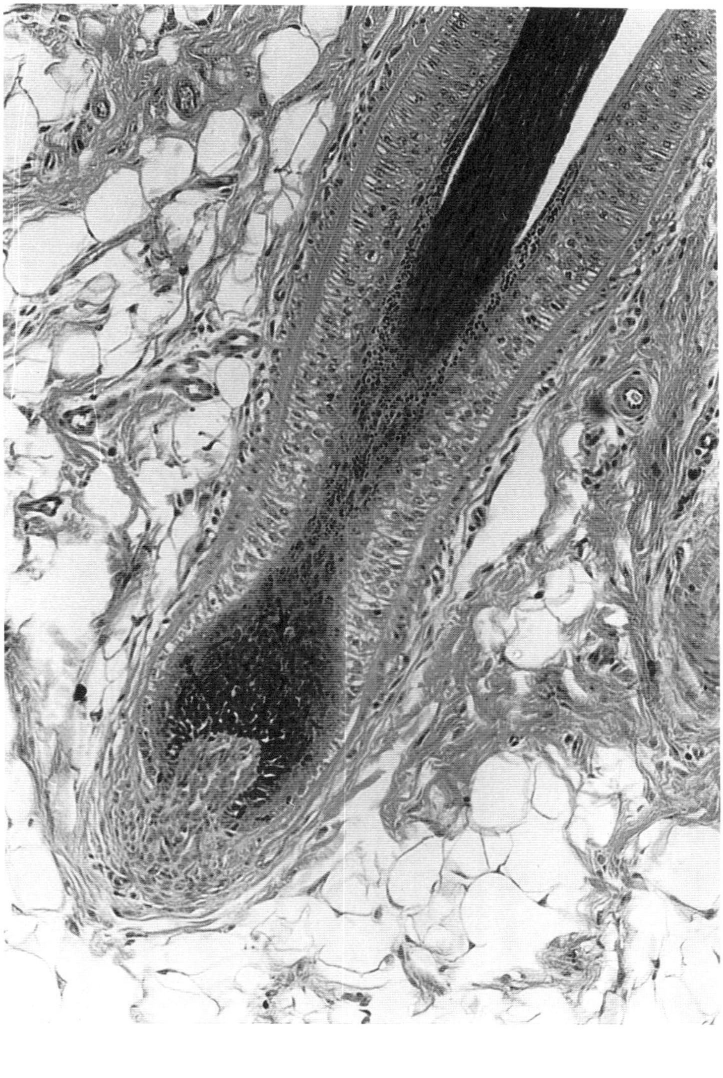

Fig. 1.14. Hair bulb.

the cortex from which they ascend in single rows. They are cuboidal and their cytoplasm appears to be packed with deeply staining basophilic granules. In the upper part of the hair bulb these presumptive cells of the cuticle are arranged with their long axis radially to the hair bulb, but as they ascend, their long axis tilts upward so that they overlap (imbricated) becoming progressively flattened and scale like. The scales do not completely encircle the hairs, the free lips are slightly raised (more pronounced in secondary hairs) and point towards the hair tip. The free edges of the cuticular cells of primary hair are serrated. Those of secondary hairs are dentate.

Cyclical activity of hair follicles

In some mammals, the hair is replaced in a wave pattern which moves over the body. In dogs and cats, it is apparently replaced in a mosaic pattern. However, there are two periods of maximum replacement in the year — spring and autumn. The cycle is apparently controlled by the photoperiod.

The cycle of activity of the follicles is anagen–catagen–telogen (the resting stage) (Fig. 1.15). The upper part of the compound follicle is the only part which is permanent, the lower half disappearing during the telogen phase of the cycle of activity (Fig. 1.16). The individual follicles of compound follicles may show variable activity, with active follicles sharing a common pilary canal with an inactive hair. Hairs which have been engaged in active growth in the anagen stage finally show signs of passing into catagen. The melanocytes in the papilla stop synthesizing melanin with subsequent lightening of pigmentation of the shaft of the hair follicle. The middle part of the bulb becomes constricted, the base of the hair becoming club shaped and keratinized. The club hair does not immediately fall out but may remain in the follicle for a considerable period. The follicle is now in the catagen stage (Fig. 1.15). During catagen, the lower end of the follicle below the club becomes thickened and corrugated. As this occurs, the upper end of the follicle containing the club hair is pulled upwards in the dermis towards the surface. When catagen has been completed, the follicle enters the telogen stage which may be of variable length. The melanocytes in the hair follicle in the telogen stage do not produce tyrosinase (precursor of melanin). The follicle containing the club hair is now in the middle and upper dermis whilst beneath it a new dermal papilla has formed. This will have received melanocytes from the previous dermal papilla. The anagen stage is complete when the dermal papilla has come to rest at its lowest point in the dermis or subcutis.

The rate of hair growth is variable, secondary hair growing

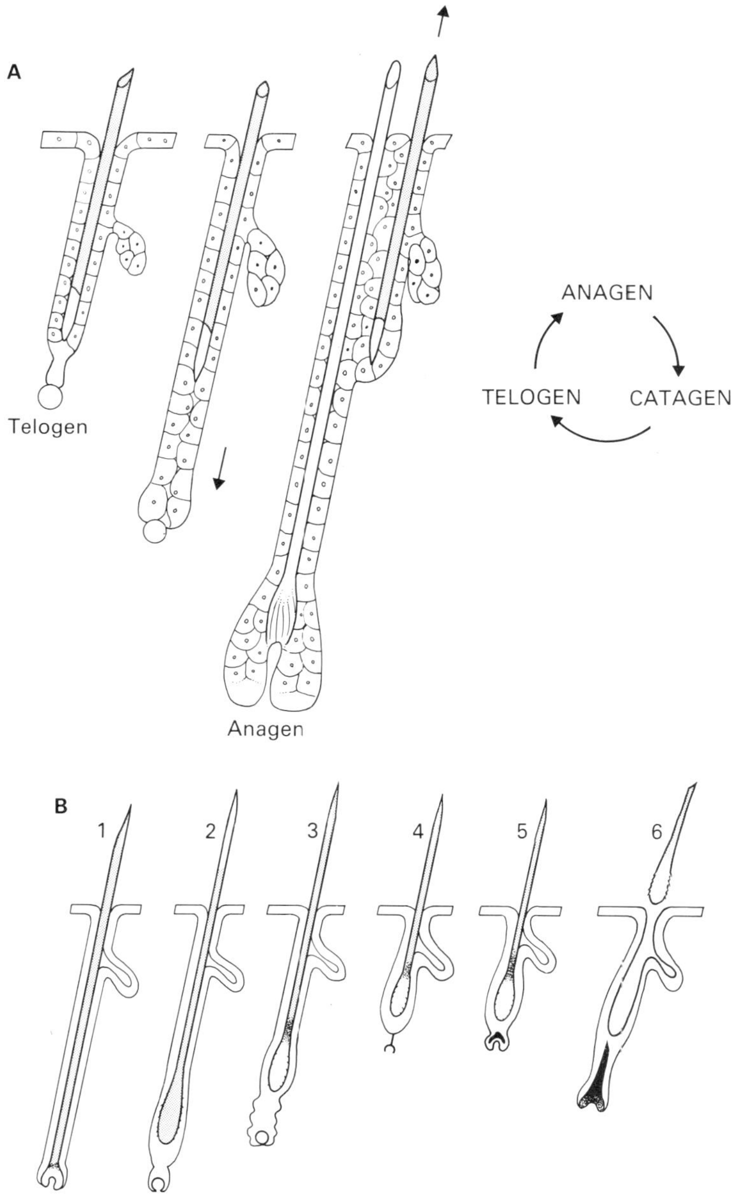

Fig. 1.15. A Changes in the hair follicle during the activity cycle.
B The sequence of events during the activity cycle.

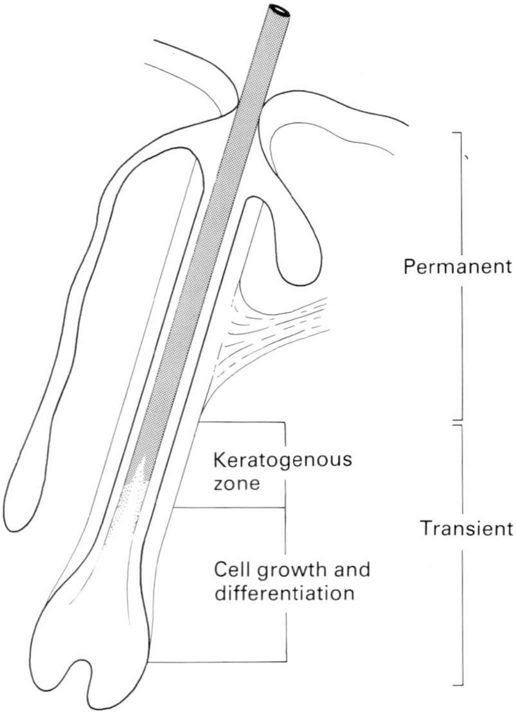

Fig. 1.16. At telogen — the resting stage of the activity cycle — the lower part of the follicle disappears.

at a slower rate than primary hair as might be expected. Baker (1974) reported a range of 270–313 μm for the daily growth rate of adult feline primary hair and a range of 239–280 μm for secondary hair.

Melanin

The actual colour of the hair is determined by the amount of melanin produced by the melanocytes which are situated at the apex of the active anagen hair follicle. If little or no pigment is produced, the hair will be grey or white. In some breeds, melanin may be produced at genetically regulated intervals; thus, the hair may be banded throughout its length as in tabby cats or have a white tip as in the Alsatian dog (agouti type).

There are two classes of melanin, both formed by the action of tyrosinase:

1 Eumelanin — black–brown.
2 Phaemelanin — yellow–red.

The variation in coat colour is entirely due to the differences in quantity of these two pigments in the hair. Galbraith (1964) and Cleffmann (1964) reported the production of the agouti band in the hair of mice. Here most of the melanocytes in the dermal papilla produce eumelanin. However, there is an interval in which phaemelanin melanocytes at the apex of the papilla produce phaemelanin in the absence of eumelanin production and a band of light-coloured hair results. The actual mode of control of melanin production is not known. It is probable that banded hair colour in cats and dogs is produced in the same way.

Specialized structures of the skin

The lips

The skin here is thick and often heavily pigmented whilst the upper lip has a medial area contiguous with the muzzle with a distinct groove (the philtrum) extending part way between the nostrils. In the bulldog type, this groove may be exaggerated, appearing as a hare lip. Whilst the lateral borders of the upper lip are firm, those of the lower lip are flaccid and denticulated posteriorly in dogs but not in cats. The lips themselves contain no sebaceous glands, but large sebaceous glands are arranged about the hairs bordering the lips. The epidermis is very thick and there is marked rete peg formation. Melanin pigment granules may be present throughout the epidermis so that the lip may be black and pigment may extend into the buccal cavity. Alternatively, they may be heavily pigmented, pink coloured or non-pigmented according to breed.

There may be a lateral skin fold below the lower lips; this is particularly marked in the spaniel breeds and generally so in brachycephalic dogs. Because of its proximity to the mouth, this skin fold is particularly predisposed to dermatitis.

The external nares

The nares may or may not be pigmented according to breed. No sebaceous glands or hairs are present, the moist surface being maintained by the activity of the nasal glands which are placed lateral to the external nares. The epidermis is very thick and the surface made up of roughly oval plaques of variable size separated by lipidaceous material (Fig. 1.17).

Rete peg formation is very marked. Sensory nerves are located deep in the dermis, having a zigzag course before ending in the epidermis.

The foot pads

The flexural surfaces of the feet have hairless thick pads. The metacarpal and tarsal foot pads are largest, somewhat heart-shaped and situated behind the smaller, oval digital pads. They may or may not be pigmented. The forelimbs have an additional pad, the carpal pad, located medially and distal to the accessory carpal bone. The epidermis is very thick and heavily keratinized, the free surface is somewhat denticulated, the stratum corneum is particularly thickened. The pad is made up of a large number of peg-shaped masses bound together which interdigitate with the dermis (Fig. 1.18). The very thick epidermis of the foot pad shows the clear division of the various strata constituting it (resembling the human epidermis) (Fig. 1.19): the malpighian layer covered by the stratum corneum, with the former layer subdivided into: (1) the germinal basal layer; (2) the stratum spinosum consisting of a number of layers of polyhedral cells resting on and surmounted by (3) the stratum granulosum in which the keratinocytes are becoming flattened, nucleated cells with distinctly basophilic-staining keratohyaline granules within them. This last layer merges imperceptibly into the very thick stratum corneum in which the outlines of individual cells are lost. Some authors recognize a stratum lucidum at the junction of the stratum granulosum and the stratum corneum.

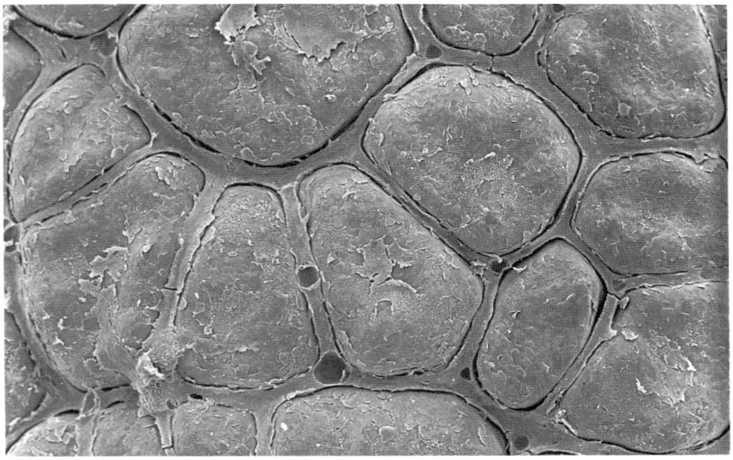

Fig. 1.17. The epidermis of the external nares.

The cells of the basal layer — the basal keratinocytes — are cylindrical in shape, arranged with their long axis at right angles to the basal membrane beneath them. The cells above them in the stratum spinosum are polyhedral in shape and become progressively flattened towards the stratum corneum. In the lower layers, these cells are seen to have interconnections, i.e. desmosomes. However, tissue processing causes some

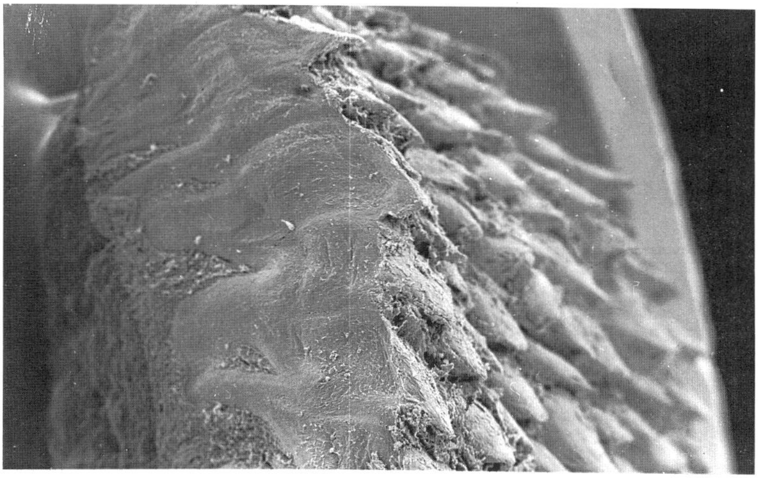

Fig. 1.18. Scanning electron micrograph of section through foot pad.

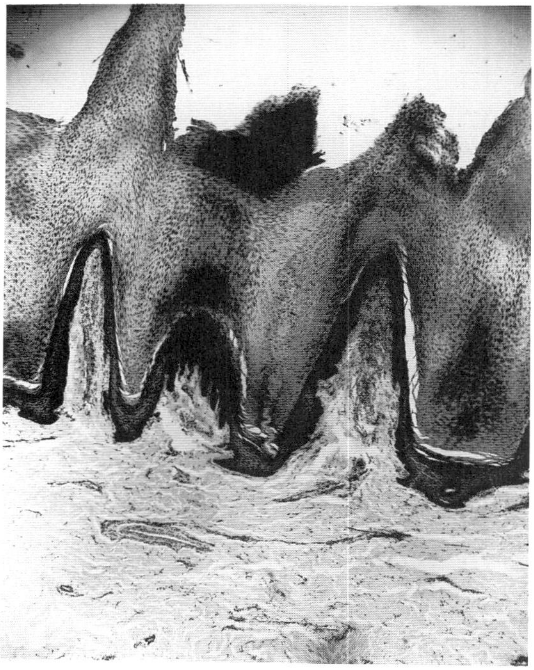

Fig. 1.19. Vertical section through foot pad.

cell shrinkage so that there is apparent separation between the cells.

The epidermis and dermis of the foot pad in an average-sized normal dog are each approximately 2 mm thick. The subcutis of the pads contains numerous merocrine glands with an overall fusiform shape of approximately 1.5 mm in length. From each gland passes a vertical duct entering the epidermis at the lowest point of a peg and then following a tortuous route to the surface (Fig. 1.20(a)). This duct is keratinized throughout the epidermis and in the upper part of the dermis (Fig. 1.20(b)).

The sweat glands are of the typical eccrine type with a narrow lumen and single layer of cuboidal secretory epithelium which is surrounded by a single layer of myoepithelial cells. The dermis of the foot pads contains numerous lamellar corpuscles — these are the mechanoreceptors and are of two types. Firstly, Meissner's corpuscles located in the dermis near the epidermis and directed vertically towards it: secondly, Pacinian corpuscles which are situated deep in the dermis in skin over weight-bearing surfaces.

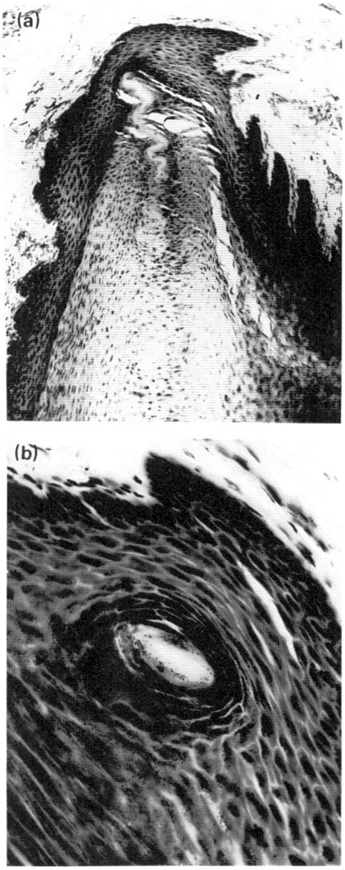

Fig. 1.20. (a) Longitudinal section through foot pad showing the route of the merocrine gland duct through the dermis and epidermis, (b) transverse section of merocrine gland duct in the epidermis of a foot pad showing keratinization.

Scrotal skin

The skin over the scrotum is relatively hairless, thin and somewhat wrinkled. The epidermis is thick and there is prominent rete peg formation. The basal layer is often heavily pigmented. The dermis is thin and characteristically contains smooth muscle fibres.

The claws

These are hollow, cone-shaped structures composed of hard keratin, the proximal ends of which are constructed to fit into the distal crescent-shaped inguinal crest. The claw is formed by the coronary band, which is most active dorsally so that growth produces a natural curve. Without continued wear the claw will eventually pierce the foot pad. The dew claws also grow continuously and may pierce the skin; older dogs with long hair are particularly at risk in this respect as the long hair hides the claws.

The palpebral margin

The skin of the eyelids is thin with a non-specialized structure.

However, the palpebral margins are thicker, the epidermis being made up of many layers of cells which are usually pigmented. The meibomian glands, which are very large sebaceous glands, are arranged in a single lateral row and discharge their contents into the palpebral margin at a visible puncta. Above them is a row of large follicles each of which contains a single large hair — the eyelash.

Embryology of the skin

See Table 1.2 for the embryonic origin of epidermis.

Initially in fetal life, the epidermis is a single layer of cells. Subsequently two layers develop: an inner layer of cuboidal cells — the stratum germinativum — upon which rests the outer layer, the periderm. Later, a third layer, placed between the periderm and stratum germinativum, is developed. This is the stratum intermedium which is composed of large, clear, vacuolated cells. At 38 days the cells of the periderm are not yet producing keratohyalin (Fig. 1.21).

Development of the hair is well established in the foetus of 38 days. The epidermis is several cells thick and the dermis is

Table 1.2. Embryonic origin of epidermis

Ectodermal	The majority of cells, the basic unit of which is the keratinocyte
Mesenchymal	Langerhans' cells, Merkel cells
Neurectodermal	Melanocytes

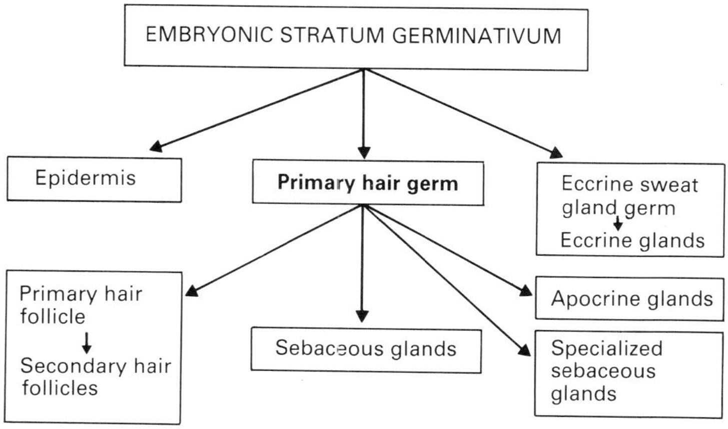

Fig. 1.21. Embryology of the skin.

very cellular with numerous mesenchymal cells. A stratum corneum is absent. The epidermis consists of approximately five layers of cells, the outer layers having a clear cytoplasm whilst the basal cells are smaller with more deeply staining cytoplasm. At intervals, there are seen to be aggregations of cells (hair germs) projecting into the dermis from the epidermis. These are produced at an obtuse angle and will form the primary follicles. Sebaceous glands are formed as buds from the upper third of the developing follicle. Just beneath the gland precursor is another protrusion and this will later be the site for the arrector pili muscle. Circumanal glands develop in the same way, with buds enlarging and differentiating from primary hair germs (Baker, 1967a). A crescent of cells beneath the advancing column will form the dermal papilla. At the 40th day of gestation, orientation of the cells of the hair follicles becomes more obvious (Fig. 1.22). Five days later, hair formation enclosing the dermal papilla is well advanced. Development of the primary follicle precedes that of the lateral follicles which are also formed as outgrowths from the epidermis. The primary follicle does not usually form hair buds.

Subcutaneous fat develops from the dermal mesenchymal cells in the second half of fetal development. At the 56th day of gestation, the primary follicles contain well-developed hairs but the secondary follicles do not.

At birth the dermis appears to be packed with well-developed primary follicles which are in the anagen stage. Development of the secondary follicles is also well advanced. The epidermis is now quite thin.

Postnatal development of cat skin is similar to that of the dog (Baker, 1966). On the first day of life there is an arrangement of triads of simple follicles. The triad contains a large

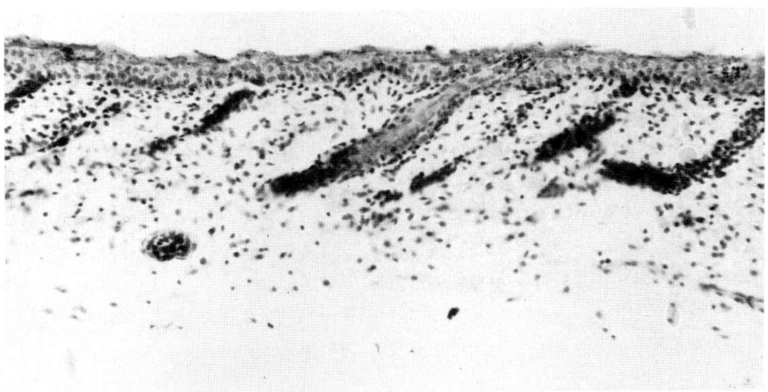

Fig. 1.22. Skin at 40 days — the hair follicles have extended into the dermis.

primary follicle bounded laterally by two smaller follicles which are producing further secondary follicles. Subsequently, the compound follicle is formed from buds which are produced from the secondary follicle just below the sebaceous gland. Thus, a number of hairs are formed which share a common pilary canal in their upper third. Further budding continues for some weeks after birth.

Skin at birth

The skin is covered with well-developed hair. The epidermis presents an even layer without ridge formation and four to five cells thick. The outlines of the cells of the basal layer and upper layer are not easily distinguishable and spinous processes are not apparent. The nuclei of the basal layer are large and vesicular; nucleoli are not seen but scattered chromatin is visible. At birth, melanin is apparent in pigmented cells in the epidermis as well as in the follicle and hair bulb. Pigmented cells are not seen in the dermis.

Above the upper layer of cells is a thin line of eosinophilic granules which constitutes the stratum granulosum and is presumably composed of keratohyalin. A thin stratum corneum is present.

The dermis is very cellular and crowded with hair follicles. Fibroblasts and mast cells are present. The latter are most numerous at birth, decreasing in numbers until puberty and thence remaining constant until senility, when there is again a decrease (Baker, 1967b).

Lovell (1955) reports that the skin of the newborn dog has a preponderance of argyrophilic fibres, the numbers of which decrease with age. He found little elastic tissue present at birth, but the amount increased with age. The collagen bundles are fine and no division between a reticular and papular layer is present. The subcutaneous layer contains much fat.

Numerous capillaries are visible, associated mainly with the hair follicles. At birth, a definite triad of follicles is seen. The triad consists of a large central primary follicle bounded on either side by smaller lateral primary follicles. In some cases, two lateral primaries may be present on one side, and another variation is the presence of a secondary follicle associated with a lateral primary. Developing simple sebaceous glands are seen as buds in the upper third of the follicle; the central primary, and occasionally the lateral primaries, may bear such buds. Some primary follicles are also associated with patent apocrine glands, which as yet are simple tubes opening into the primary follicles above the sebaceous glands.

The primary follicles are arranged at an angle of approximately 60° to the epidermis. In sections showing follicles cut transversely, an occasional primary follicle shows the arrangement by which secondary follicles are formed. These appear as strands of intensely basophilic cells, often with melanocytes, running deeply into the dermis from their point of origin just below the sebaceous glands of the primary follicles (Fig. 1.23). In the lip the sinus hairs are already well developed, although the sinuses themselves are still very cellular and contain no blood cells. Arrectores pilorum muscles are better developed in this region at this age than they are elsewhere in the skin; they appear as strands of spindle-shaped cells, two or three cells thick, in association with the sinus hairs.

At birth, the eyelids are still fused and remain so for 8 or 9 days. It might be supposed that the eyelids adhere solely because of the presence of gland secretions, but in fact this is not so. At birth, the eyelids are fused by a bridge of living cells. At 4 days of age, the outer surface of the fused part is becoming keratinized and begins to separate. However, throughout the fused areas the cells are large and viable, with vacuolated cytoplasm. Keratinization is not observable in the inner two-thirds of the fused junction at 4 days of age. It would appear that keratinization of the fused area is responsible for causing separation of the two eyelids. Melanocytes are present in the basal layer of the fused area and are actively

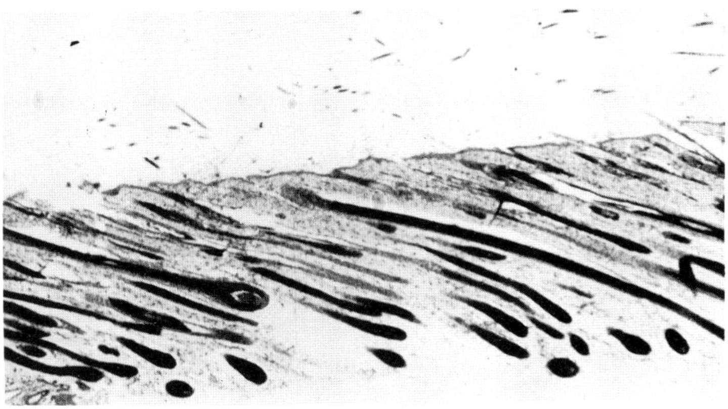

Fig. 1.23. Skin at birth — the secondary follicles and apocrine glands are growing into the dermis.

producing pigment at this age. The epidermis is not ridged, as it will be later at the palpebral margin. The meibomian glands are comparatively large and multilobed structures at 4 days of age, and holocrine breakdown is just beginning in the cells bordering the main collecting duct. Mitosis has been observed on several occasions in the cells lining these glands. The conjunctival surface is composed of two rows of cuboidal cells supporting a single layer of flattened cells with fusiform, deeply staining nuclei. This layer is non-keratinized and melanocytes are absent.

Skin at 3–4 weeks of age

At this stage, the follicle is compound and each follicle contains three to four hairs. The epidermis is two to three cells thick and the stratum corneum is well formed. The dermis is less cellular than at birth but many fibroblasts are still present. Each primary follicle can be seen to be giving rise to two or three secondary follicles which arise as projections from the upper third of the primary follicle above the sebaceous gland ducts.

Skin at 8–10 weeks of age

The dermis is less cellular and the epidermis has two to three cell layers. Sebaceous glands are becoming larger and show signs of budding to form a lobed structure. Some of the secondary follicles now show formation of more hairs; these appear as two to three small hairs arranged in a crescent about the central or lateral primaries. In a transverse section, these are seen to arise on the same side in each follicle group. Subsequently, secondary follicle formation continues until puberty, when six to 10 hairs may occupy a single follicle (Lovell, 1955). The epidermis of the mature, hairy skin is thin, usually not more than two to three cell layers being present.

Occasional follicles in the catagen phase are seen in the first few weeks of life. Lovell (1955) reports no replacement during the first 7 months of life.

Sebaceous and apocrine glands are active at birth but both are of the simple type. The arrector pili muscle is slender at birth and is still so at 70 days; it joins the follicle in its lower third, passing between the secondary follicle. Melanocytes are carried down into the dermis by the growth of both the primary and secondary follicles: however, they are not formed in the stratum germinativum but originate in the neural crest, from which they migrate in early fetal life with the nerves of the skin (Rawles, 1947; DuShane, 1948).

References

Allen T.D. (1977) Cell stacking, shape, and epidermal proliferative unit concept. *Journal of Anatomy* **124**, 4–83.

Allen T.E. & Bligh J.A. (1969) A comparative study of the temporal patterns of cutaneous water loss from some domesticated mammals with epitrichial sweat glands. *Comparative Biochemistry and Physiology* **31**, 347–363.

Baker K.P. (1966) Post-natal development of the dog's skin. *British Veterinary Journal* **122**, 344–347.

Baker K.P. (1967a) The histology and histochemistry of the circumanal hepatoid glands of the dog. *Journal of Small Animal Practice* **8**, 634–647.

Baker K.P. (1967b) Senile changes of dog skin. *Journal of Small Animal Practice* **8**, 39–53.

Baker K.P. (1974) Hair growth and replacement in the domestic cat. *British Veterinary Journal* **130**, 327–335.

Baker B.B., Maibach H.I., Park R.D., McFarland L.Z. & O'Brien, T.R. (1973) Epidermal cell renewal in the dog. *American Journal of Veterinary Research* **34**, 93–94.

Breathnach A.S. (1980) Branched cells in the epidermis, an overview. *Journal of Investigational Dermatology* **75**, 6–11.

Briggaman R.A. & Wheeler C.E.J. (1975) The dermal-epidermal junction. *Journal of Investigational Dermatology* **65**, 71–84.

Brown A.G. & Iggo A. (1967) A quantitative study of cutaneous receptors and afferent fibres in the cat and rabbit. *Journal of Physiology* **193**, 707–733.

Cashman D.C., Laryea J.U. & Weissman B. (1969) The hyaluronidase of rat skin. *Archives of Biochemistry and Biophysics* **135**, 387–395.

Cauna N. (1973) The free penicillate nerve endings of the human hairy skin. *Journal of Anatomy* **155**, 227–228.

Cauna N. (1976) Morphological basis of sensation in hairy skin. In *Progress in Brain Research* Vol. 43 (Eds Iggo. A. & Ilyusky O.B.) pp. 35–45. Elsevier, Amsterdam.

Cleffmann D.G. (1964) Function specific changes in the metabolism of agouti pigment cells. *Experimental Cell Research* **35**, 590–600.

DuShane G.H. (1948) The development of pigment cells in vertebrates. In *The Biology of Melanomas*, p. 1. New York Academy of Science.

Edelson R.L. & Fink J.M. (1985) The immunologic function of the skin. *Scientific American*, 34–41.

English K.B. (1974) Cell types in cutaneous Type I mechanoreceptors (Haarscheiben) and their alterations with injury. *American Journal of Anatomy* **141**, 105–126.

English K.B. (1977) Morphogenesis and denervating atrophy of Haarscheiben. *Journal of Investigational Dermatology* **69**, 58–67.

Epstein W.L. & Maibach H.L. (1964) Cell proliferation and movement in human hair bulbs. In *Advances in Biology of Skin Hair Growth* Vol. 9 (Eds Montagna W. & Dobson R.L.). Pergamon, Oxford.

Galbraith D.B. (1964) The agouti pigment pattern of the mouse, a quantitative and experiential study. *Journal of Experimental Zoology* **115**, 71–90.

Gray W.R., Sandberg L.B. & Foster J. (1973) Molecular model for elastin structure and function. *Nature* **246**, 461–464.

Greaves (1987) In *Dermatology in General Practice* Vol. III (Eds Fitzpatrick T.B., Eisen A.Z., Wolff K., Freedburg I.M. & Austen K.F.) pp. 74–78. McGraw-Hill, New York.

Halliday G.W., McArdle J.P., Knight B.A. & Muller H.K. (1986) New methodology for assessment of the Langerhans' cell network. *Journal of Pathology* **148**, 127–134.

Hughes H.V. & Dransfield J.W. (1959) The blood supply to the skin of the dog. *British Veterinary Journal*, 299–310.

Isitor G.N. (1979) Origin and early development of canine circumanal glands. *American Journal of Veterinary Research* **40**, 487–492.

Lichtenstein J.R. (1979) Basement membranes. In *Dermatology in General Practice* (Eds Fitzpatrick T.B., Eisen A.Z., Wolff K., Freedburg I.M. & Austen K.F.). McGraw-Hill, New York.

Liotta L. (1980) Metastatic potential correlates with enzymatic degradation of basement membrane collagen. *Nature* **284**, 67.

Lovell R.J.E. (1955) *Veterinary Anatomy — Histological and Histochemical Studies of Growth Changes of Canine Skin*. Master's thesis, Iowa State College.

Mann S.J. & Straïle W.E. (1965) Tylotrich (hair) follicle: association with a slowly adapting tactile receptor in the cat. *Science* **147**, 1043.

Mathieson J.M. & Pearce R.H. (1963) The glycosaminoglycan of the ground substance of rat skin. *Canadian Journal of Biochemistry* **41**, 2327–2325.

Nilsson B.Y. (1970) The tactile organ on the cat's foreleg. Structure and function of a group of functionally coordinated mechano-receptors. *Dissertations Abstracts International* **31B**, 3678.

Partridge S.M. (1962) Elastin. *Advances in Protein Chemistry* **17**, 227–302.

Rawles M.E. (1947) Origin of pigment cells from the neural crest in the mouse embryo. *Physiology and Zoology* **20**, 248.

Reinits K.G. (1960) The acid mucopolysaccharides of the sexual skin of apes and monkeys. *Biochemical Journal* **74**, 27–38.

Schiller S., Slover D. & Dorfman A. (1962) Effect of the thyroid gland on metabolism of acid mucopolysaccharides in skin. *Biochimica et Biophysica Acta* **58**, 27.

Schiller S. *et al.* (1963) Mucopolysaccharides in relation to growth and thyroid hormones. *Journal of Chronic Diseases* **16**, 291–294.

Schiller S., Blumen Krantz N. & Dorfman A. (1965) Effect of prednisolone and hydrocortisone on distribution of polysaccharides in skin. *Biochimica et Biophysica Acta* **101**, 135–137.

Schummer A, Wilkens H., Vollmerhaus B. & Habermehl K.H. (1981) *The Anatomy of the Domestic Animal* Vol. III. Paul Parey, Berlin.

Silberberg I., Baer R.L., Rosenthal S.A., Thorbecke G.J. & Beresowsky V. (1975) Dermal and intramuscular Langerhans' cells at sites of passively induced allergic contact sensitivity. *Cell Immunology* **18**, 435–453.

Stingl G., Wolf-Schreiner, Pinchler W.J., Gschnait F. & Knapp W. (1977) Epidermal Langerhans' cells bear Fc and C3 receptors. *Nature* **268**, 245–246.

Straile W.E. (1960) Sensory hair follicles in mammalian skin: the tylotrich follicle. *American Journal of Anatomy* **106**, 133–141.

Strickland J.H. & Calhoun M.L. (1963) The integumentary system of the cat. *American Journal of Veterinary Research* **24**, 1018–1029.

Uitto J.I. (1979) Collagen. In *Dermatology in General Practice* (Eds Fitzpatrick T.B., Eisen A.Z., Wolff K., Freedburg I.M. & Austen K.F.) pp. 164–180. McGraw-Hill, New York.

2 / Clinical Examination and Laboratory Procedures

Skin disease is so common that familiarity may predispose to a superficial examination. This is a mistake; it is essential that a thorough, step-by-step procedure be made in every case, the client being fully informed as to the necessity of this procedure if the patient is to be helped.

The basic steps are as follows:

1 Obtaining and recording the clinical history. During this time the clinician observes the patient which then has time to accustom itself to its new surroundings.

2 The general clinical examination. Skin lesions may be the visible signs of systemic disease. It is a mistake to examine only the skin.

3 The dermatological examination.

4 The use of diagnostic and laboratory aids.

5 The deductive process.

6 The diagnosis.

Case history

Obtaining and interpreting the case history are the first steps towards the diagnosis. The clinician's aim is to obtain all the relevant past information by posing a number of questions; this must be complete and therefore it is helpful to fill in a case-history chart (Fig. 2.1). The clinical record should include body outlines for recording the distribution of the lesions. The length of time the complaint has been present will indicate an acute or chronic problem. Seasonality may suggest association with specific allergens.

Housing and bedding

Association with possible allergens is of relevance here: animals sleeping in bedrooms or even beds may be unduly exposed to house-dust mites which produce a most potent allergen. Close proximity to epoxy resins or garage material, will have relevance to contact-allergic dermatitis. Animals sleeping on hay or straw or in dusty food stores may be in contact with large numbers of forage mites or may perhaps be exposed to fomites contaminated with large animal ringworm spores or hyphae, and hounds exercised on earthed paddocks may be exposed to hookworm larvae.

Some dogs spend long periods in their owner's car. Here they may be in contact with potential contact allergens in car upholstery (particularly leather) and rubber matting. For the

OWNER	NAME			ADDRESS			
	HOME PHONE NO.	BUSINESS PHONE NO.		Prev. Attendance	Animal's Name or Number		
ANIMAL	SEX	AGE	SPECIES	BREED	COLOUR/MARKINGS	WEIGHT	
ATTEN-DANCE	DATE:	HOUR:	ADMITTANCE ☐	DISCHARGE	DATE:	HOUR:	
PRIMARY COMPLAINT							
REFERRED BY	NAME			REPLY SENT	PRIMARY CLINICIAN		
	ADDRESS			PHONE	ATTENDING CLINICIAN		

THIS HISTORY IS TO BE COMPLETED IN FULL. Ring appropriate signs. IN EMERGENCIES, FILL IN AFTER EMERGENCY CARE.

IMMUNIZATION State age, none or ? — Initial: C.D. C.V.H. Lepto.con/ict. Other (specify)
Repeats: C.D. C.V.H. Lepto.con/ict.

PREVIOUS ILLNESS OR INJURIES: (specify age, or none)

	Duration		Duration
		LENGTH OF TIME OWNED:	
DIET: nature / daily amount — meat/fish veg.		LIQUID: type	
carbohyd. other		INTAKE: daily consumption	
APPETITE: N – anorexic – inappet. – variable – fair – good – excessive		THIRST: N – decreased – increased – excessive	
RESPIRATION: N – hypernoeic – dyspnoeic – abdominal – thoracic		NASAL DISCHARGE: (nature)	
COUGH: none – dry – productive – persistent – intermittent – When seen?			
FAECES: N – hard-formed – soft – liquid – blood – mucus. Colour		DEFAECATION: difficulty – pain Frequency	
URINATION: N – frequent – incontinent – difficulty – pain – haematuria			
VOMITION: none – occasional – frequent – persistent – retching only. VOMITUS: character & when seen?			
TEMPERAMENT: N – unreliable – listless – lethargic – excitable – neurotic			
NERVOUS: ataxia – paraplegia – chorea – convulsions – nystagmus – fits.			
SKIN: N – puritus – lesion – alopecia – abnormal pigment – ectoparasites. Site			
SEXUAL: Fertility: proven – apparent infertile – unknown/ / Libido: N – none excessive – unknown			
OESTRUS: age of onset: Last oestrus Duration		Intervals (regular?)	
Pseudo-preg: yes/no Last litter (date) No. of litters		DISCHARGE: none: vulval: preputial	

A

Fig. 2.1. A Case history chart. **B** Clinical examination chart.

same reason potential allergens in toys played with habitually should be assessed.

Contacts

This information is recorded to assess if other animals (including humans) developed skin lesions shortly after these were observed on the patient. *Sarcoptes scabiei* var. *canis*, for example, readily produces an irritant papular rash in contact with humans, whilst urticarial wheals (hives) result from flea bites.

Ringworm and lice are also easily transmitted. Although animals may not develop disease themselves, they may act as carriers to others in the same household.

NAME OR NO.

CODE: N – Normal Detail all abnormalities X – Not examined

ATTITUDE: CONFORMATION:

WEIGHT: NUTRITIONAL STATUS:

SUPERFICIAL LYMPH NODES: CHARACTER OF HAIR COAT:

TEMP: PULSE RATE: RESP. TYPE & RATE:

EYES: ( )

MUCOUS MEMBRANES: ( )

EARS: ( )

SKIN and APPENDAGES: ( )

ALIMENTARY SYSTEM: ( )

RESPIRATORY SYSTEM: ( )

CARDIOVASCULAR SYSTEM: ( )

URINARY SYSTEM: ( )

GENITAL SYSTEM: ( )

MUSCULOSKELETAL SYSTEM: ( )

NERVOUS SYSTEM: ( )

RADIOLOGICAL SUMMARY and DETAILS OF EXAMINATIONS:

B

Age

Ectoparasitism is generally more common in young animals less than 1 year old, although older animals are also infested, this situation is often overlooked. Juvenile demodicosis with its characteristic distribution is seen in dogs less than 6 months old. Sarcoptic mange occurs particularly in unweaned litters. Flea hypersensitivity, whilst sometimes occurring in the first year of life, most commonly occurs in older animals. Similarly, contact-allergic and atopic dermatitis, which require a latent period, are seen most commonly in adult more than 1 year old.

Sex

Pruritus, with or without alopecia, may be a clinical sign of diabetes mellitus which is more common in female dogs and male cats.

Sertoli-cell tumours with associated feminization occur in male dogs; ovarian imbalances, hyperoestrogenism and hypo-oestrogenism are seen in bitches. Removal of the gonads may initiate skin disease and the condition of the genitalia should be determined at the clinical examination.

Therapy

It is relevant to determine if any therapy has been given to the patient recently. Corticosteroids are too wildly used in veterinary practice and may mask pruritus, long-term therapy can produce marked systemic and dermatological changes. Antibiotics may initiate anaphylactic and allergic reactions whilst sulphonamides may produce skin eruptions.

In many cases the owner has consulted a number of clinicians prior to the consultation and the range of medication given must be recorded. For example, a course of parasiticidal baths responsibly given should eliminate the possibility of ectoparasitism with the exception of demodicosis (unless the appropriate medication has been given for sufficient time), or drugs may have been given in an uncontrolled manner for a prolonged period with the development of iatrogenic disease. (Medicated baths may have been prescribed but inefficiently executed.) Drug reactions may cause a number of disease manifestations and therefore all medication should be recorded. Response to corticosteroid therapy may suggest allergic disease or autoimmune skin disease.

Feeding

The clinical history should record the diet. An imbalanced diet could be related to essential fatty acid deficiency with an associated seborrhoeic dermatitis. Food allergy, although not common, does occur and a previous examining clinician may have prescribed a non-allergic diet for possible food-allergy dermatitis; however, commonly these are not strictly enforced, thus non-improvement does not necessarily preclude the diagnosis. All foods given, including titbits, need to be recorded: the problem of the determination of food allergy in the straying, foraging dog is a very real one. Appetite can be important: polyphagia may indicate diabetes mellitus or hyperadrenocorticism; decreased appetite may indicate hypothyroidism or systemic disease with associated skin manifestations.

The fluid intake should be assessed. Polydipsia may indicate hyperadrenocorticism or diabetes mellitus.

Duration and season

Pruritic diseases of recent origin are most likely to be parasitic in origin. However, pruritic diseases of long duration may also be parasitic even if treatment has been given by a previous clinician. Flea hypersensitivity is more prevalent during the warmer months of the year; seasonal recurrent dermatitis is a characteristic of this very common disease. Seasonal pollenosis has not been recorded in Europe, but conjunctivitis, rhinitis and sneezing of a summer seasonal type do occur and may possibly be related to pollen allergy. Reactions to midges and other biting flies will be seen during the seasons when adult flies are on the wing.

Exercise tolerance

Diminished activity and lethargy occur in a number of cases of hypothyroidism, while physical weakness is characteristically seen in hyperadrenocorticism.

Sexual activity

Lack of libido is a feature of the male feminizing syndrome as is hypothyroidism.

Breed

There is a definite breed predisposition to certain skin diseases (Table 2.1).

The clinical examination

The patient will have been presented for examination with a specific complaint. The veterinarian should determine when a problem was first apparent, what the lesions, if any, were like at that time, and how the condition has progressed since.

Table 2.1. Skin diseases associated with breed

Breed	Disease
Bulldogs	Tail-fold pyoderma Facial fold pyoderma
Collies	Autoimmune disease
Dachshund	Acanthosis nigricans Regional follicular dysplasia Sternal callus
Dalmatian	Bronzing syndrome
Alsatian	Autoimmune disease Perianal fistula Pituitary dwarfism
Doberman	Generalized demodicosis Flank sucking Colour-mutant alopecia
Golden retriever	Lick granuloma
Great dane	Acne Lick granuloma Dermoid cyst
Irish setter	Colour-mutant alopecia
Irish terrier	Foot pad hyperkeratosis
Irish wolf hound	Hygroma
Keeshond	Keratoacanthoma
Labrador retriever	Lick granuloma Supracaudal gland alopecia
Malamute	Zinc-deficiency dermatosis
Norwegian elkhound	Keratoacanthoma
Pekingese	Facial fold pyoderma
Poodle	Epiphora
Rhodesian ridgeback	Dermoid sinus
Shar Pei	Seborrhoea, fold dermatitis
Siamese cat	Regional alopecia, demodicosis Facial leucotrichia Psychosomatic dermatosis
Shetland sheepdog	Autoimmune disease
Siberian husky	Zinc-responsive dermatosis
Staffordshire bull terrier	Interdigital pyoderma Supracaudal gland alopecia
Scottish terrier	Atopy

A general impression should first be obtained by commencing the examination at a distance: is the animal active or lethargic? Is there evidence of systemic disease? Has it been well cared for? Is it well nourished? Is there obesity or thinness? Following this, the overall distribution of the lesions should be determined and documented.

Examination should be made in good lighting with the patient as relaxed as possible for convenience of examination. A useful source is a loop light around a magnifying lens with an extendable adjustable arm. All parts of the body surface should be examined, including the natural orifices, the mucous membranes, and the nails and pads.

The following should be assessed:

1 Is there pruritus?

2 Palpation. Is the skin dry or moist, pliable or inelastic? Is there obesity, excoriation or scaliness?

3 What is the hair like? Is it brittle or broken? Is there hair loss?

4 Examination of lesions. What is their type? Are they grouped?

5 What is the distribution of the lesions? Several conditions have a characteristic pattern of distribution.

First the head is examined with the pinnae, external auditory meatus, eyelids and eyes, mouth and nostrils. The position of any lesions and their nature is recorded on the skin chart. Examine the dorsum then the lateral surfaces. Turn the animal over on its back and examine ventral trunk, external genitalia and perineum. The legs and feet should also be examined. The state of the hair is assessed and combings and brushings are removed for examination. The surface of the skin is examined minutely for abnormalities, with the hair turned back. The skin's texture should be determined together with the degree of elasticity. Observation of specific signs are encircled or otherwise noted on the examination chart (Fig. 2.2).

A fine-toothed comb is a valuable asset — the presence of the large mites, fleas, lice and ticks is quickly indicated. Brushing on to a dark surface is helpful and the brushings may be collected on to paper for subsequent examination in the laboratory.

The palpation of the skin assesses temperature and the degree of hydration and elasticity. Whether the skin is thinned or thickened can be determined. Close inspection with palpation and olfaction determines whether the skin is unduly dry or moist and the presence of abnormal odour. Decrease or

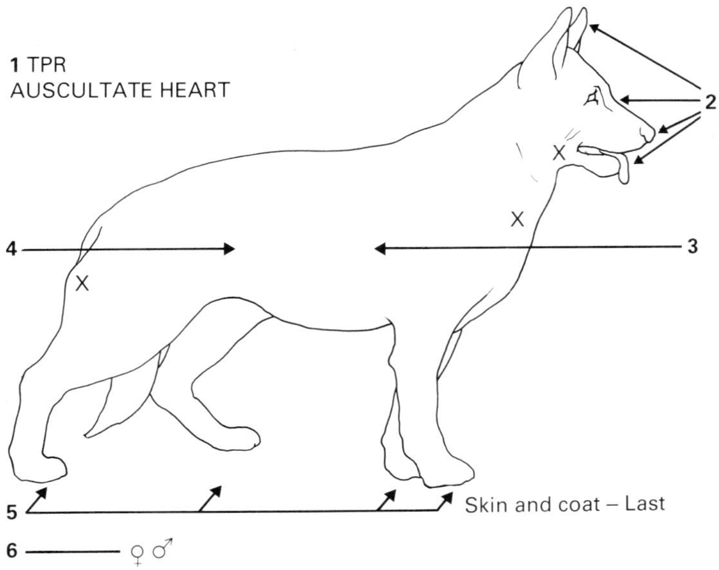

Fig. 2.2. Sequence of clinical examination. X = lymph nodes.

increase in pigmentation is assessed. The state of the hair — evidence of licking, self-excoriation, depilation — is obvious.

Morphology and distribution of lesions

An essential part of any dermatological investigation is an appreciation of the nature of the presenting lesions. The morphology of lesions (see Glossary) is, in many diseases, characteristic, as is their distribution about the animal's skin and appendages (see Fig. 2.3, pp. 46–49).

PRIMARY LESIONS

Specific pathological processes attributable to the disease from which the patient is suffering may be clinically diagnostic, e.g. blisters, bullae or erosions of autoimmune disease.

Many primary lesions are missed in veterinary practice because self-trauma and other changes supervene before the patient is presented for examination.

SECONDARY LESIONS

The initiation of behavioural changes due to discomfort or the progress of the disease to a spontaneous secondary stage may give rise to secondary lesions, e.g. chronic lichenification of self-trauma due to scratching, licking and rubbing or the spontaneous, secondary ulceration due to the foreign body reaction in calcinosis cutis of hyperadrenocorticism. In many instances these are the initial lesions observed by the clinician. (See Table 2.2.)

DISTRIBUTION OF LESIONS

Generalized

Skin lesions, depending on their aetiology, may commonly be generalized. This situation can readily result from an initial localized diseased area from which centrifugal spread takes place, as in fungal infection. Alternatively, generalized involvement of the skin may occur by mechanical spread through self-trauma, environment or similar process or by the whole of the skin being the target organ as in allergic disorders or in haematogenous spread of infection.

Localized

Skin lesions may be localized as in the manifestation of lesions at mucocutaneous juctions in some forms of autoimmune disease, flank alopecia in hormonal disorders or the discrete isolated lesions of bacterial infection in interdigital pyoderma.

Symmetrical

The symmetrical distribution of skin lesions, particularly bilateral alopecia, is characteristically seen in endocrine disorders

Table 2.2. The nature of primary and secondary lesions. Morphology of lesions is described in the Glossary.

Primary lesions	Secondary lesions
Macules	Scale
Patches	Crust
Papules	Excoriation
Pustules	Lichenification
Wheals	Erosion
Vesicles	Ulcer
Bullae	Fissure
Nodules	
Tumours	

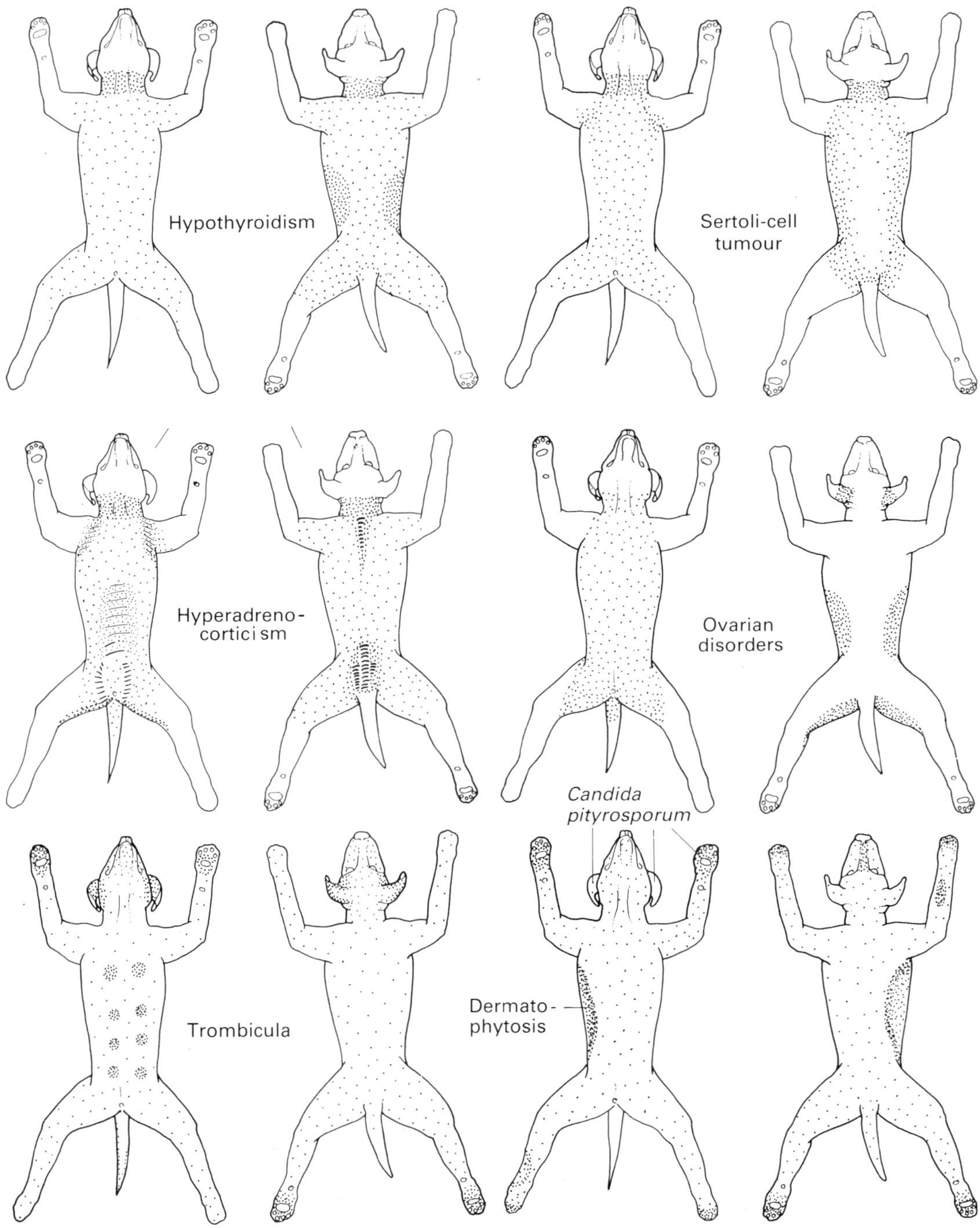

Fig. 2.3. Skin charts showing distributions of lesions characteristic of various diseases.

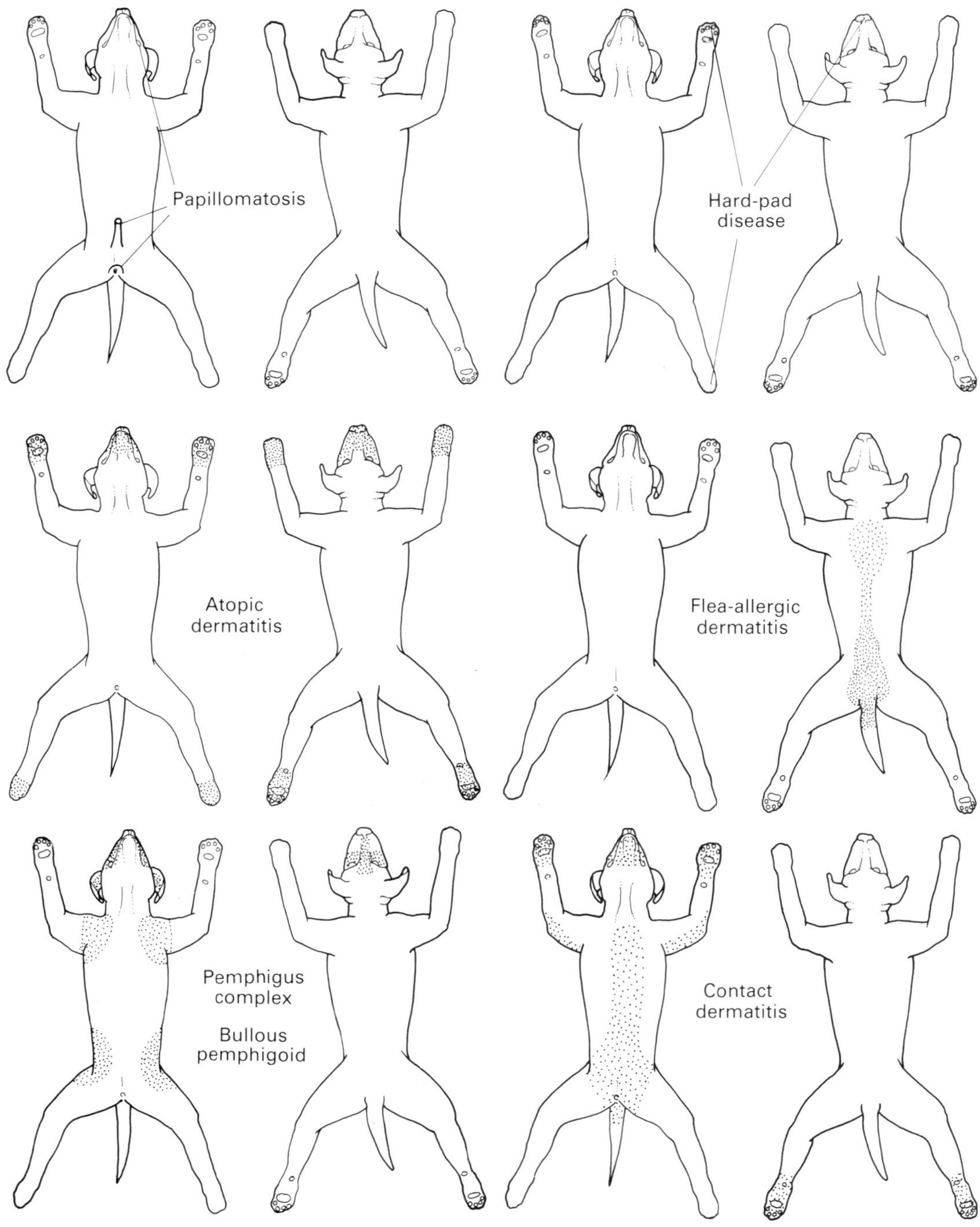
Papillomatosis
Hard-pad disease
Atopic dermatitis
Flea-allergic dermatitis
Pemphigus complex
Bullous pemphigoid
Contact dermatitis

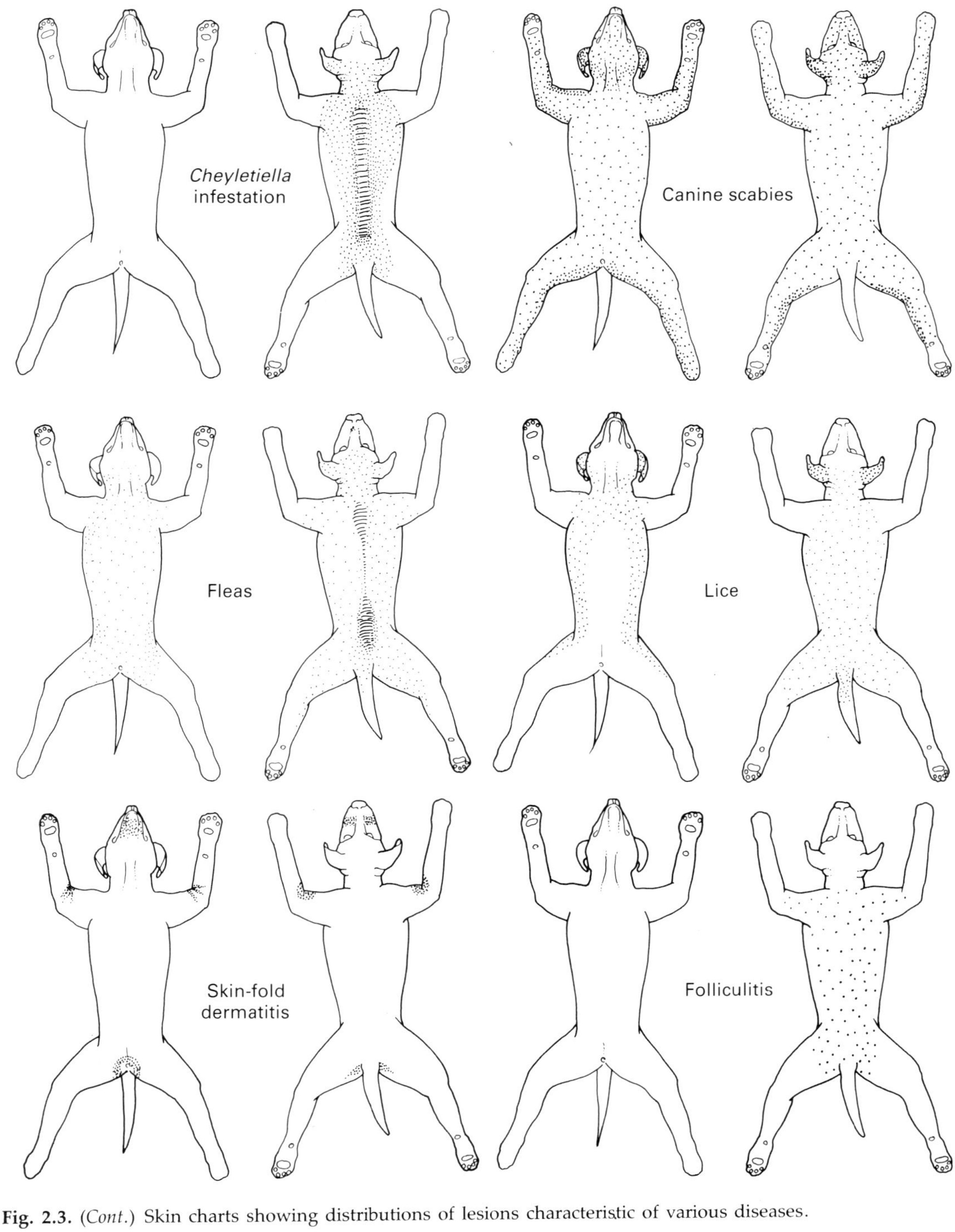

Fig. 2.3. (*Cont.*) Skin charts showing distributions of lesions characteristic of various diseases.

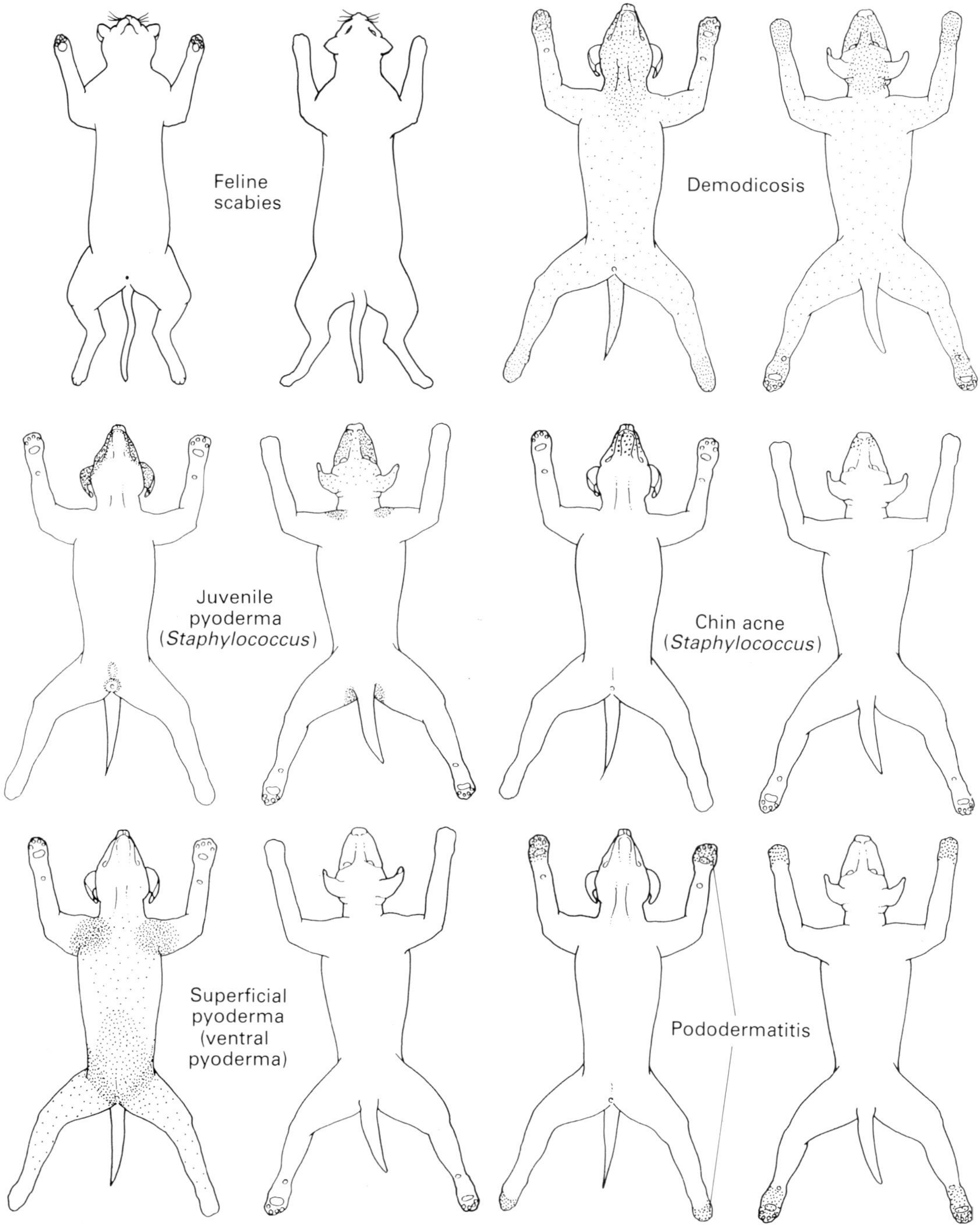
Feline scabies
Demodicosis
Juvenile pyoderma (*Staphylococcus*)
Chin acne (*Staphylococcus*)
Superficial pyoderma (ventral pyoderma)
Pododermatitis

of the dog and cat. It occurs less commonly in infectious disease although in some cases the configuration can be almost pathognomonic, e.g. *Microsporum canis* of the limbs in cats, sarcoptic scabies infestation of the fringe of the pinnae of dogs.

Asymmetrical

Skin lesions associated with acquired infectious agents are more commonly asymmetrical in distribution, as opposed to the symmetry of lesions of functional origin whether physiological or immunological.

THE CONFIGURATION OF LESIONS

Many terms have been given to indicate the description of the outline of lesions:

Annular lesions

Lesions are in the form of a ring which may be eroded, crusted, erythematous or otherwise affected by a pathological process. The central area may show minimal change from normal.

Linear

Lesions following a line — claw scratches, eosinophilic granuloma complex of cats (linear granuloma).

Serpiginous

Serpentine or snake-like lesions in some neoplastic and autoimmune skin diseases.

Arciform

Having an arch-like or crescentic outline, seen where other lesions are likely to be annular and certain of them are incomplete, e.g. epidermal collarettes, circular lesions of superficial pyoderma.

Skin testing

These procedures have a place in the diagnosis of atopic dermatitis, flea allergy and bacterial hypersensitivity. With practice it is a reliable diagnostic aid.

However, false positive reactions do occur while some hypersensitive animals will give no reactions. The intradermal injection is more reliable than the prick or scratch test.

There is no standardization of allergens used in veterinary dermatology, an obvious disadvantage. Protein nitrogen (PN) units are used and various weight/volume concentrations. Whatever the practitioner decides upon, he or she should stick to one so that a standardized procedure can be followed. For standard intradermal testing two controls are used, the vehicle alone, phosphate-buffered saline (PBS, negative control), and a 1 : 1000 solution of histamine sulphate (positive control).

Food extracts give relevant intradermal reactions in anaphylaxis but not in food allergy.

Commercial extracts are available. These may be given as scratch or prick tests or by the injection of extracts by syringe into the skin. They are expensive and have the disadvantage of a comparatively short shelf life. It is possible to prepare extracts in the practice laboratory. The vehicle is PBS (pH 7.4) containing 0.5% phenol and 0.005 Tween 80. The latter prevents the adhesion of the test ingredient to the sides of the vial where it is unavailable. Individual test substances are weighed and the correct volume of the vehicle for a final 1 : 1000 concentration estimated for intradermal testing. For the prick test and scratch test, concentrations of 1 : 100 are used.

A little of the vehicle is added to weighed specimen (say 0.5 g) and the mixture is ground for 5 minutes in a Gratling tube. The remaining volume is then added, well mixed and filtered through a filter funnel containing a No. 20 Whatman paper. Some of the filtered extract is then taken up in a 20 ml syringe and passed through a millipore filter containing a sterile 0.22 μm millipore filter disc. It is collected in a sterile vial which is then labelled to identify the contents and the date added. The extracts should be kept in the cool compartment of a refrigerator.

Intradermal skin testing

Intradermal testing is time consuming; a quiet, orderly procedure is essential, and for that reason intradermal testing should be undertaken when the clinician can devote sufficient time for the procedure.

In human medicine, both scratch and intradermal tests are used. In veterinary practice the latter is more successful. Animals for challenge should not have received corticosteroid therapy within the previous 48 hours. Many dogs will lie quietly on their side with minimal restraint for the test procedure, others will require short-acting anaesthesia or xylazine immobilization.

An area of the lateral abdomen immediately posterior to the last rib is clipped with a No. 20 blade fitted to an Aesculap clipper or similar. Loose hair is removed lightly with cotton wool or a soft brush. Cleaning with spirit is not indicated because the surface should be disturbed as little as possible. Allergic skin may react with erythema or oedematous swelling if too vigorously rubbed. Sites are marked with a felt-tipped pen 2 cm apart in the manner indicated in Fig. 2.4.

Compromise may be necessary with regard to size or position of the prepared area in some cases. In severely allergic skin, much, if not all, may exhibit papular excoriation and erythema. In this case, small areas may be selected and tests undertaken at intervals.

Minimal restraint of the patient is desirable. Test solutions are taken up in 1 ml graduated syringes fitted with No. 26 standard wire gauge (s.w.g.) needles, 15 mm in length. Intradermal injections (0.05 ml) are made under each spot, recording these on a test sheet (Fig. 2.5).

Examination of the sites should be made at 15 minutes, 1 hour and 24 hours subsequent to the test. All sites are examined and the greatest diameter of each wheal measured. These are compared and recorded on the test chart, the reaction at the site of the (PBS) control must be subtracted from positive reaction sites. If there is no reaction at the histamine site, the test should be repeated on another day. Positive reactions are erythematous and comparatively large.

Prick test

A drop of the test solution is placed on the clipped skin and a minute intradermal injection is made using a stylet (available

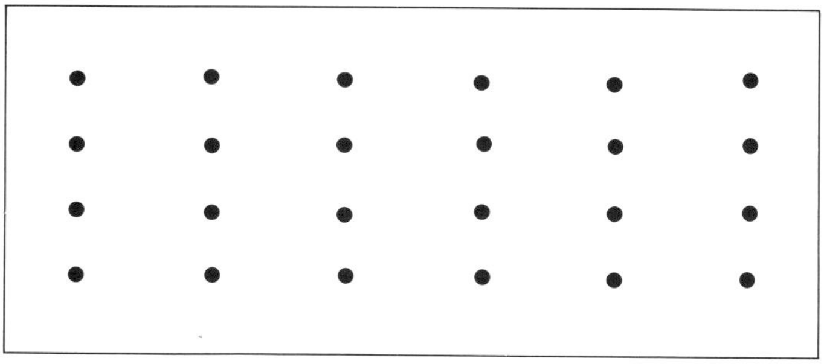

Fig. 2.4. Arrangement of test sites for intradermal tests.

INTRADERMAL TEST RECORD

NAME: CASE NO:

Add E for erythema DATE:

	Control	Hist.	Flea test	House dust	Moulds Beef Milk
15 min 1 hr 24 hrs					
15 min 1 hr 24 hrs					
15 min 1 hr 24 hrs					
15 min 1 hr 24 hrs					
15 min 1 hr 24 hrs					

Fig. 2.5. Chart for recording results of intradermal tests.

from allergen manufacturers). The test is read at 20 minutes, 1 hour and 24 hours and compared to the sites of the PBS control and the histamine control.

Scratch test

A drop of the test solution is placed on the clipped skin and a superficial scratch 0.5 cm in length is made through it. The site is again read as for the prick test and compared to the sites of the negative and positive controls.

The patch test

This is used for the diagnosis of contact-allergic dermatitis.

The veterinary dermatologist can only envy the ease with which the technique can be performed on human skin. There are many problems facing the veterinary clinician; the impregnated patch and control patch (vehicle alone) must remain exactly in position for at least 48 hours without disturbance and the sites then examined daily for 3 days.

Test allergens in petrolatum or aqueous solution are applied individually to gauze pads 2.5 cm in diameter, placed on the clipped normal skin of the flank and taped in position.

Positive reactions are shown as erythematous, thickened areas. The reaction is a delayed hypersensitive reaction and a comparatively long time-scale with *exact* positioning is essential. The preparation may be a primary irritant at the dilution used; prepared solutions should therefore be screened on the skin of a normal dog.

The allergen test must be available in solution.

Standard weights (1 : 1000 in PBS) are ground in a mortar and pestle for 5 minutes and left for 1 hour before filtering and storing at 4 °C.

Laboratory procedures

Parasitic infestation

Superficial ectoparasite infestation may be confirmed by an examination of the coat and skin macroscopically or by taking brushings or skin scrapings for microscopic investigation.

COAT BRUSHINGS

A fine-toothed brush or comb is required and a hand-magnifier. Lice, fleas, *Cheyletiella* and some sarcoptic infestations may be detected.

A collection of hair and skin debris is made by standing or sitting the patient on a large sheet of paper, smooth side uppermost, and either brushing material out using a coarse brush (hair-dresser's styling brush) or by firmly and briskly rubbing the tips of the fingers over the animal, particularly the dorsum from neck to tail root.

Dandruff, hair, flea faeces and debris from both coat and skin fall onto the paper for collection and further examination. Hair retained in the brush should be added to this.

Dandruff and hair on close examination under the low magnification of a hand lens can reveal *Cheyletiella* mites, and ova may be seen attached singly to hairs. Crust and debris examined in wet preparations identifies *Cheyletiella* species and also *Sarcoptes* and other surface mites trapped in the coat.

The examination of teased-out hair tufts placed between two microscope slides at a magnification of up to ×25 can be of value in revealing *Cheyletiella* ova in those cases where mites and dandruff are sparse. The examination of hair plucked from an alopecic or excoriated area is helpful; microscopic examination on a slide under a cover slip may reveal split and broken hairs as a result of licking or self-excoriation in pruritic or psychosomatic conditions. Hairs from animals with hormonal alopecia will have club roots with normal hair tips.

SKIN SCRAPINGS

A scalpel blade, scissors, microscope slides and cover slips, potassium hydroxide (6% KOH) solution, mineral oil, pipettes, envelopes or small plastic bijou bottles are required for this procedure.

An area of active disease is chosen and the surrounding hair clipped away before the surface of the skin is scraped using a scalpel blade; representative samples are collected from a number of sites.

It is essential always to take adequate material. Scrapings may be taken dry, i.e. without moistening the skin surface, or wet using either KOH solution (6%) or mineral oil.

The value of KOH solution is that it is keratolytic and softens the skin surface. It does, however, kill mites in time. The use of mineral oil is preferred by some, since in this medium mites may often be seen to be alive.

The transmission of wet material to the laboratory should be in sealed, rigid plastic containers, particularly if the blade is to be sent; dry material can be dispatched in a paper envelope. All specimens should be clearly labelled for their identification by the laboratory.

Microscopic examination

Potassium hydroxide solution. A small portion of the scraping, taken either dry or using 6% KOH solution, is placed on a glass microscope slide. One or two drops of KOH solution are added, it is covered with a coverslip, warmed gently in the Bunsen flame and gentle pressure is then applied to the coverslip to spread the material and so make a thin preparation, thus making examination more straightforward. Microscopic examination is then carried out. With experience, warming will be found to be unnecessary: excessive warming will produce a mush. Concentration techniques of sedimentation and sugar flotation can also be used with KOH macerates.

Mineral oil. The mineral oil scraping or dry material is placed on a microscope slide, one or two drops of mineral oil are added, a coverslip is applied and light pressure applied to spread the preparation. No warming is required before microscopic examination. Mineral oil has the disadvantage of producing artefacts indiscernable from dermatophyte spores to the inexperienced.

Use of the microscope. In the examination of material for parasites and also fungal infection (ringworm), correct use of the microscope is essential, use the low power objective first.

Specimens mounted in wet preparation are virtually transparent. It is essential therefore that only moderate illumination is used, with some adjustment to increase refraction, i.e. by adjustment of light intensity (rheostat) or by the use of the condenser.

Fungal infections

SKIN SCRAPINGS

Required: scalpel blades, epilation forceps, glass microscope slides and coverslips, envelopes, KOH solution, lactophenol cotton blue, Quink, Wood's lamp.

For cultural identification: neutral Sabouraud's medium, mycobiotic medium, dermatophyte test medium (DTM) are used.

Where appropriate, the hair around the site to be sampled can be clipped to allow for easier access to the infected area. Material for investigation for dermatophyte infection is obtained by epilation of affected hairs identified under the Wood's lamp or of suspect hairs from the active fungal growth area, often best seen at the periphery of the lesion. Scrapings may be collected from the periphery and also the centre of the lesion without moistening the skin. The material obtained by both techniques should be transferred to a paper envelope, sealed and labelled for forwarding to the laboratory.

Examination of specimens under the Wood's lamp, where

appropriate, can identify the greenish fluorescence of *Microsporum canis* infection in a high proportion of cases (approximately 60%). Hairs so identified may be transferred directly to the chosen mounting fluid on a microscope slide or, alternatively, dealt with as for non-fluorescent ringworm specimens, i.e. they are examined microscopically according to the techniques indicated.

Microscopic examination

Potassium hydroxide — wet preparations. One or two drops of a 6% KOH solution are placed on a glass microscope slide. The specimen is placed in the solution and a coverslip is applied, after which the slide is warmed gently, avoiding boiling the specimen. Light pressure to the coverslip spreads the preparation and aids examination. This should be with moderate illumination and adjustment of the optical system to produce some refraction. Hairs with hyphae and arthrospores can then be visualized.

Potassium hydroxide and Quink. Using the above technique but adding 1 part of a 1.2% solution of permanent black Super Quink to 2 parts of the 20% KOH solution stains the hyphae and arthrospores making them more readily identifiable.

CULTURAL EXAMINATION

Fresh, non-fixed material is obtained for the inoculation of culture media or for biological confirmation by animal inoculation in cases of systemic mycoses with skin signs.

Material obtained by dry scraping or epilation is applied to the culture medium by pressing it onto the surface to ensure close contact prior to incubation.

Sabouraud's medium

This supports both pathogens and contaminating fungi. Where contaminants are present, their overgrowth of pathogenic species may lead to a negative or indeterminate result. Neutral Sabouraud's medium should be used (Emmons *et al.*, 1977). It should be incubated at 27° and 37° (enriched with yeast at this temperature). It is best put up as a slope in a Universal glass container fitted with a lid, not tightly screwed, and placed on its side during incubation.

Mycobiotic medium

This contains antibiotic and cyclohexamide to inhibit bacteria and contaminant fungi respectively and enables the pathogens to grow more freely and thus increases the likelihood of cultural confirmation of dermatophyte infection.

The incubation of these two media at 27 °C for 1 to 3 weeks should show colonial growth on which fungal identification can be made by means of lactophenol cotton blue wet preparations of samples of the colonies to determine hyphal and conidial characteristics and colony colour and morphology.

Dermatophyte test medium

This is the equivalent of mycobiotic medium with the addition of phenol red indicator.

Inoculation of slopes of medium in universal bottles at room temperature with the cap released allows growth to take place which, should it be of a pathogen, causes a colour change from amber to deep red. Care should be exercised in using this technique since failure to follow the instructions for use implicitly can lead to erroneous results.

Biopsy

Histopathological investigation of fungal infection may be required where lesions are deep seated or where investigation techniques already employed have failed to confirm the diagnosis.

Staining of sections by silver or periodic acid–Schiff (PAS) methods allows visualization of fungal elements should they be present.

Direct impression smears

For the rapid evaluation of pustular lesions and the differentiation of infected from non-infected bullous lesions, direct impression smears may be employed. They are of value also for the rapid demonstration of yeast cells in swabs from the external auditory meatus.

These may be prepared by: pressing a clean, grease-free microscope slide onto the fresh surface exposed by removal of a scab or opened pustule; scraping the exposed tissue with a blade and smearing the material collected; smearing a swab obtained as for bacterial culture below; or after obtaining the contents of a lesion by aspiration by syringe and needle.

Smears are fixed in alcohol and dried. Staining by Gram's method or Diff Quik gives a preparation which, when examined under the microscope, should aid the differentiation of important infective, non-infective and neoplastic diseases. Toluidine blue 1% is of value for the visualization of mast cell granules, which it stains purple (metachromasia).

Bacterial infection

Required:
Curved scissors
Cotton wool swabs and applicators
Transport medium
Clean, grease-free microscope slides
Sterile needles and forceps
1% alcohol
Diff Quik or Gram stain
Culture media.

Smear preparations and cultural investigation for organisms taken from skin lesions are important in the determination of the causal organisms of the patient's skin disease as well as for prognosis and therapy.

The choice of a new lesion is important so that fresh material may be obtained free from contamination, e.g. intact pustules or adherent crusts.

Preparation of the site prior to sampling is important: the surrounding hair should be clipped away and the area cleansed with 70% alcohol, paying particular attention not to rub or abrade the site causing rupture of the lesion.

Pustules are opened using the point of a sterile needle and the surrounding skin is squeezed to express a bead of pus which is absorbed onto a sterile swab. Lesions covered by crust should have this lifted by using sterile forceps and the exposed lesion swabbed. The sample so obtained is then treated as in the case of pustular lesions. This swab is placed in its tube and passed directly to the practice laboratory or, if for a commercial laboratory, it is placed in transport medium and posted.

Virus infections

Although only rarely necessary, samples may be required for

laboratory investigation for viral infection. Before forwarding to the laboratory, their requirement for tissue or blood samples should be ascertained and also the method of preservation and transport.

Biopsy

When a biopsy study is indicated, it can be of great value, but is often neglected, abused or misapplied, e.g. in acanthosis and lesions associated with chronic pruritus.

Reasons why skin biopsies are needed in diagnosis:

1 Primarily to note histopathological change which may confirm a clinical diagnosis.

2 To provide information on which to base a prognosis.

3 To provide information on which to base therapy and to monitor its efficacy, e.g. in cases of neoplasia.

4 To aid diagnosis by providing uncontaminated specimens of deep-seated infection for cultural purposes.

5 To allow immunohistochemical techniques to aid diagnosis, e.g. in bullous diseases where fluorescent antibody studies may be helpful.

Laboratory investigations may be required in some patients but should supplement and not replace the clinical examination.

Veterinary dermatological histopathology is relatively poorly developed compared with human medicine and there are few pathologists with an expertise in the interpretation of the disease processes in animal skin.

Therefore, before embarking on biopsy techniques, be sure that the laboratory to which the specimens are forwarded is competent to provide the service required.

Some hospital pathology departments will accept animal tissue for report. Where there is a pathologist with an interest in the comparative field the service can be admirable, but one must always remember that human and animal tissues do not always show similar changes in comparable clinical conditions.

TECHNIQUE

The site of the biopsy must be carefully chosen; the technique must be adequate, the fixative appropriate and the clinical history sufficiently detailed. The laboratory facility required for processing must, because sections of skin are often difficult to cut, offer high-quality cutting and staining. The equipment for biopsy is shown in Table 2.3.

The dermatologist should, whenever possible, personally examine the sections and in the ideal situation discuss them with the pathologist in the light of their knowledge of the patient.

CHOICE OF SITE

A fully developed lesion characteristic of the clinical condition should be included. The edges of ulcerated or bullons lesions should always be included in the biopsy. Small lesions may be totally excised using an elliptical approach approximately 1.5 × 0.5 cm. Alternatively a Keyes biopsy punch up to 8 mm diameter may be used, or a disposable punch, or even a high-speed rotary punch. Full thickness skin including the subcuticular fat layer should be taken. To prevent curling, the specimen is placed on a piece of firm blotting paper before fixation.

ANAESTHESIA

Depending on the site:

1 Local anaesthesia using lignocaine by subcutaneous field block, avoid damaging tissue.

Table 2.3. Biopsy equipment

Technique	Equipment
Punch biopsy	Curved scissors Keyes punch, disposable punches up to 8 mm diameter Syringes 2 ml Hypodermic needles 25–21 gauge × 12.7/20.3 cm (5/8″) Haemostats Suture material Suture needles Needle holder Fine scissors Fine forceps Gauze swabs Aeroplast dressing Strips of thick filter or blotting paper 0.5 × 2.5 cm Universal bottles of 10% buffered formalin solution
Excision biopsy	Equipment as above, but the punches are replaced by No. 10 or No. 22 scalpel blades with handles
Impression smear	Clean, grease-free slides Sterile scalpel blades No. 10 or No. 22

2 Sedation with acetyl promazine and lignocaine locally.
3 General anaesthesia.

The skin surface should not be rubbed when cleansing the site as this removes essential information, i.e. the superficial layers.

FIXATION

For most routine preparations, 10% buffered formalin is suitable, or a non-formaldehyde alternative; for special techniques the laboratory should be consulted. The appropriate volume of fixative for proper fixation is essential — at least 10 × volume of specimen. Frozen sections may be required for some procedures, e.g. fat stains, immunohistochemistry, and special arrangements for preservation need to be made, e.g. liquid nitrogen, storage at −70 °C, Michel's holding solution.

PROCESSING

This may be automatic or manual; hand processing is often necessary for better results.

STAINING TECHNIQUES

Haematoxylin and eosin (H & E), Giemsa (thionin, toluidine blue), PAS, Gram ZN, Von Kossa. Direct immunofluorescence or enzyme techniques may be employed.

INTERPRETATION

The first essential is a detailed knowledge of the normal for the species and even the breed.

Nearly all current histology textbooks base their information on paraffin sections, and the true anatomy of the epidermis, especially of the stratum corneum, is ignored.

There are many basic pathological changes in the skin and for these the reader is referred to Muller *et al.* (1989), Lever (1983), and to Bostock and Owen (1975).

References

Bostock O. & Owen L.N. (1975) *A Colour Atlas of Neoplasia in the Cat, Dog, and Horse*. Wolfe Medical Publications, London.
Emmons C.W., Binford C.H., Uta J.P. & Kwow-Chung K.J. (1977) *Medical Mycology*, 3rd edn. Lea & Febiger, New York.
Lever W.F. (1983) *Histopathology of the Skin*, 6th edn. Lippincott, London.
Muller G.H., Kirk R.W. & Scott D.W. (1989) *Small Animal Dermatology*, 4th edn. W.B. Saunders, London.

3 / Heritable Defects

Heritable defects in dogs are usually rare; however, atopy is relatively common and is inherited.

Many of the rarer defects result from a single mutant gene (heterozygous) and the condition is termed dominant. If the mutant gene must be present in the double (homozygous) state to produce disease, the condition is termed recessive or, more correctly, autosomal recessive. Sex-linked skin disease (congenital alopecia) has been reported in dogs (Thomsett, unpublished data). For this the gene must be present on the X chromosome.

The more grotesque dog breeds have been produced by inbreeding; these animals often demonstrate mutant conditions.

Ehlers–Danlos syndrome (cutaneous asthenia)

A disease of apparent increased elasticity associated with fragility of the skin has been reported in cats and dogs and resembles the Ehlers–Danlos syndrome of humans. In humans, at least eight varieties have been reported (Pinnell & McCusick, 1979), four of which have been described as being a result of abnormal collagen biosynthesis (Pinnell, 1978).

The disease has been reported in a number of widely different breeds. It is very rare.

CLINICAL SIGNS

The defect may not be noticeable in young animals until the skin is injured or subjected to surgery. Then cuts which would produce only small openings in normal animals produce extensive tears as a result of increased skin fragility. However, there is little bleeding. Hegreberg *et al.* (1970a) reported a tensile strength of affected canine skin of 89 lb/in^2 compared to the normal of 2610 lb/in^2. The skin shows hyperextensibility but recoils quickly. However, in older dogs it may hang in loose folds. Abnormal joint mobility is not seen in affected cats and dogs. In mature cases there will be a history of abnormal tearing of the skin as a result of minor injury, with numerous scars (Fig. 3.1).

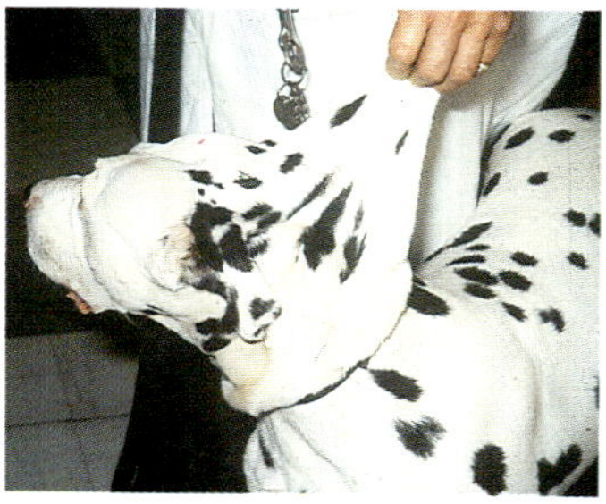

Fig. 3.1. Ehlers–Danlos syndrome in the Dalmatian.

A diagnosis is made on clinical examination. Histological examination may be helpful in some cases — the collagen, when stained by conventional methods, appears broken and shortened (Hegreberg *et al.*, 1970b).

THERAPY

There is no treatment. The owner must be advised about the nature of the abnormality, and breeding of the subject must be avoided. Injuries to the skin are obviously to be avoided; removal of the hind claws in cats is advisable to prevent self-trauma.

Congenital ichthyosis (fish-scale disease)

(Fig. 3.2)

This is a rare, congenital disease of dogs in which the skin is much thickened and fissured and is very scaly in appearance. It is rare but has been reported in dogs and cattle (Julian, 1960). It resembles human ichthyosis, which is transmitted by an autosomal recessive gene. There is extensive scaliness of the skin, the scales projecting above the surface. These scales easily detach and there is marked seborrhoeic odour. The hyperkeratinization is particularly marked on and about areas where the epidermis is normally thick, e.g. the foot pads and perioral region.

Examination of a skin biopsy reveals marked hyperkeratinization, numerous mitotic figures in the epidermis and follicular plugging with some hair loss.

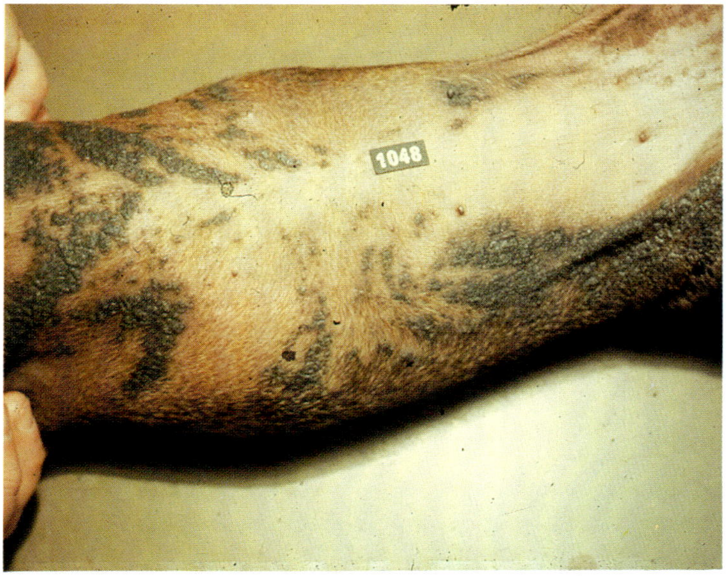

Fig. 3.2. Congenital ichthyosis in a miniature dachshund.

DIAGNOSIS

This may be distinguished from other conditions characterized by seborrhoea with marked skin thickening in that it is present from birth. Zinc hyperkeratosis, although not present at birth, has some similarities but there will be response to zinc sulphate oral therapy over a prolonged period.

THERAPY

If presented when young, euthanasia is advisable to prevent the possible transmission of this most undesirable trait.

If therapy is requested, the owner should be instructed concerning the nature of the condition. Life-long skin care will be essential using keratolytic shampoos (selenium sulphide) or 2.5% benzoyl peroxide washes. Goldsmith and Boden (1972) have used propylene glycol under occlusion for the treatment of human ichthyosis.

Epitheliogenesis imperfecta (aplasia cutis)
(Fig. 3.3)

A rare, congenital absence of areas of skin and mucous membrane that has been reported in puppies (Gupta, 1973; Hewitt *et al.*, 1975), lambs, calves and foals, probably transmitted by an autosomal recessive gene. It is characterized by the patchy absence of areas of the epidermis revealing the reddening underlying dermis. Secondary infection with septicaemia may lead to death at an early age. The epidermis and epidermal appendages (hair follicles, glands) are absent from the ulcerated areas. Gupta (1973) observed the condition in a beagle puppy, whilst Hewitt *et al.* (1975) observed it in one puppy in a litter of eight labradors. A genetic study was not conducted.

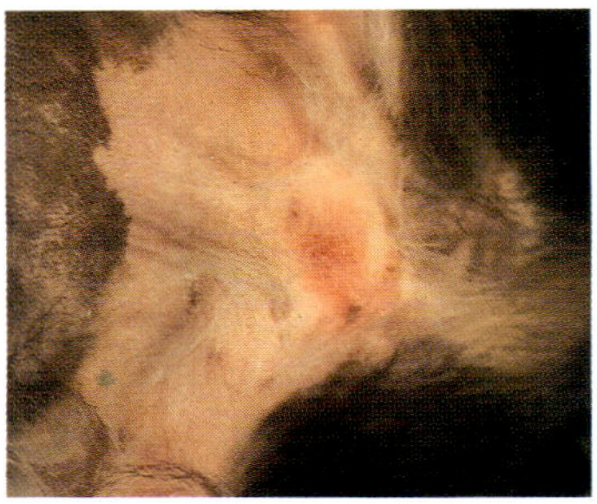

Fig. 3.3. Epidermolysis bullosa in the collie.

THERAPY

As with other undesirable traits, euthanasia or neutering is advisable to prevent continuation. If the defects are relatively small surgery may be indicated.

Epidermolysis bullosa

A rare, hereditary disease which may be congenital, characterized by the formation of blisters and subsequent loss of the associated epidermis following minor trauma. It has been reported in cattle (Bassett, 1987), sheep (McTaggart *et al.*, 1974), and collie dogs (Yager & Scott, 1985). In humans, the term refers to a group of disorders in which dominant and recessive forms exist. The cause is not known. The term epidermolysis is unfortunate, for actual lysis of the epidermis is not seen, cleft formation being usually at the epidermal junction.

CLINICAL SIGNS

In the canine the disease has only been reported in Shetland sheepdogs and collies. Clinical signs appear in the first 6 months of life. Initially, there is erythema and blister formation; healing produces crust formation. As the dog matures there is patchy alopecia, ulceration and plaque formation with scarring, particularly of the extremities and over pressure points. Pruritus is absent, affected animals are otherwise normal and there may be periods of remission. In active phases, blisters may be produced by rubbing the skin with a finger tip for 1 minute: erythema and blistering occur at the site within 15 minutes.

DIAGNOSIS

The differential diagnosis includes other bullous diseases. Positive diagnosis is dependent on histopathology. The biopsy should be taken to include a fresh lesion. Cleft formation below the epidermis occurs, with associated hydropic degeneration of cells of the basal layer. There is little or no associated inflammatory reaction and immunofluorescence of immune complexes is not seen.

THERAPY

Minor trauma should be avoided and affected animals should not be bred. Remission may occur without therapy. In the active phase, prednisolone 1 mg/kg orally is given daily, diminishing the dose to a minimum constant while maintaining a good response. A guarded prognosis should be given.

Vitiligo (Fig. 3.4)

Depigmentation of hair may be hereditary, acquired or idiopathic. Hereditary vitiligo has been described in North

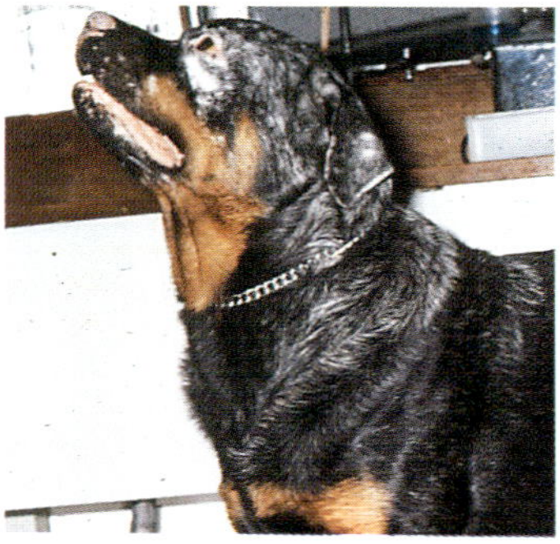

Fig. 3.4. Focal vitiligo in a Rottweiler (acquired).

America, with local loss of hair pigment in the Belgian tervuren dog (Mahaffey *et al.*, 1978) and in India in the German shepherd dog (Sen & Ansari, 1971). Pigment loss in the former most commonly affected the face and buccal cavity; the loss usually occurred in early adulthood without apparent loss of health.

Acral mutilation syndrome

This is a very uncommon condition which has been reported in pointers (German and English) in Germany (Pivnik, 1973; Cummings *et al.*, 1981). Clinical signs are first seen between 3 and 5 months of age. Several puppies of either sex in a litter may be affected. There is licking and biting of the paws, which feel cool. Severe self-mutilation may be seen; paronychia occurs. There is loss of sensation, affected animals walking on their mutilated feet.

The diagnosis is on the clinical signs and breed disposition, with the histopathology showing degenerative changes in myelinated and non-myelinated nerve fibres (Cheville, 1968). Death is inevitable at an early age.

Rubra pilaire (red-hair syndrome)

This condition was reported in France in 1979 in dogs with poor nutrition — diets high in protein of low biological value. The first sign was redness of the hairs of the feet, with progression to involve the ventral surface of the body, the face and the ears. Some dogs had gastrointestinal signs, with dermatitis and pruritus developing later (Dorchies *et al.*, 1979).

Diagnosis is made on the history, clinical signs and the finding of elevated indican levels (Griess *et al.*, 1981). Correction of the diet is necessary (decrease protein but of high biological value). Tetracycline therapy has been given orally for 8 days with yoghurt for 12 days.

Progressive nasal depigmentation has been reported in some large breeds of dogs. The black pigmentation of the external nares is normal at birth but lessens with age, to brown. The aetiology is not known, pigmentary changes are not apparent elsewhere and no therapy is satisfactory: in some cases normal pigmentation returns.

Pili torti

This condition involves abnormalities of the hair shaft with rotation of the long axis (Fig. 3.5). A number of variants occur in humans. Clockwise rotation has been reported in a litter of kittens in England, and as far as is known it has not been reported elsewhere (Geary & Baker, 1986). In humans, this inherited condition is associated with marked systemic defects and mental disturbance. All the kittens in the above record died within 2 months of age.

Twisting of hair shafts around their long axes gives rise to the condition termed 'pili torti' (Fig. 3.6). The defect is usually noted in infancy or childhood resulting from hair fragility. Mental retardation may occur and a number of cases have been reported in association with sensory deafness. Both associated syndromes are inherited as autosomal recessives. The scalp hair becomes more normal as childhood passes.

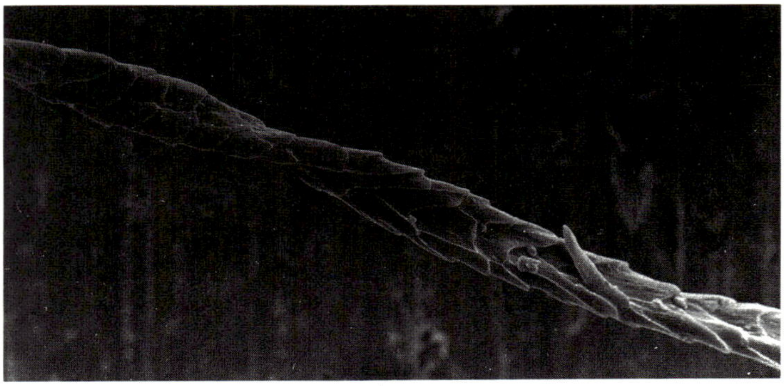

Fig. 3.5. Scanning electron micrograph of secondary hair displaying pili torti.

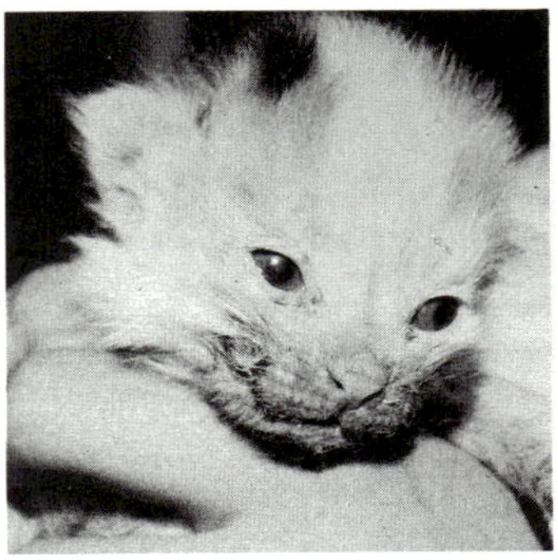

Fig. 3.6. Pili torti in 3-week-old kitten with fine alopecia and dermatitis of the extremities.

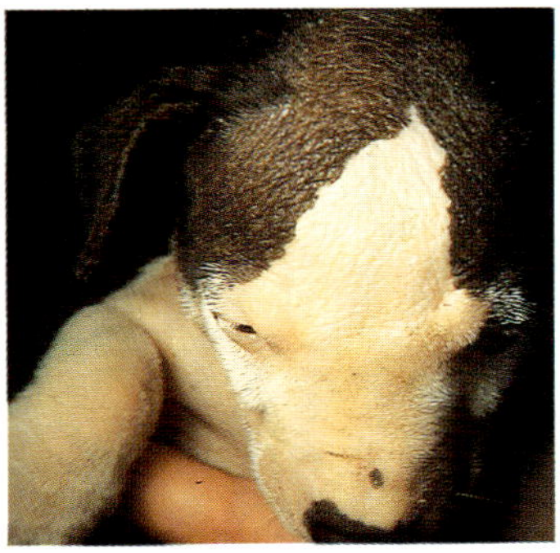

Fig. 3.7. Congenital hypotrichosis. Head of Jack Russell terrier puppy.

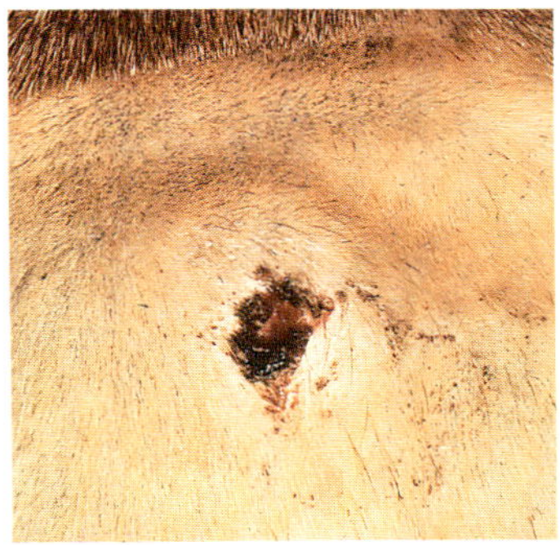

Fig. 3.8. Rhodesian ridgeback with a dermoid sinus.

Feline alopecia universalis

Naturally hairless cats, so-called 'sphinx cats', are being bred (Warner, 1976). They are grotesque and are a most undesirable development of the cat breeders' fancy; they are unquestionably the least handsome of cats. These animals have no primary hair and the whiskers are absent; there is a fine covering of secondary hairs and the skin is oily (Eisenman, 1970).

Canine hairless breeds

The breeding or continuation of any breed which is partially or completely hairless is to be discouraged. Unfortunately there are a number of breeds in which breed standards define partial or complete hairlessness as essential requisites for breeding recognition. These are the Chihuahua, the Mexican hairless breed (Xoloitzcuintl), and the Chinese crested dog. Regular bathing of the Chinese crested dog with a mild shampoo is essential to prevent objectionable skin odour, a little body oil being added to the rinsing water.

Congenital hypotrichia has been reported by Thomsett (1961) in a male whippet which showed patchy alopecia at birth, continuing when the dog was presented for examination at 6 months of age (Fig. 3.7). Hair was absent for many parts of the body, the remaining areas being covered by sparse hair. Hair follicles were reduced in number or absent from the hairless area on histopathological examination. The dog was otherwise normal. At 2 years of age there was no change, previous and subsequent litters were normal and there was no history of similar abnormality in the ancestors of the dam and sire, which were normal.

Dermatomyositis

A rare, mild to severe condition developing in collies aged 2–6 months has been reported (Haupt *et al.*, 1983; Hargis *et al.*, 1983, 1984). The initial lesions are alopecia, erythema, exfoliative dermatitis, ulceration (sometimes vesiculation) on the head (perioral, bridge of nose, lips, inner aspects of pinnae) and over bony prominences of the distal extremities. Subsequently, there is myositis with reduction in the mass of the temporalis muscle and in severely affected animals there may be generalized reduction in muscle mass (Werner *et al.*, 1985; Yager *et al.*, 1985).

In mild cases, healing occurs but with permanent skin changes — small foci of alopecia and hypopigmentation or hyperpigmentation of the bridge of the nose.

Biopsy of affected muscles reveals myositis with thickening of the intima and media of the arteries of affected animals. The aetiology is not known. Therapy is prednisolone by mouth reducing as the clinical signs are controlled. A guarded prognosis should be given.

Uveodermatological syndrome (Harada's disease)

A rare disease reported in the Japanese Akita dog, possibly hereditary with dermatitis and uveitis (Asakura *et al.*, 1977; Bussanich *et al.*, 1982; Romatowski, 1985; Fukui & Furukawa, 1986). It was recently reported in a female Japanese Akita in the UK (Cottrell & Barnett, 1987). The condition resembles the Vogt–Koyanagi–Harada syndrome of young adult people. This has three phases: meningoencephalitic, ophthalmic and the dermatological phase.

In the cases reported in dogs, there has been depigmentation of the lips and eyelids and ulceration of the lips with severe uveitis and vision impairment.

Dermoid sinus of the Rhodesian ridgeback

The Rhodesian ridgeback dog has a prominent ridge along the dorsal line of the back extending from the posterior cervical to sacral region, formed by hair growing in an opposite direction to the adjacent hair. A small percentage have an associated dermoid sinus anterior and posterior to the area of the ridge; there may be one or more sinuses (Fig. 3.8). The entrance of the sinus has darkly pigmented hair projecting through it. From the orifice, the sinus extends towards the vertebral column and ends blindly. Mann and Stratton (1966) describe and illustrate three types of sinus; Lord *et al.* (1957) describe a fourth type where the sinus extends to and is attached to the dura mater of the spinal cord (Fig. 3.9) similar to human pilonidal sinus.

Histopathology reveals the sinus to be lined by skin containing active hair follicles and sebaceous glands. With maturity there is accumulation of sebum and scale. Bacterial infection leads to pyoderma. The only therapy is surgical excision (Hofmeyr, 1963).

The breed society encourages breeders to destroy puppies

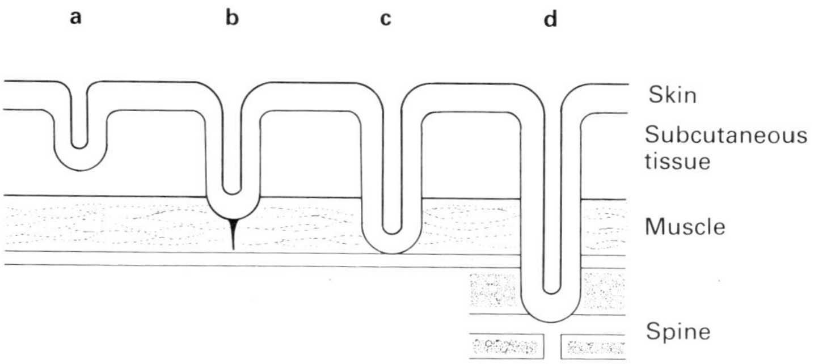

Fig. 3.9. Diagrammatic separation of various types of dermoid sinus of the Rhodesian ridgeback.

with the defect at birth; the parents of affected animals and their siblings should not be bred from. Mann and Stratton (1966) present some inheritance data and suggest that the dermoid sinus factor may be inherited by a single recessive gene.

Pedal hyperkeratosis of Irish terriers

Excessive keratin develops with age on the foot pads of this breed, producing horny excrescences which are displaced laterally by pressure around the pads. These may be 1 cm in length. Shearing may cause fissuring of the dermis with associated pain.

The excessive keratin should be trimmed regularly.

Congenital black-hair dysplasia

This is a rare, congenital, follicular dysplasia confined to the black hair of the pelage reported in various breeds and some cross breeds. Affected hair is shortened, fractures easily and is associated with scale.

There is no treatment. Affected animals should not be bred.

Dysplasia of black hair follicles has been reported in a litter of bearded collies (Harper, 1978). A litter of apparently normal puppies was produced by parents with normal pelages. Four weeks after birth alopecia of the pigmented areas developed; this was of variable intensity in both brown and black puppies of both sexes. The skin in the affected cases was dry and scaly and the remaining hair was brittle.

Histopathologically, the follicles in pigmented areas showed abnormally dense accumulations of pigment in the melanocytes. These follicles were dilated and plugged with fragments of heavily pigmented hair.

Lethal acrodermatitis in bull terriers

A lethal syndrome in bull terriers with progressive acrodermatitis (dermatitis surrounding all the orifices of the body) diarrhoea, pneumonia and abnormal behaviour has been reported in the USA in 17 related puppies (Jezyk *et al.*, 1986).

Although resembling human acrodermatitis enteropathica, it does not respond to therapy with high doses of zinc sulphate. Histopathologically there is parakeratosis, hyperkeratosis and superficial bacterial infection.

Colour mutant alopecia (blue dog disease)

Colour mutant alopecia is a hereditable condition of blue colour mutants, first observed in blue Doberman pinschers, it also occurs in fawn Irish setters, blue dachshunds, blue chows, blue whippets, blue great Danes, blue standard poodles and red and fawn Doberman pinschers.

The defect does not become noticeable for several weeks subsequent to birth; however, some dogs do not develop defects in the blue-haired areas until they are mature adults. The first sign is pityriasis in the blue areas where the hair is dry, brittle and lustreless. Alopecia develops and may be extensive in the blue areas. With maturity the skin in the blue areas feels rough because of the formation of papules which are actually cystic hair follicles. Secondary pyoderma may occur but otherwise colour mutants are normal (Austin, 1975). The disease is not associated with hypothyroidism or zinc deficiency, thyroxine therapy and zinc therapy are of no benefit.

The diagnosis may be confirmed by the histopathology and resembles that in pinnal alopecia. The differential diagnosis is demodicosis and dermatophytosis. These should be eliminated by the routine examination of skin scrapes and hair plucks.

THERAPY

No therapy will reverse the cystic follicular degnerative changes. However, selenium sulphide or other antiseborrhoeic washes are beneficial at 4-day intervals adding bath oil to the rinsing water. Benzoyl peroxide shampoos should be used initially if pyoderma is present.

Pinnal alopecia

An hereditary alopecia of the pinna is seen in mature dachshunds and miniature Yorkshire terriers.

The terminology is inexact for, although fine alopecia with associated hyperpigmentation is first seen in these breeds on the pinna, it also develops over pressure points and intermittently along the dorsum of the tail. Alopecia develops in both sexes after puberty and is progressive and non-responsive to therapy. It is to be distinguished from other dermatoses associated with alopecia of the pinna, seborrhoea and demodicosis. The histopathology is charactersitic: many follicles are cystic and hyperkeratinized whilst the hair bulbs show dysplasia with intensive melanocytic activity, the dermis contain numerous macrophages stuffed with melanin.

There is no therapy yet available.

Canine cyclic neutropenia (grey collie syndrome)

An autosomal recessive condition of grey collies with fatal termination at an early age was reported by Cheville (1968).

Affected puppies are stunted and develop systemic signs of disease by 3 months of age: diarrhoea, pyrexia and lameness is seen. Characteristically, the planum nasale is unpigmented and the coat is silver-grey at birth. Episodic neutropenia and neutrophilia is reported at intervals on average of 11.5 days until death occurs.

References

Asakura S., Takahashi K. & Onishi T. (1977) Vokt–Koyanagi–Harada (uveitis diffusa acuta) in the dog. *Japanese Veterinary Journal* **673**, 445–455.

Austin V. (1975) Blue dog disease. *Modern Veterinary Practice* **56**, 34.

Bussanich M.N., Rootman J. & Dolman C.L. (1982) Granulomatous panuveitis and dermal pigmentation in dogs. *Journal of the American Animal Hospital Association* **18**, 131–138.

Bassett H. (1987) A congenital bovine epidermolysis bullosa resembling epidermolysis simplex of man. *Veterinary Record* **121**, 8–11.

Cheville N.F. (1968) The grey collie syndrome. *Journal of the American Veterinary Medicine Association* **152**, 620–630.

Cottrell B.D. & Barnett K.C. (1987) Harada's disease in the Japanese Akita. *Journal of Small Animal Practice* **28**, 517–522.

Cummings J.F., de Lahunta A. & Winn S.S. (1981) Acral mutilation and nociceptive loss in English pointer dogs. *Acta Neuropathologica* **53**, 119.

Dorchies P., Griess D., Franc M., de Lahitte J.D. (1979) Le syndrome rubra-pilaire ou maladie des poils roude du chien. *Revue de Medecine Veterinaire* **130**, 1371–1372.

Eisenman W.D. (1970) The sphinx cat (hairless). *Cat Fancier News* **3**, No. 5.

Ferrer L., Durall I., Closa J. & Mascort J. (1988) Colour mutant alopecia in Yorkshire terriers. *Veterinary Record* **122**, 360–361.

Fukui M. & Furukawa T. (1986) On the canine fundus abnormalities in Japan. *Transactions of the 17th Annual meeting of the American College of Veterinary Ophthalmologists and the Scientific Programme of the International Society of Veterinary Ophthalmologists*, New Orleans, Louisiana, 1976.

Geary M.R. & Baker K.P. (1986) The occurrence of pili torti in a litter of kittens in England. *Journal of Small Animal Practice* **27**, 85–88.

Goldsmith L.A. & Boden H.P. (1972) Propylene glycol with occlusion in ichthyosis. *Journal of the American Medical Association* **220**, 579–589.

Griess D., Guagere E. & Veau P.K. (1981) Variations de l'indecamenie et di'indicanurie dans le syndrome rubra pilaire du chien. ll etude experimentale. *Revue de Medecine Veterinaire* **132**, 797–804.

Gupta B.N (1973) Epitheliogenesis imperfecta in a dog. *American Journal of Veterinary Research* **34**, 443–444.

Hargis A.M., Prieur D.S., Haupt K.H. & Collier L.L. (1983) Post mortem findings in a Shetland sheep dog with dermatomyositis. *Veterinary Pathology* **23**, 509–511.

Hargis A.M., Haupt K.H., Hegreberg G.A., Prieur D.J. & Moore M.P. (1984) Familial canine dermatomyositis. Initial characteristics of the cutaneous and muscular lesions. *American Journal of Pathology* **116**, 234–244.

Harper R.C. (1978) Congenital black hair dysplasia in bearded collie puppies. *Veterinary Record* **102**, 87.

Haupt K.H., Prieur D.J., Hargis A.M., Cowell R.L., McDonald T.L., Werner L.L. & Everman I.F. (1985) Familial canine dermatomyositis. Clinicopathologic, immunologic and serologic studies. *American Journal of Veterinary Research* **46**, 1870–1875.

Haupt K.H., Prieur D.J., Moore M.P., Hargis A.M., Hegreberg G.A., Gavin P.R. & Johnson R.S. (1983) Familial canine dermatomyositis. Clinical, electrodiagnostic and genetic studies. *American Journal of Veterinary Research* **46**, 1861–1869.

Hegreberg G.A., Padgett G.A., Gorham J.R. & Henson J.B. (1970a) A hereditable connective tissue disease of dogs and mink resembling Ehlers–Danlos disease of man. 1. Skin tensile strength properties. *Journal of Investigative Dermatology* **54**, 337.

Hegreberg G.A., Padgett G.A., Gorham J.R. & Henson J.B. (1970b) A hereditable connective tissue disease of dogs and mink resembling Ehlers–Danlos syndrome of man. 2. Histopathologic changes of the skin. *Archives of Pathology* **99**, 159–166.

Hewitt M.P., Mills J.H.L. & Hunter B. (1975) Epitheliogenesis imperfecta in a black labrador. *Canadian Veterinary Journal* **16**, 371–374.

Hofmeyr C.F.B. (1963) Dermoid sinus in the Ridgeback dog. *Journal of Small Animal Practice* **4** (Suppl. p.1–5).

Jesyk P.F., Hoskins M.E., Mackay-Smith W.E. & Patterson D.F. (1986) Lethal acrodermatitis in bull terriers. *Journal of the American Veterinary Medicine Association* **186**, 833–839.

Julian R.J. (1960) Ichthyosis congenita in cattle. *Veterinary Medicine* **55**, 35–41.

Lord L.H., Cawley A.J. & Gilroy J. (1957) Mid-dorsal dermoid sinuses in Rhodesian Ridgeback dogs. A case report. *Journal of the American Veterinary Medicine Association* **131**, 515–518.

Lund J.E., Gorham J.R.T. & Padgett G.A. (1970) Canine cyclic neutropenia: diagnosis and treatment. *Veterinary Medicine Review* **1**, 33–46.

Mahaffey M.B., Yarborough K.M. & Munell J.F. (1978) *Journal of the American Veterinary Medicine Association* **173**, 390–396.

Mann G.E. & Stratton J. (1966) Dermoid sinus in the Rhodesian Ridgeback. *Journal of Small Animal Practice* **7**, 631–642.

Pinell S.R. (1978) Disorders of collagen. In *The Metabolic Basis Of Inherited Disease* 4th edn. (Eds Strasburg J.B. *et al.*) pp. 1136–1394. McGraw-Hill, New York.

Pinnell S.R. & McCusick V.A. (1979) Hereditable disorders of connective tissue with skin changes. In *Dermatology in General Practice* 2nd edn., (Eds Fitzpatrick T.B., Eisen A.Z., Wolff K., Freedburg I.M. & Austen K.F.) p. 1149. McGraw-Hill, New York.

Pivník L. (1973) Zur Vergleichenden Problematic eineger Akrodystrophischer Neuropathien bei Menschen und Hunden Schweizer. *Archiv fur Neurologie Und Psychiatrie* **112**, 365–371.

Romatowski J. (1985) A uveodermatological syndrome in an Akita dog. *Journal of the American Animal Hospital Association* **21**, 777–780.

Sen S. & Ansari A.I. (1971) Depigmentation (vitiligo) in animals and its treatment with Meladinine. *Indian Journal of Animal Health* **10**, 249–251.

Thomsett L.R. (1961) Congenital hypotrichosis in the dog. *Veterinary Record* **73**, 915.

Warner M. (1976) *Cats of the World*. Bantam, London.

Werner L.L. & Evermann I.F. (1985) Familial canine dermatomyositis: clinicopathologic, immunologic and serologic studies. *American Journal of Veterinary Research* **46**, 1870.

Yager J.A. & Scott D.W. (1985) In *Pathology of Domestic Animals* (Eds Jubb K.V.F., Kennedy P.C. & Palmer W.) p. 426. Academic Press, New York.

4 / Idiopathic Abnormalities

Seborrhoeic dermatitis

Seborrhoea literally means an outflowing of sebum. However, in humans at least, there is no quantitative increase of lipids in seborrhoeic skin compared to normal skin (Burton & Pye, 1983). In the human there is an increased proportion of cholesterol, triglycerides and fatty acids, with decreases in squalene, free fatty acids and wax esters (Gloor *et al.*, 1972). Irke (1979) states that fat deficiency is a very common cause of primary metabolic seborrhoea. Seborrhoea is a poorly understood, little-researched condition which is common in dogs and less common in cats.

Generalized seborrhoeic dermatitis is characterized by a strong, rancid odour with marked exfoliation; if a hand is passed through the coat, it displaces much scale and grey, greasy marks are acquired on the hand. The scale is grey–yellow in colour and of variable size. There is some superficial resemblance to lice and nits. Areas of skin folds show erythema and brushing produces a shower of scale. It may be primary or secondary to a number of other diseases.

If pruritus is marked, primary ectoparasitism should always be suspected.

AETIOLOGY

The aetiology of primary seborrhoea is not known. There is an apparent defect of keratinization with changes in quantitative sebum production. Baker (1972) reported an increased turnover time for epidermal cells of dry skin compared to the normal time of 8 weeks.

Mammalian sebum is implicated in epidermal permeability, chemical defence and control of the skin surface micropopulation. In cattle and sheep it provides a physical barrier at the cell margins of the outer stratum corneum (McEwan-Jenkinson & Lloyd, 1979). Garthwaite *et al.* (1982) demonstrated several imunologically active proteins (including IgA) on the surface of canine stratum corneum and considered that they may prevent desiccation and form a protective layer.

Ihrke *et al.* (1978) state that the increased incidence of pyoderma in seborrhoeic dogs relates to the inflammatory changes due to the seborrhoea, pruritus and resulting self-trauma in the presence of large numbers of pathogenic bacteria. However, normal dog and cat skin is host to a wide range of organisms (including pathogens) and therefore some caution is necessary in commenting on the isolation of pathogens from seborrhoeic skin. Ihrke *et al.* (1978) examined cultures from the skin of normal and seborrhoeic dogs and reported significantly lower total bacterial counts on normal skin compared to seborrhoeic skin; in the former the flora consisted primarily of coagulase negative *Staphylococcus aureus* whilst in the latter the flora was composed predominantly of *S. aureus* coagulase positive. They did not report the isolation of yeasts (Baker, unpublished data), however, examined cultures from 10 skin sites predisposed to seborrhoea and isolated yeasts in two of the 10 areas; numerically they ranked 11th of the organisms isolated. *Streptococcus faecalis* and *Streptococcus intermedius* were the only organisms consistently isolated from all 10 areas. There is some evidence that fungal pathogens are incriminated in the aetiology of human seborrhoea; for example, ketoconazole is of therapeutic benefit (Ford *et al.*, 1984).

It is possible that seborrhoea is an accelerated disorderly exfoliation of keratinocytes associated with altered composition of epidermal lipid (Figs 4.1 and 4.2).

Seborrhoea may be classified as primary and secondary (Table 4.1).

HISTOPATHOLOGY

The histopathology of primary seborrhoeic dermatitis is not diagnostic. The epidermis is much thickened with moderate parakeratosis, with papilliform extensions into the upper dermis where there are marked cellular infiltrates of neutrophils, mast cells, plasma cells, lymphocytes and histiocytes. The follicles show hyperkeratosis and there is some resulting hair loss. There is sebaceous-gland hyperplasia (Fig. 4.3).

Table 4.1. Classification of seborrhoea

Primary	Secondary
Idiopathic (Disturbed metabolism/ catabolism of epidermal lipids?)	Ectoparasitism — the most important cause Allergy Autoimmune disease Neoplasia Primary essential fatty acid deficiency Zinc deficiency Vitamin A deficiency Secondary malabsorption

Primary idiopathic seborrhoea

Here no cause can be determined. Whilst cocker spaniels and springer spaniels are reported as being particularly predisposed, there is no statistical evidence to support this.

Secondary idiopathic seborrhoea

Many conditions are associated with secondary seborrhoea;

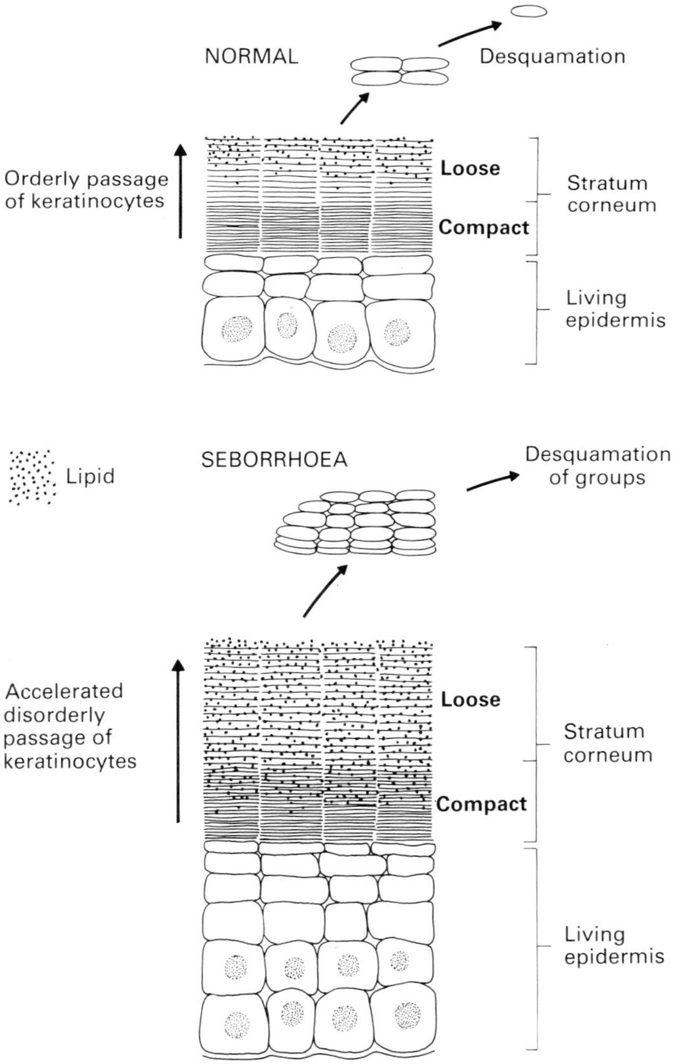

Fig. 4.1. Diagrammatic representation of the possible sequence in ordered and disordered exfoliation of the stratum corneum.

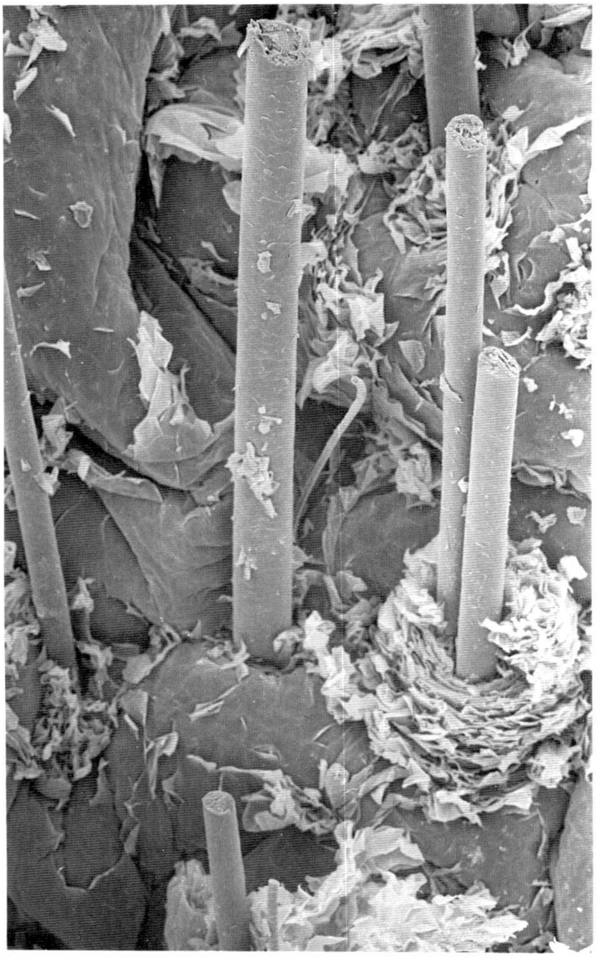

Fig. 4.2. Interscapular skin of a normal young dog, keratinocytes exfoliated singly.

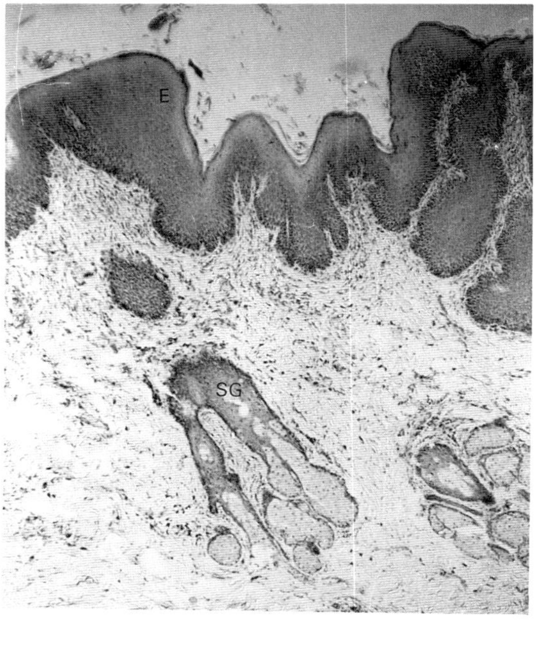

Fig. 4.3. Moderate inflammatory infiltrate in the dermis. E = epidermis, SG = sebaceous gland.

ectoparasitism, endocrine diseases, malabsorption diseases, deficiency diseases, atopy, autoimmune diseases and neoplasia. Of these, the most important is ectoparasitism. Generalized demodectic mange, sarcoptic mange, pediculosis, chronic flea hypersensitivity and cheyletiellosis are the most common causes.

Hypothyroidism, diabetes mellitus, ovarian imbalance and the male feminization syndrome may exhibit variable degrees of seborrhoea. Where intestinal absorption is abnormal due to liver disease, endocrine pancreatic disease or intestinal disease, seborrhoea may occur. It also accompanies diets low in fat, protein and zinc.

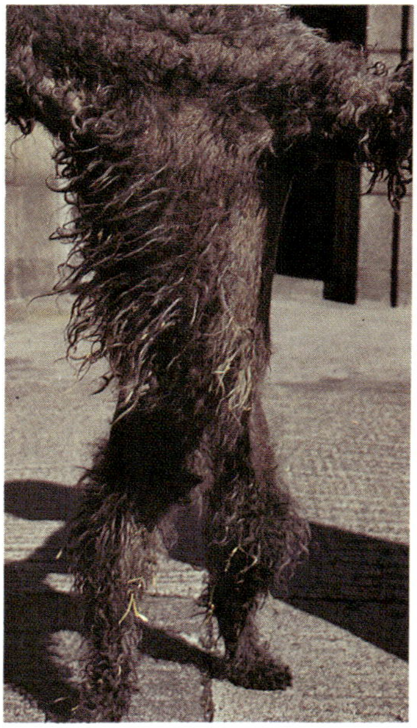

Fig. 4.4. Seborrhoea oleosa in an Irish water spaniel.

CLINICAL SIGNS

Two types of seborrhoea have been described, seborrhoea sicca and seborrhoea oleosa. In the first the coat is dry and the surface of the skin is variably covered with fine white-grey scale. In the latter the coat is oily to the touch and there is much yellowed scale, the hair may be stuck by scale and, with growth of the hair, these matted areas are carried upwards and resemble nits (Fig. 4.4). In both forms the characteristic seborrhoeic odour is apparent. However, there is often considerable overlapping between the two forms, so that clear distinction is not always possible. Seborrhoea sicca is the most usual type in cats.

When generalized, the whole body may be affected with more severe signs in the skin folds, flexures, axillary, inguinal, interdigital and perineal regions and the external auditory meatuses (Figs 4.5–7). There may be variable hair loss. Pruritus may or may not be a feature of seborrhoea; marked pruritus with seborrhoea usually indicates ectoparasitism and there may be self-trauma.

Focal pyoderma of a superficial type is seen often with collarette formation. These lesions may be distributed on the dorsal and ventral trunk.

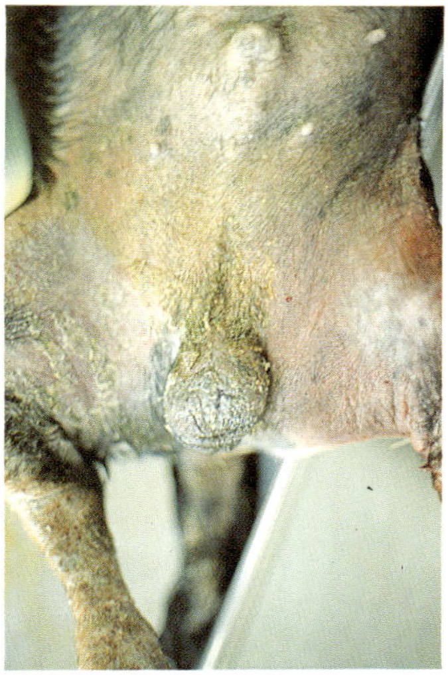

Fig. 4.5. Seborrhoea in a Jack Russell terrier.

DIAGNOSIS

The investigation should include a thorough history with assessment of diet: deficiency disease can produce seborrhoea.

Determine if the oestrous cycles are normal, and if the animal's human and animal contacts are normal. As ectoparasitism is so often related to seborrhoea-associated pruritus,

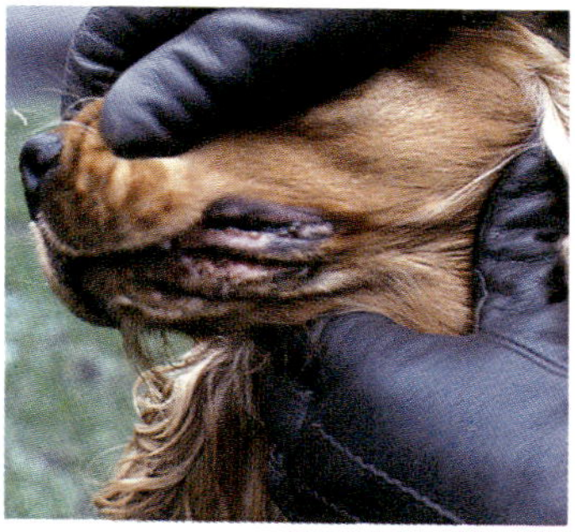

Fig. 4.6. Seborrhoeic dermatitis of the lips of a cocker spaniel.

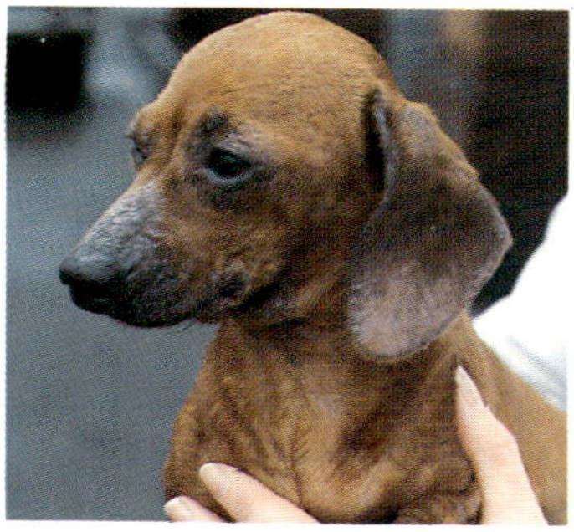

Fig. 4.7. Seborrhoea in a miniature dachshund.

the health of contacts is of obvious importance.

The general clinical examination must be thorough. Abnormal faeces may indicate malabsorption or hepatomegalic liver disease. Obesity is often related to seborrhoea. Lethargy and bradycardia may indicate seborrhoea secondary to hypothyroidism; polydipsia and polyphagia can suggest seborrhoea secondary to hyperadrenocorticism.

Examination of the skin should include noting the distribution and type of the lesions (Fig. 4.8), e.g. atopy will have a characteristic distribution with pruritus. Close examination should be made with brush and comb and skin scrapings scrutinized for the presence of ectoparasites or parasitic fungi.

Biopsy examination will show the nature of the histopathology and indicate the presence or absence of autoimmune disease.

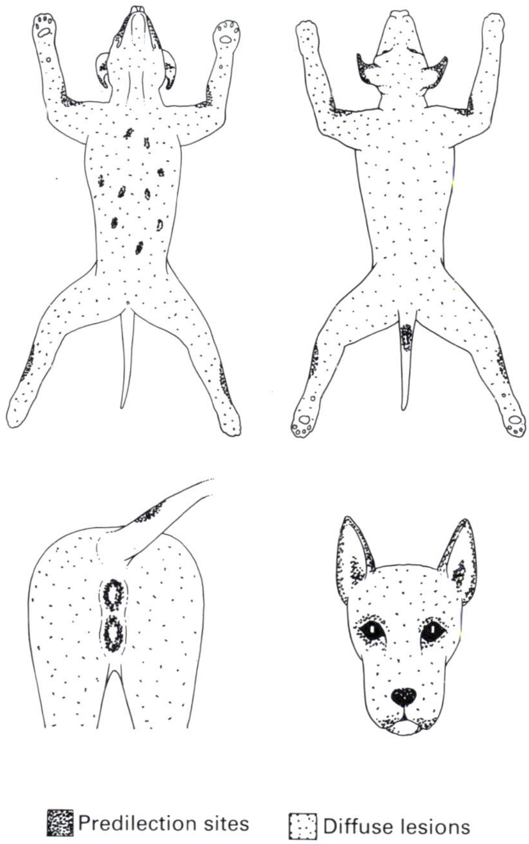

Fig. 4.8. Distribution of the lesions of seborrhoeic dermatitis in dogs.

Laboratory examination should include investigation for hypothyroidism and hyperadrenocorticism, diabetes mellitus and zinc deficiency, whilst intradermal tests and elimination diet should be undertaken if allergy is suspected.

Dietary investigations may reveal deficiency whilst the possibility of an associated malabsorption may be indicated by weight loss, ravenous appetite and abnormally fatty faeces. The evaluation of liver enzymes will be helpful to eliminate liver disease. Examine the serum zinc level if zinc deficiency is suspected.

THERAPY

Apart from therapy for the causes of secondary seborrhoea, specific therapy for the seborrhoeic state is asepsis and hydration achieved by frequent washing with mild shampoos, which may contain keratolytics if the seborrhoea is severe. These may be coal-tar based; preparations containing salicylic acid are useful and selenium sulphide base shampoos also have a place. Whichever preparation is used, rinsing with tepid water containing a hydrating oil is indicated; baby oil is relatively cheap and perfectly satisfactory. Its purpose is to seal water into the stratum corneum by forming an impervious barrier. Drying should be accomplished with a hair dryer or by patting dry, not rubbing, with clean towelling.

Clinical trials with shampoos containing 2.5% benzoyl peroxide indicate it to be a valuable therapeutic aid in primary seborrhoea and secondary seborrhoea. The addition of sunflower oil in primary seborrhoea is beneficial; 10 ml daily should be adequate for a dog of 60 kg body weight.

Local seborrhoea

SUPRACAUDAL GLAND SEBORRHOEA

Both dogs and cats have well-developed, large sebaceous glands on the dorsum of the tail. In the dog, these are grouped together in the anterior third whilst in cats they are diffusely arranged along the length of the tail.

In male dogs and male cats (particularly of some breeds, e.g. Labrador, Staffordshire bull terriers) these may become large and prominent with associated hair loss and the presence of localized seborrhoea. In male cats the term stud tail is used. Male cats may develop a localized area of seborrhoea of the submental gland with secondary pyoderma.

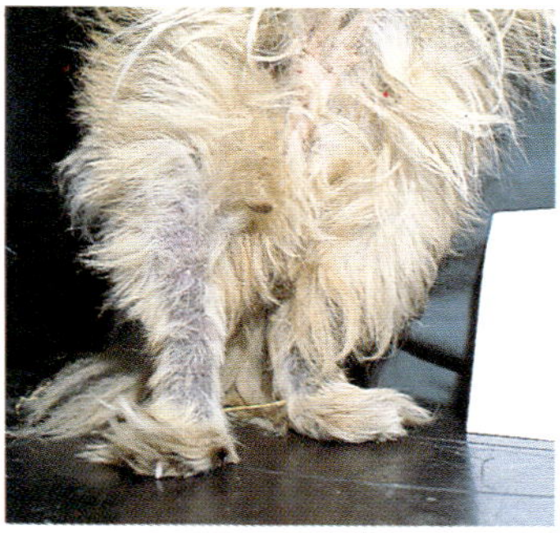

Fig. 4.9. Seborrhoea with hyperpigmentation in the Pekingese.

PINNA HAIR DYSPLASIA

Flop-eared dogs, particularly short-haired dachshunds and Yorkshire terriers, in middle and old age may develop greasy tufts along the margins of the ear. These may be detached easily with a few hairs leaving a ragged margin which does not bleed. Usually the condition is accompanied by patchy alopecia of the pinna with marked hyperpigmentation (Fig. 4.9). The histopathology is follicular dysplasia with active hyperpigmentation. The aetiology is not known.

MINIATURE SCHNAUZER SYNDROME

The schnauzer breed, particularly the miniature variety, has an inherited predisposition to the formation of multiple comedones along the dorsal midline of the trunk. These may be felt as a roughened area of skin. Initially the comedones, although unsightly, cause no clinical signs. However, they may rupture into the dermis and provoke a chronic inflammatory response. The differential diagnosis is flea hypersensitivity, which has a similar corporeal distribution. However, this is markedly pruritic. Close clipping of the skin will reveal the characteristic comedones, with some quite large cutaneous horns.

Eosinophilic granuloma complex

Chronic, moist, exuberant, circumscribed granulomata of unknown aetiology of the skin are fairly common in cats and rare in dogs. In the former, three types are recognized:

1 Eosinophilic ulcer (rodent ulcer), eosinophilic granuloma.
2 Eosinophilic plaque.
3 Linear granuloma.

The description 'eosinophilic' is unfortunate, although firmly established in the literature. Lesional eosinophilia is seen only in oral linear granulomata and eosinophilic plaques, whilst eosinophilia is not usually seen in the blood of affected cases.

The lesions themselves vary from red to brown to yellow and may be frankly ulcerative or granulomatous.

It is possible that eosinophilic plaque and linear granuloma are the visible response of skin repeatedly licked as a result of pruritus; both are commonly observed in cats with allergic and psychogenic dermatoses.

Eosinophilic granuloma

This is a chronic, circumscribed, ulcerated lesion usually immediately lateral to the nasal labial groove of middle-aged cats which are more usually female (Figs 4.10 and 4.11). There may be associated lesions on the hard palate, lower lip and the skin. Occasionally bilateral ulceration of the upper lip is seen. The lesion is red to brown in colour (Baker, 1965).

Scott (1978) stated that lesions cannot be transmitted to other cats by tissue homogenates or cell-free extracts, but Baker (1965) reported the rapid development of rodent ulcer in a cat sharing a common feeding bowl with a chronically affected cat.

The lesion is not painful to the touch although there is associated swelling. The histopathology is of an ulcerating dermatitis with numerous neutrophils, plasma cells and mononuclear cells. Peripheral to the lesion, the epidermis shows pseudocancerous hyperplasia, and occasionally squamous-cell carcinomata develop here.

The differential diagnosis is squamous-cell carcinoma, which is distinguishable by the histopathology.

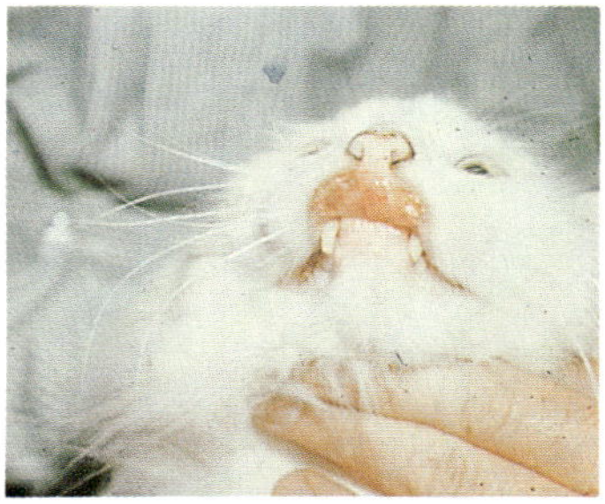

Fig. 4.10. Eosinophilic granuloma of the upper lip, resembling squamous-cell carcinoma.

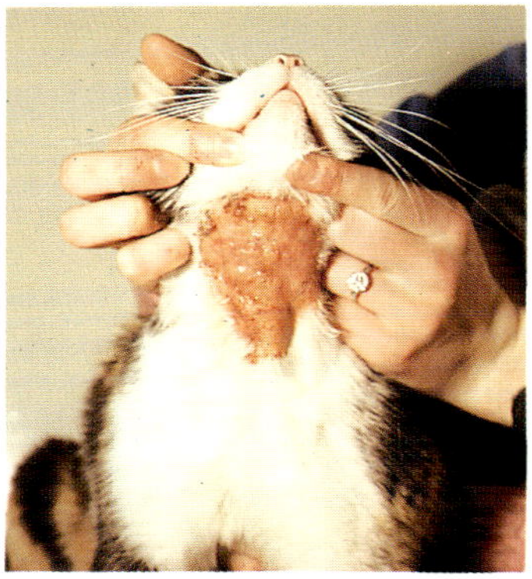

Fig. 4.11. Eosinophilic granuloma.

Eosinophilic plaque (lick granuloma)

These are raised ulcerated granulomatous lesions, usually multiple, which are more often found on the inner aspects of the thighs, ventral abdomen and perineum (Fig. 4.12). They are of variable size (usually 2–3 cm in diameter) and often grouped together, most commonly seen in middle-aged female cats. They are usually pink to red in colour but may be yellow and are typically located in areas accessible to licking. The associated hair is obviously moist through licking. They may be associated with allergic dermatitis. The differential diagnosis is neoplastic which can be distinguished by histopathological examination; characteristically in eosinophilic plaque the dermis contains large numbers of eosinophils with numerous mast cells. Latimer and Dunsten (1986) reported eosinophilic plaque as a pruritic periocular blepharitis in a neutered 6-year-old male cat with histological features of eosinophilic plaque: subsequently, similar lesions developed on the cheek and chin. Eosinophilic granuloma is considered to be implicated in the aetiology of chin-oedema (fat-chinned cats) by Muller *et al.* (1989).

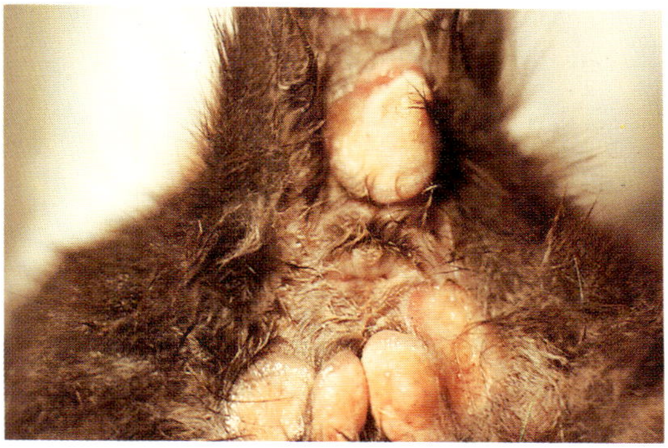

Fig. 4.12. Eosinophilic plaque.

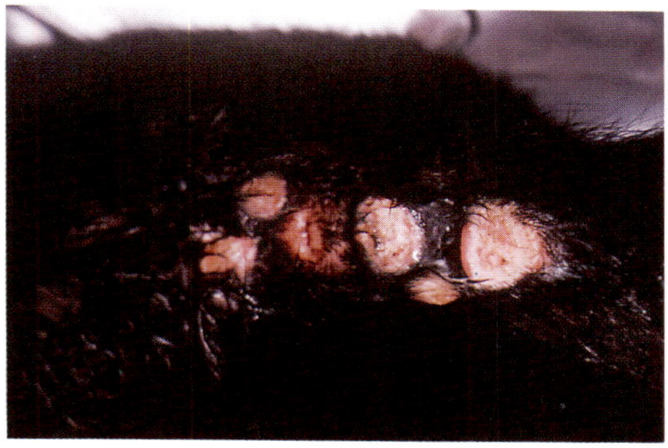

Fig. 4.13. Linear granuloma.

Linear granuloma

This variant of the eosinophilic granuloma complex differs in that it affects younger cats (average age 1 year), is located on the posterior aspect of the thigh, and is an elongated pink to yellow lesion not associated with pruritus (Fig. 4.13). It may be associated with ulcerated areas in the mouth. Histopathologically, there is a chronic inflammatory dermatitis with degenerative changes in the collagen with associated foreign-body giant cells. Marked dermal infiltration of eosinophils may or may not be seen.

THERAPY

The eosinophilic granuloma complex responds well to anti-inflammatories. Rodent ulcers may be removed surgically and heal well with a good cosmetic effect even when large. As eosinophilic plaque and linear granuloma may be associated with allergic dermatitis, therapy should include measures to contain or prevent this. Some cases may also be seen in psychotic dermatoses, and the appropriate therapy routine is necessary.

The lesions of eosinophilic plaque and linear granuloma are aggravated by licking, therefore an Elizabethan collar should be used, at least in the initial stages. Corticosteroid therapy or progestogen therapy gives good results.

Prednisolone 2 mg/kg is given orally for 5 days, decreasing to alternate-day therapy and then to zero with remission. There may be individual variation in response to prednisolone and larger doses may be necessary initially. Megestrol acetate

(Ovarid, Pitman Moore) is also effective, although this drug is not licensed for use in cats in the USA. It is given orally at an initial dose rate of 5 mg daily, decreasing with response (which is rapid) to 5 mg alternate-day therapy for 1 week, then 5 mg on two occasions during 1 week followed by 5 mg given weekly until the lesions have finally resolved, when therapy should be continued for a further 2 weeks at the same dose rate. This drug is effective for the treatment of psychotic dermatoses often associated with eosinophilic granuloma. It therefore has a dual function, whilst the cause of the psychosis is removed if this is possible.

Plasma cell pododermatitis (feline pododermatitis)

A rare disease of unknown aetiology affecting the foot pads of cats. These are initially swollen and painless, and later ulceration develops with pain.

CLINICAL SIGNS

The disease has been reported in a number of widely separated countries. Owners usually present the case (usually a mature adult) because they have observed that the foot pads, particularly the metacarpal and metatarsal pads, have gradually increased in size over a period of weeks or months, although the cat is otherwise apparently normal. Examinations reveal that the pads are large, soft and painless, the overlying epidermis appearing thinned and dry. As the lesions develop, the pads become tense, and palpation may be resented. Subsequently, there is rupture of the epidermis with the exudation of a pink granulomatous mass (Fig. 4.14). There is now pain and there may be lameness. The associated lymph nodes are moderately enlarged. There may be lymphocytosis and hyperglobulinaemia with failure to isolate feline leukaemia virus (Gruffyd-Jones *et al.*, 1980).

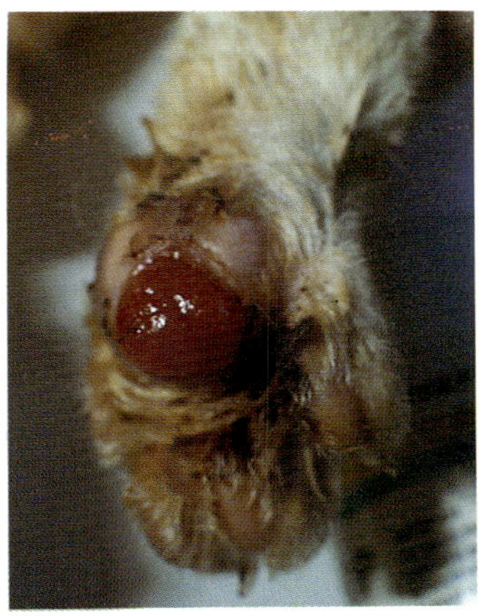

Fig. 4.14. Feline plasma-cell pododermatitis. The epidermis has ruptured releasing a granulomatous mass.

HISTOPATHOLOGY

Biopsy examination shows an enormous number of plasma cells in the affected areas, many containing Russell bodies (Fig. 4.15). An associated inflammatory response is present if there is secondary bacterial invasion. Medleau *et al.* (1982) report deposition of immunoglobulins at the basement membrane of the epidermis.

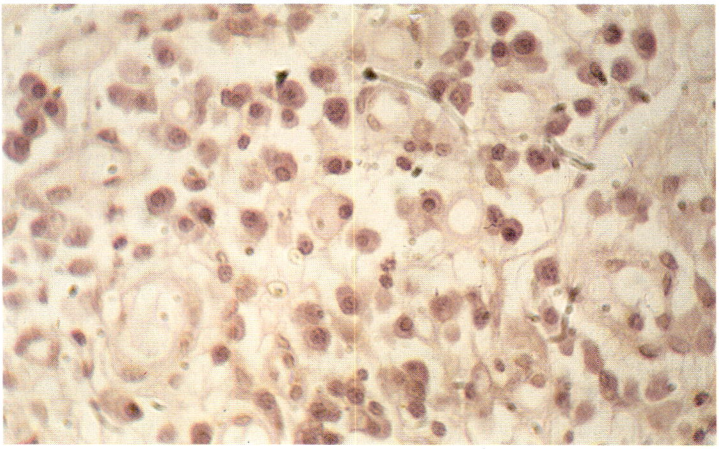

Fig. 4.15. Histology of feline plasma-cell pododermatitis. There is an enormous number of plasma cells, many containing Russell bodies.

DIFFERENTIAL DIAGNOSIS

The differential diagnosis should include contact dermatitis, feline calicivirus and feline rhinotracheitis virus infection, and neoplasia. Reaction of the feet to irritant chemicals produces ulceration rapidly with marked lameness and there may be lesions on the tongue and lips as a result of licking the irritant. The two viral infections are associated with systemic signs and lesions elsewhere on the body. Neoplasia is distinguishable on histopathological examination.

THERAPY

In three cases recently treated in the Clinic of the Faculty of Veterinary Medicine, Dublin, good response, although slow, was obtained using megestrol acetate 5 mg daily for 1 week then 5 mg on alternate days for 1 week, followed by 5 mg twice weekly for 2 weeks. Medleau *et al.* (1980) used aurothioglucose 1 mg/kg intramuscularly at weekly intervals for 8 weeks then twice monthly for 1 month, subsequently once monthly in their reported case, following surgery. A variable response has been reported using prednisolone by mouth. Other therapy has involved surgery, bandaging or plastering.

Hairy tongue

This is a hypertrophic condition of the filiform papillae in the anterior central two-thirds of the tongue. The hairs are actually conical piles of parakeratotic cells. It is rarely seen. Thomsett (unpublished) observed the condition (Fig. 4.16) in an otherwise normal spaniel in the Royal Veterinary College Clinic, London.

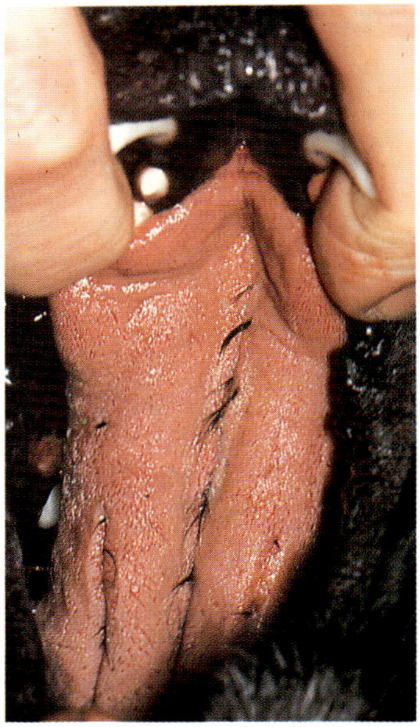

Fig. 4.16. Hairy tongue.

Subcorneal pustular dermatosis

A rare, chronic and recurrent pustular disease of dogs of unknown aetiology with sterile pustules in the stratum corneum containing numerous neutrophils (Baker, 1980).

CLINICAL SIGNS

There have been too few cases reported to indicate age or sex predisposition. Although apparently healthy, patients have recurrent crops of small vesicles or pustules predominantly on the trunk. These may enlarge but are of short duration and rupture to leave circular, dry, scaly crusts (Fig. 4.17). Peripheral spreading results in macules with collarettes. There may or may not be pruritus. Established cases may have an extensive seborrhoeic dermatitis.

HISTOPATHOLOGY

The histopathology is subcorneal pustules containing predominantly neutrophils without bacteria or evidence of

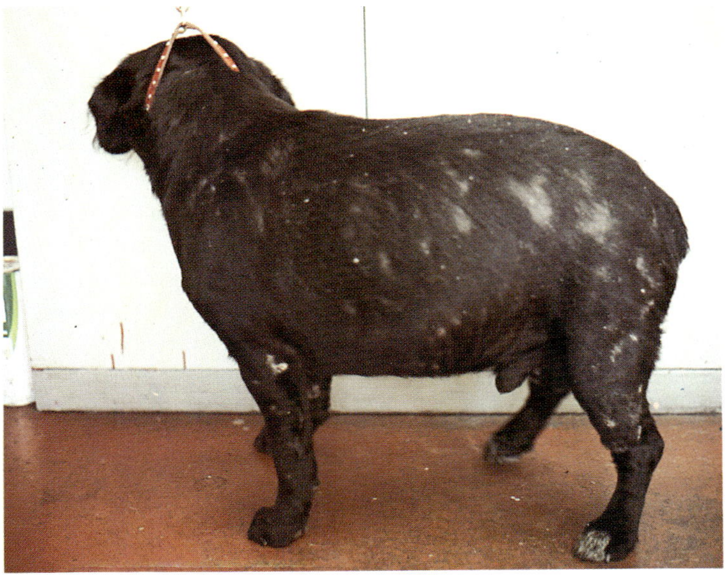

Fig. 4.17. Subcorneal pustular dermatosis

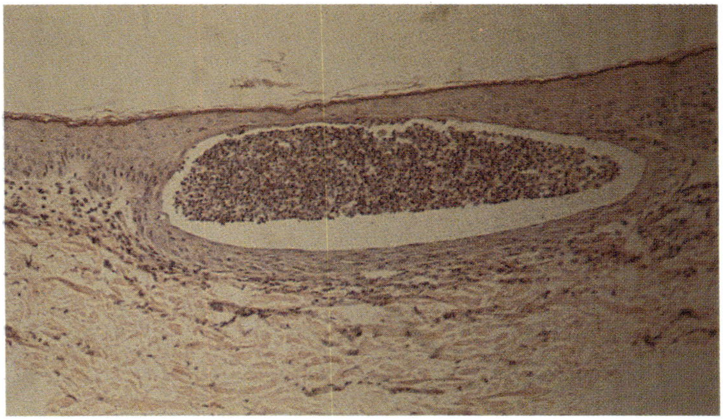

Fig. 4.18. Pustule of subcorneal pustular dermatosis containing neutrophils.

acantholysis (Fig. 4.18). The underlying epidermis is little affected although diapedesis is seen and a perifollicular neutrophilic infiltrate is present. Tests for immunoglobulins in the epidermis are negative.

DIFFERENTIAL DIAGNOSIS

The differential diagnosis is seborrhoeic dermatitis, demodectic mange, pemphigus foliaceus and bacterial pyoderma. Examination of the pustules fails to reveal numerous bacteria, absence of immunofluorescence in the epidermis distinguishes it from pemphigus, and the histopathology is characteristic.

THERAPY

Dapsone by mouth is specific for this disease. The dose rate is 2 mg/kg daily. The response may be slow and resolution may not be effected for 4 weeks; thereafter dosing is constrained for 1 month and then according to progress. In some cases the drug may be withdrawn.

Dapsone is potentially hepatotoxic and the clinician must examine the case regularly during dapsone therapy for signs of drug-related disease. A guarded prognosis should be given as there may be relapses.

Acanthosis nigricans (frictional acanthosis)

This is a relatively common canine condition of multiple aetiology associated with lesions of the axillary and inguinal regions and flexural areas. These show hypermelanotic pigmentation, lichenification and alopecia. It is most commonly seen in smooth-coated dachshunds (Fig. 4.19).

It is to be distinguished from the disease of the same name of humans, which is often associated with adenocarcinoma of the stomach.

Primary acanthosis nigricans is seen most commonly in smooth-coated dachshunds which are not necessarily obese and have normal thyroxine levels, suggesting a genetic predisposition.

Secondary acanthosis nigricans is seen in other breeds associated with obesity, seborrhoeic dermatitis, allergy hypothyroidism and hyperadrenocorticism.

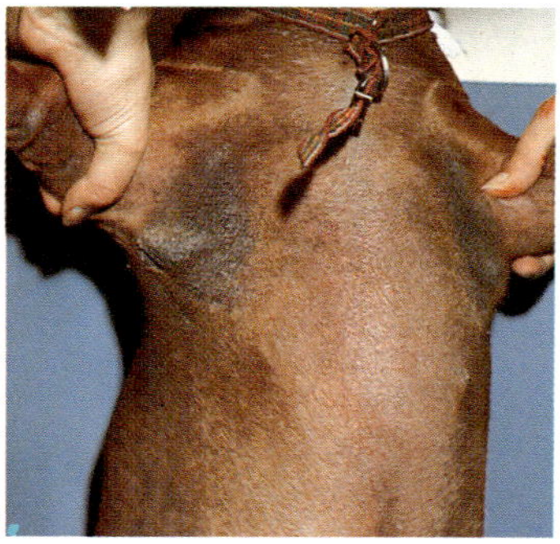

Fig. 4.19. Acanthosis nigricans in a dachshund. There is hypermelanosis, lichenification and alopecia.

CLINICAL SIGNS

Hyperpigmentation with associated alopecia and thickening of the skin is usually first observed in the axilla. Subsequently, these may be spread to other areas of the skin having skin flexures. Often the skin is seborrhoeic and has the characteristic odour. Pruritus is not associated with idiopathic acanthosis nigricans but commonly occurs in the secondary conditions.

The histopathology is not specific.

As this condition is often secondary to numerous diseases the primary disease must be ascertained and the appropriate therapy given.

THERAPY

When there is obesity, the weight must be reduced. Numerous methods of therapy have been used for this condition. Prednisolone 1 mg/kg daily may be given for 7 days, then reduced, according to the response, to alternate-day therapy until control has been achieved; the drug is then withdrawn. Keratolytic preparations like selenium sulphide or Pragmatar ointment (Smith Kline & French Ltd); these are may be helpful applied topically to the affected areas. There are several reports in the literature indicating the value of melatonin given subcutaneously daily for 5 days then once weekly according to the response (Rickards, 1966; Kirk, 1979). Scott and Walton (1985) report improvement in eight smooth-coated dachshunds treated with vitamin E by mouth (DL-α-tocopherol acetate, 200 i.u. twice daily, 2 hours before or after a meal). Six owners indicated that improvement of the affected areas was noticeable within 60 days of the commencement of therapy. The authors reported that therapy had been maintained from 6 months to 3.5 years without side effects.

Nodular panniculitis

This is a very rare, sterile, localized inflammatory reaction of subcutaneous fat reported in dogs and cats. The aetiology is unknown, possibly multifactorial (Edgar & Furrow, 1984). It is to be distinguished from infectious panniculitis and panniculitis associated with vitamin E deficiency in combination with diets containing excessive fat.

CLINICAL SIGNS

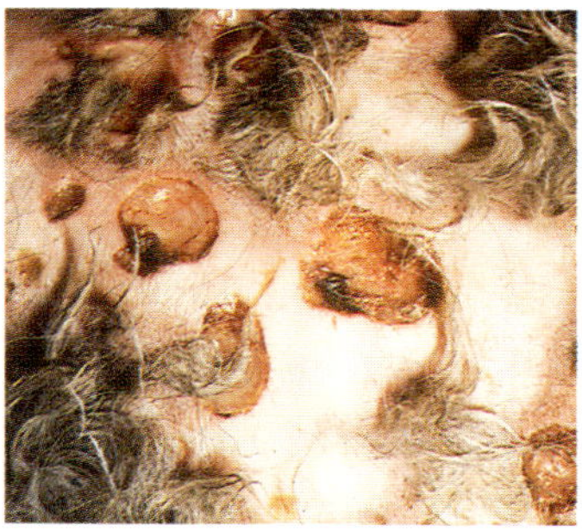

Fig. 4.20. Nodular panniculitis.

The nodules (of variable size, 5 mm to 3 cm) are usually multiple, located in the subcutis, ulcerated and may have a thick, sanguinous discharge (Fig. 4.20). They may or may not be painful on palpation and there is a tendency for individual healing. Most reported cases have systemic signs, poor appetite, fever or lethargy.

DIAGNOSIS

The differential diagnosis is neoplasia, chronic pyoderma and cysts. For diagnostic purposes a complete nodule should be removed for histopathological examination and submitted to fat staining and Gram stains for bacteria. The histopathology is a sterile area of fat necrotic tissue associated with acute inflammatory cells.

THERAPY

A good response may be expected to oral prednisolone therapy 2 mg/kg daily. A response is obtained within 7 days, when dosage can be reduced to zero within a further 7 days. Therapy may be required to be repeated.

Lentigo

A lentigo is a black, sharply defined, pigmented macule of variable size (1–3 cm) in the skin of dogs and is of unknown aetiology. It is rare. The macules are usually multiple (lentigines) and are easily observable on the comparatively hairless ventral abdomen of affected dogs (Fig. 4.21). The skin is thickened in the pigmented area but is not noticeably raised above the surrounding area, as there are no associated clinical signs.

The histology is an increase in thickness of the epidermis, the keratinocytes of which are packed with melanin granules.

Lentigines are not themselves of clinical significance but are to be distinguished from melanomata. This can only be determined by histological examination.

No therapy is required.

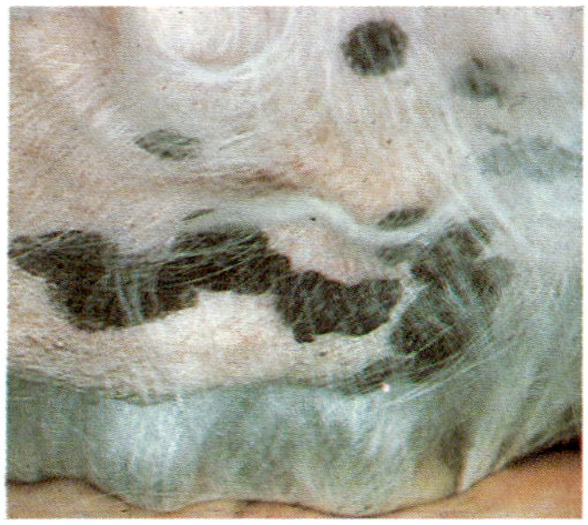

Fig. 4.21. Lentigines.

Sterile pyogranuloma (canine pododermatitis)

This is a rare, sterile, chronic granulomatous reaction of adult dogs most commonly affecting the feet and face. The lesions are firm and painless; all four feet may be grossly enlarged with 'webbing' in which the plantar surfaces of the digits are continuous and no longer separated. There is some associated alopecia and there may be ulceration and erythema. The aetiology is not known. Special staining of affected tissue does not reveal pathogens or foreign bodies in the affected dermis, the histopathology being a sterile granuloma. The differential diagnosis should include bacterial pyoderma and demodectic mange, which in some cases may be associated with gross enlargement of the feet. However, pustules are present in which numerous *Demodex canis* mites may be demonstrated.

THERAPY

A guarded prognosis should be given; some cases will respond well to prednisolone (2 mg/kg daily for 3 weeks).

Canine eosinophilic granuloma

This is a rare chronic inflammatory disease, most usually involving the hard palate and tongue of otherwise normal dogs. Occasionally, numerous non-pruritic plaques and nodules are found on the ventral abdomen. The aetiology is not known. The lesions, which are painless, show collagen degeneration with infiltration of eosinophils. Madewell *et al.* (1980) reported a predisposition to the condition in Siberian huskys. The diagnosis is confirmed by histopathological examination.

THERAPY

Prednisolone by mouth (2 mg/kg daily) will give a good clinical response within 3 weeks. Further therapy is not usually required.

Discoloration of hair

Continued licking of the skin as a result of persistent pruritus (e.g. in acral lick granuloma) will result in dark brown discoloration of the associated hair. A similar effect is observed in 'tear streaking' in dogs with persisting epiphora: in some breeds, the conformation of the eyelids produces ectropion or entropion so that most mature adults with comparatively lighter-coloured hair below the eyes will show hair discoloration. It is common for exhibitors of such dogs to mask this effect prior to showing by dusting the area with powder; for example, boric powder is used in white Maltese terriers.

It has been assumed that the discoloration resulted from the effect of bacterial action. However, examination by the scanning electron microscope reveals the hair to be covered by an amorphous brown sheath beneath which the hair cuticle appears undamaged with only a very small number of bacteria present. Probably the effect is produced by the degradation of protein contained in saliva or tears (Baker, unpublished observations).

References

Baker B.B., Maibach H.I., Park R.D., McFarland L.Z. & O'Brien T.R. (1972) Epidermal cell renewal in the dog. *American Journal of Veterinary Research* **34**, 93–94.

Baker K.P. (1965) Eosinophilic granuloma of cats. *Irish Veterinary Journal* **19**, 13–15.

Burton J.L. & Pye R.J. (1983) Seborrhoea is not a feature of seborrhoeic dermatitis. *British Medical Journal* **286**, 1169–1170.

Edgar T.P. & Furrow R.D. (1984) Idiopathic nodular panniculitis in a German shepherd. *Journal of American Animal Hospital Association* **20**, 603–606.

Ford G.P., Farr P.M., Ive F.A. & Shuster S. (1984) The response of seborrhoeic dermatitis to ketoconazole. *British Journal of Dermatology* **3** (Suppl. 26), 9.

Garthwaite G., Lloyd D. & Thomsett L.R. (1982) Localisation of immunoglobulins and complement (C3) at the surface within the skin of dogs. *Journal of Comparative Pathology* (1983) **93**, 185–193.

Gloor M. (1972) Über Menze und zusammersetzung der Hautober Flächenlipide beim Sogennanten Sorborischen. *Ekzem Dermatologie Monatssch* **158**, 759–764.

Gruffydd-Jones T.J., Orr C.M. & Lucke V.M. (1980) Food pad swelling and ulceration in cats: a report of five cases. *Journal of Small Animal Practice* **21**, 381–389.

Ihrke P.J., Schwartzman R.M., McGinley B.S., Horwitz L.N. & Marples R.R. (1978) Microbiology of normal and seborrhoeic canine skin. *American Journal of Veterinary Research* **39**, 1481–1489.

Ihrke P.J. (1979) Canine seborrhoeic disease complex. *Veterinary Clinics of North America* **9**, 93–106.

Kirk R.W. (1979) Acanthosis nigricans. *Veterinary Clinics of North America* **9**, 49.

McEwan-Jenkinson D.M. & Lloyd D.H. (1979) The topography of the skin surface of cattle and sheep. *British Veterinary Journal* **135**, 376–379.

Madewell B.R., Stannard A.A., Pulley L.T. & Nelson V.G. (1980) Oral eosinophilic granuloma in Siberian husky dogs. *Journal of the American Veterinary Medical Association* **177**, 701–703.

Medleau L., Kaswan R.L., Lorenz M.D. & Dawe D.L. (1982) Ulcerative dermatitis in a cat: immunofluorscent findings and response to cyrosurgery. *Journal of the American Animal Hospital Association* **18**, 449–451.

Muller G.H., Kirk R.W. & Scott D.W. (1989) *Small Animal Dermatology*, 4th edn. W.B. Saunders, London.

Rickards R.A. (1966) A new treatment for canine melanosis. *Modern Veterinary Practice* **47**, 38.

Scott D.W. & Walton D.K. (1985) Clinical evaluation of oral vitamin E for the treatment of primary acanthosis nigricans. *Journal of the American Animal Hospital Association* **21**, 345.

5 / Disorders Associated with Pathogens

5.1 Viruses

Viral skin diseases of dogs and cats are very rare. In the following list only the first three conditions are of importance.

1 Canine oral papillomatosis.
2 Canine distemper.
3 Feline orthopox (cowpox) infection.
4 Feline leukaemia. Immunosuppressive effect of virus allows skin lesions to develop.
5 Feline herpes virus infection. Herpetic ulcers generalized over the body and limbs.
6 Feline calicivirus infection. Vesicular lesions of oral mucosa, erosions of feet.
7 Feline sarcoma virus. Cutaneous fibrosarcomata.

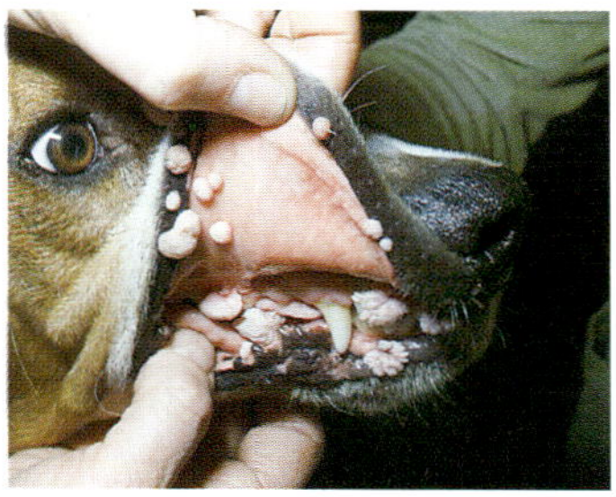

Fig. 5.1. Oral papillomatosis of the beagle. Multiple verrucose warts on oral mucosa.

Canine oral papillomatosis

The causal agent of canine oral papillomatosis is DNA papovavirus. This contagious disease is confined to young dogs of any sex or breed.

Following an incubation period of approximately 30 days, affected animals develop white plaques which progress to cauliflower-like masses, some pedunculated, others sessile, on the mucous membrane of the mouth (Figs 5.1 and 5.2), pharynx and occasionally the eyes, as well as the mucocutaneous junction of prepuce and vulva.

Within the oral cavity, papillomatous masses may cause difficulty in eating, particularly swallowing, and can give rise to persistent oral mal odour.

In most cases the disease is self-limiting but occasional persistent infection can occur, possibly due to immune defects or immunosuppression.

Where treatment is required, surgical excision, removal by thermocautery or cryosurgery is effective.

Infectious viral papillomatosis has not been recorded in cats.

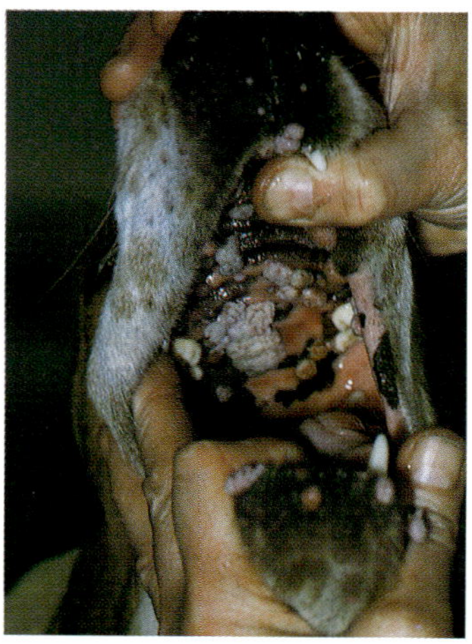

Fig. 5.2. Oral papillomatosis of the beagle. Lesions on hard palate.

Canine distemper (hard-pad disease)

The virus, after an initial incubation of 7–21 days, causes a severe illness involving the respiratory, gastrointestinal and nervous systems.

Bronchopneumonia, diarrhoea and vomiting, encephalitis, chorea and paralysis are common sequelae.

Skin changes in the form of hyperkeratosis affect the epithelium of the metacarpal, metatarsal and digital pads as well as the epithelium of the nose (Fig. 5.3).

Characteristic changes are marked cornification of the bearing surface of the pads to form corn-like masses and excessive cornification of the papillae of the pads so that at the periphery of the pad there may be fissuring. A similar change affects the nasal epithelium.

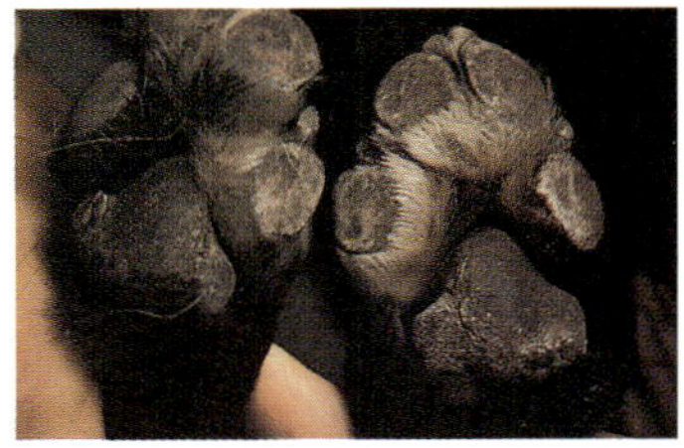

Fig. 5.3. Canine distemper with hyperkeratosis of the pads.

DIAGNOSIS

Since hyperkeratosis does not usually manifest itself until the systemic signs already described have become established, there should be little difficulty in diagnosis.

TREATMENT

There is no specific therapy. Once affected dogs have reached the stage of hyperkeratosis, concurrent neurological signs have become established and the prognosis is poor.

Orthopox virus (cowpox) infection of cats: feline poxvirus infection

The infection of domestic cats and some wild felidae in captivity with a virus considered to be cowpox was first recorded in the 1970s.

Domestic cats between 2 months and 12 years of age have been seen to be affected.

A variety of systemic signs have been recorded involving the respiratory and alimentary tracts with associated loss of appetite, fever and lethargy.

The most commonly recorded sign has been the development of skin lesions, ranging from papules to ulcers, on the face, limbs, body and foot pads (Fig. 5.4).

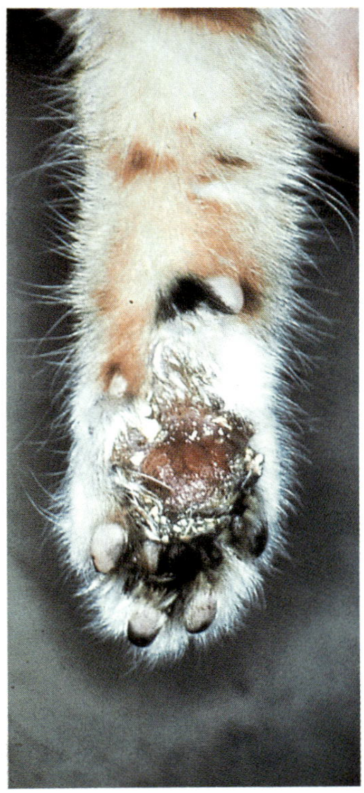

Fig. 5.4. Cowpox (orthopox) infection of cats with erosive lesion on pad. (Courtesy of Professor C.J. Gaskell.)

DIAGNOSIS

This depends on demonstrating the viral agent by serology and virus isolation.

Histopathological examination of lesion biopsy shows changes characteristic of poxvirus infection, particularly the presence of large eosinophilic intracytoplasmic inclusion bodies (Figs 5.5 and 5.6).

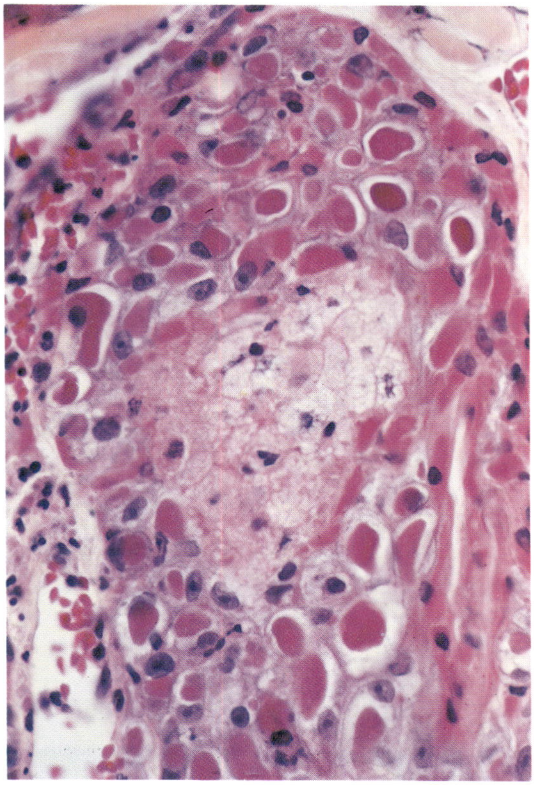

Fig. 5.5. Cowpox infection of cats. Intracytoplasmic eosinophilic inclusion bodies in follicle epithelium of cheetah.

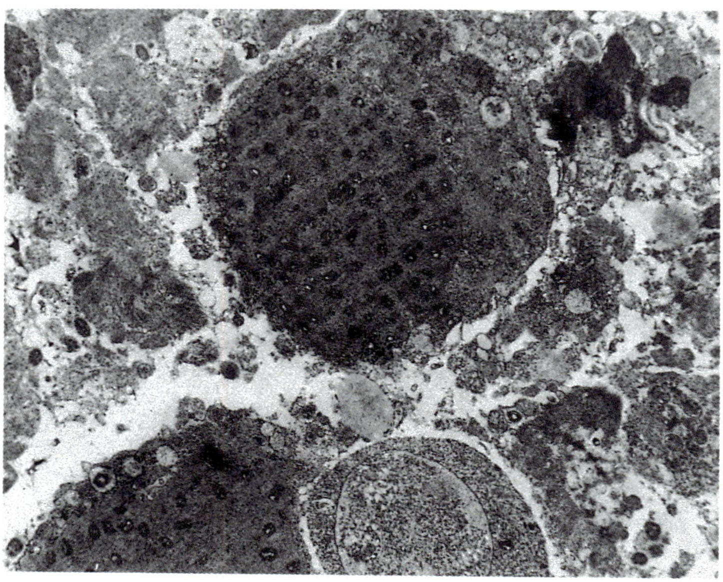

Fig. 5.6. Intracytoplasmic inclusions in feline epidermal cells showing individual virions. (Courtesy of Dr D. Baxby.)

TREATMENT

There is no specific therapy. Where necessary treatment is symptomatic. Spontaneous recovery usually takes place in 1–2 months.

5.2 Bacteria

Primary defence mechanisms of the body are the physical barriers to infective organisms, preventing their access to the surface of the skin. At this level, a combination of the physical and biological defences will, in normality, prevent colonization by pathogens and subsequent disease.

The ability of the epidermis to protect against infection is determined by the integrity of the stratum corneum. Consisting of a mass of densely packed, flattened keratinized squamous cells, its surface is covered and its interstices permeated by a lipid/aqueous barrier carrying inorganic salts and fatty acids together with other substances, e.g. immunoglobulins IgA, IgG, IgM and IgE, which it is considered also play a protective role.

In addition, the skin surface is populated by a normal microflora of bacteria and fungi. These are found in the outer layers of the stratum corneum, living in a symbiotic relationship and able to play a significant inhibitory role by the production of active metabolites against pathogens.

In the dog, organisms commonly present are *Staphylococcus epidermidis*, *Micrococcus* spp. and *Acinetobacter* while, in the cat, *Staphylococcus*, *Streptococcus*, *Micrococcus* spp. and *Acinetobacter* have been isolated as resident flora (Krogh & Kristensen, 1976). A variety of other micro-organisms appear on the skin surface from time to time but do not multiply.

A secondary role in infective processes may be played by organisms such as *Proteus mirabilis*, *Pseudomonas* spp. and *Escherichia coli*.

The most significant organisms isolated from infected skin lesions in small animals are coagulase-positive, penicillinase-producing staphylococci; of these, *Staphylococcus intermedius* has been shown to be of the greatest importance in dogs (Ness, 1984; Medlau *et al.*, 1986).

Pyoderma has been classified by some as surface, superficial and deep according to the depth at which the bacterial process occurs. Since surface and superficial are by definition synonymous, the conditions are more properly considered as two entities (Table 5.1):

Table 5.1. Classification of pyodermas

Superficial pyodermas	Deep pyodermas
Pyotraumatic dermatitis	Nasal
Skin-fold pyoderma	Callus
Impetigo	Interdigital
Folliculitis	Acne
Short-haired dog pyoderma	Anal furunculosis
Superficial ventral pruritic pyoderma	

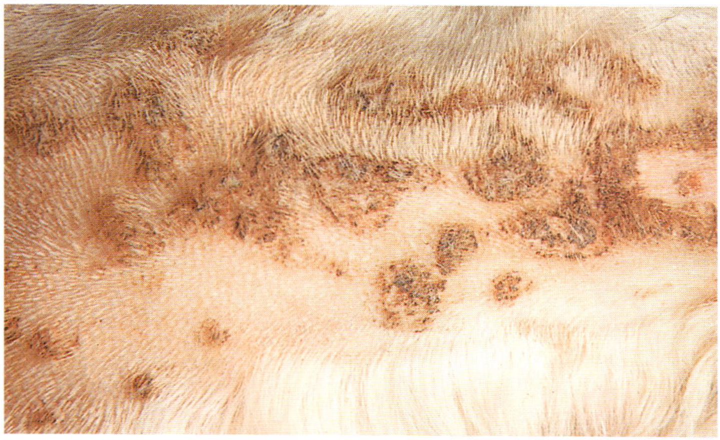

Fig. 5.7. Dog with staphylococcal pyoderma — superficial.

1 Superficial (Fig. 5.7). Those which involve the upper and outermost layers of the skin and extending to include the intact hair follicle.

2 Deep (Figs 5.8 and 5.9). Those which extend deeper than the hair follicles.

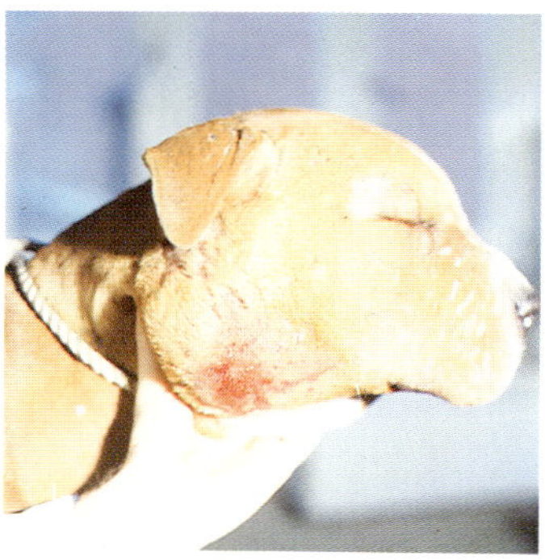

Fig. 5.8. Deep pyoderma — abscess.

Pyotraumatic dermatitis (hot spot, wet eczema)

The aetiology of this condition is often obscure and in many cases complex with allergy playing a significant role.

INCIDENCE

Although all breeds can be affected there appears to be a predisposition for those having long hair, e.g. retrievers, Scottish terriers, and for the disease to be more prevalent in periods of warm weather.

CLINICAL SIGNS

Acute in onset it is characterized by the sudden appearance of often single, exudative lesions several centimetres in diameter on the body, head or neck (Fig. 5.10). The area of accumulated exudate is often straw coloured, matting the hair, and the periphery may often be outlined by an erythematous line.

Lesions often cause discomfort or their appearance may be accompanied by mild systemic upset inducing self-trauma from scratching, biting or licking.

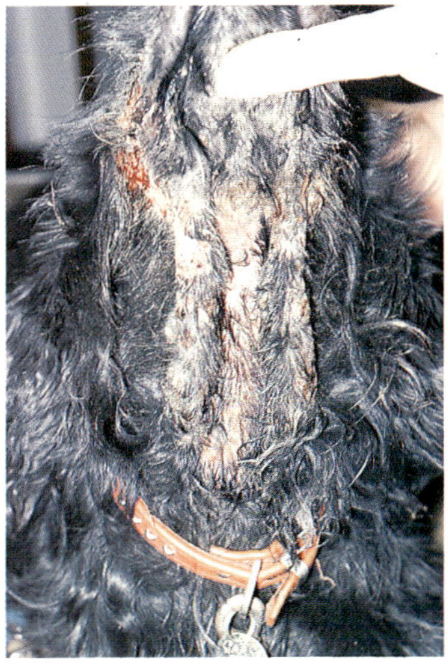

Fig. 5.9. Deep pyoderma — furunculosis.

DIFFERENTIAL DIAGNOSIS

Few conditions truly mimic this disease. Consideration should, however, be given to the possibility of dermatophyte infection, e.g. *Trichophyton mentagrophytes*, confirmed by laboratory investigation, or skin neoplasia, e.g. squamous-cell carcinoma, confirmed histologically.

Candidiasis is often quoted as a possible cause of hot-spot lesions. Although commonly reported by some laboratories as present in skin-scrape material, confirmed cases of canine exudative dermatitis due to *Candida* organisms are extremely rare.

DIAGNOSIS

The history of acute onset and the appearance of the characteristic lesions, virtually pathognomonic for this disease, should make diagnosis straightforward.

Since the aetiology may be multifactorial, the factors triggering the response may be difficult to determine.

The elimination of internal or external parasitism as contributory causes, parasitic allergy, atopy and contact sensitivity, as well as painful and infective conditions giving rise to self-trauma, is important.

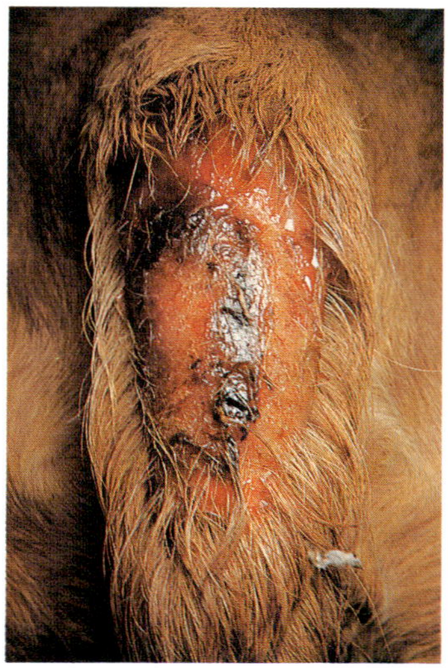

Fig. 5.10. Hot spot — pyotraumatic dermatitis.

TREATMENT

1 Eliminate the predisposing cause if it can be determined.

2 Symptomatic treatment after initial clipping away of hair at and around the lesion; if particularly painful, this procedure may necessitate mild sedation.

3 Cleanse with warm antibacterial solutions, e.g. 0.5% Hexetidine, Dermisol solution, 2.5% benzoyl peroxide. Dry and apply a topical glucocorticoid cream.

4 A short course (5 days) of oral or short-acting parenteral glucocorticoid may be indicated but should be accompanied by the appropriate antibiotic cover. Self-trauma may need to be controlled by mechanical restraint using an Elizabethan collar.

Skin-fold pyodermas

This is mostly a disease of dogs but occasionally it is seen in the cat, affecting flat-faced breeds.

The disorder is associated with either continuous or intermittent apposition of folded, hairless or hairy skin giving rise to poor ventilation and the accumulation of skin surface debris and sebaceous and apocrine secretions.

The abnormal surface microclimate allows bacteria to flourish, a process often enhanced by the presence of other secretions, e.g. saliva and tears, and complicated by the presence of food and other debris.

CLINICAL SIGNS

Areas of superficial bacterial infection are often exudative and superficially eroded with accumulations of debris matting the hair.

Facial and labial folds are often affected so severely that the lesions have a marked necrotic mal odour.

Labial-fold pyoderma (lip-fold dermatitis)

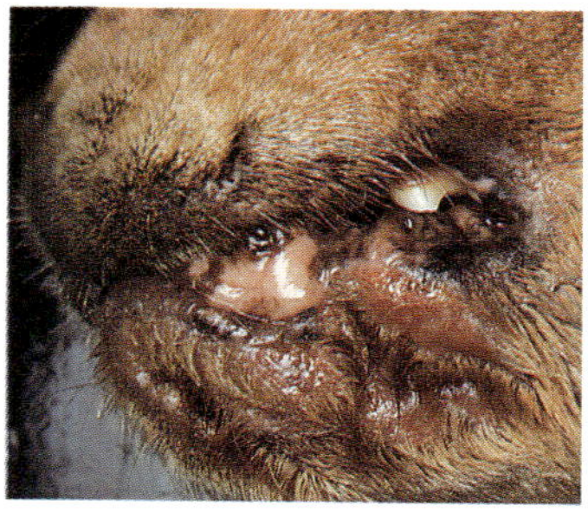

Fig. 5.11. Fold dermatitis — labial fold, spaniel.

This occurs in dogs, in particular the various breeds of spaniel and others prone to salivary seepage due to poor conformation (Fig. 5.11).

The skin of the lower jaw in the region of the canine teeth becomes superficially infected. There is associated inflammation, erosion, exudation and soiling with saliva, often contaminated with food particles.

This situation in many cases gives rise to a strong necrotic odour, often mistaken by owners as the result of dental disease from which the condition has to be differentiated.

TREATMENT

Since the condition is essentially due to an anatomical defect, ablation of the fold (where possible) provides the more lasting result. Cryosurgery may also be considered.

Medical treatment of the immediate clinical signs by the topical application of, for example, a solution of hydrogen peroxide may give temporary relief by controlling the bacterial infection. Once discontinued, the condition readily recurs.

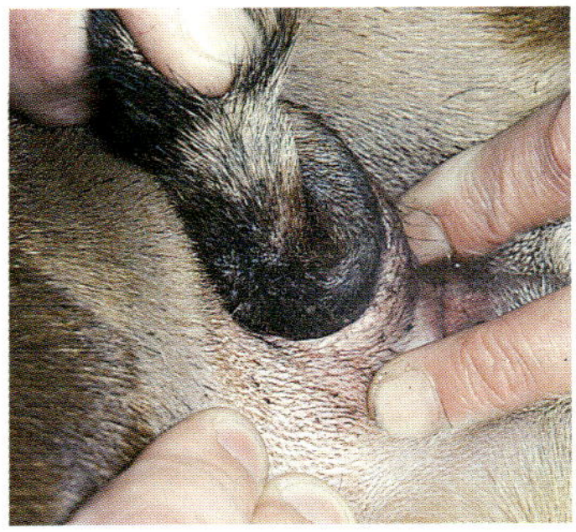

Fig. 5.12. Fold dermatitis — tail fold, bulldog.

Body-fold pyodermas

With the increase in numbers of unusual breeds having excessively folded body skin, e.g. Shar Pei, problems of body-fold pyoderma are now more common.

Surgical management is impractical and the regular application of benzoyl peroxide shampoo or other antiseborrhoeal or antibacterial preparation may be the only approach for a very persistent problem.

Other fold pyodermas

These occur particularly in brachycephalic breeds, e.g. bulldogs and Pekingese, in the *facial folds* where infection is associated with tear scalding, accumulation of skin debris and infection with subsequent discomfort leading to self-trauma to the face by scratching and rubbing. Damage to the eyelids and cornea is not uncommon.

Tail-fold pyoderma is seen in breeds having anatomically abnormal tails and tails deeply recessed into the hind quarters, e.g. bulldog, pug (Fig. 5.12).

Vulval fold pyoderma is a similar condition seen in bitches of any breed where the vulval recess is deep, allowing the accumulation of skin debris; together with skin secretion this causes inflammatory change, discomfort and self-trauma by licking.

TREATMENT

Attempts to control these conditions medically give only temporary relief. Surgical correction is often difficult.

Breeding out anatomical abnormalities and neutering bitches after their first oestrus are long-term approaches for consideration.

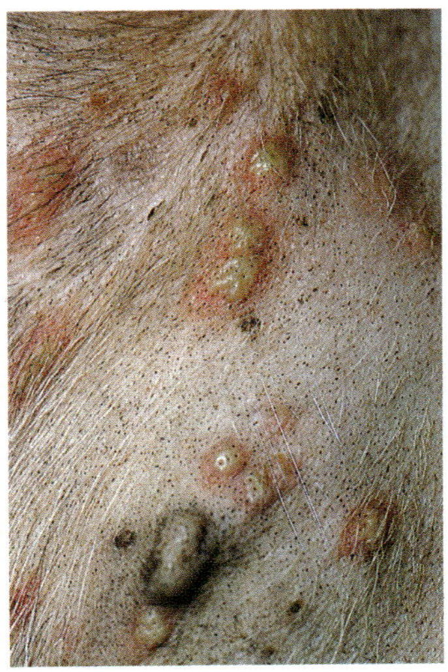

Fig. 5.13. Superficial pyoderma — puppy impetigo, medial thigh.

Impetigo (superficial pustular dermatitis) (Fig. 5.13)

Staphylococcal infection of the skin of young dogs, as in most bacterial infections, is secondary to other predisposing factors, e.g. management, infection, infestation with parasites, disordered immune responses. The differential diagnosis is parasitism.

LESIONS

These are interfollicular pustules of the fine-skinned, somewhat hairless areas of the body, axillae, ventral abdomen and inguinal region. In cats, the lesions are seen more commonly on dorsal surfaces.

At biopsy, subcorneal pustules may be demonstrated histologically and infective organisms revealed in impression smears of pustule contents.

Resolving lesions leave yellow-coloured scabs or crusts.

Muller *et al.* (1983) describe a staphylococcal disease of dogs, similar in epidemiology to impetigo and affecting the axillary and inguinal skin, where the lesion is within the hair follicle and which may be identified by the follicular pustule containing a protruding hair.

TREATMENT

Most cases require little treatment: 2.5% benzoyl peroxide shampoos may be adequate. Antibiotics against the infecting staphylococci are only required as a last resort if managemental changes do not improve the condition.

Superficial ventral pruritic folliculitis: (ventral) pyoderma (Fig. 5.14)

This is a pruritic skin disease of multifactorial aetiology particularly affecting larger breeds of dog and characterized by the presence of skin rashes ranging from papules to pustules. It affects mainly the ventral abdominal skin and also the axillae and inguinal area.

The disease has been shown to be particularly prevalent in the German shepherd breed. Ihrke (1983) listed 12 other breeds in which the disease had been recorded.

AETIOLOGY

A number of factors have been incriminated, in particular:

1 Allergy — to foods and ectoparasites.
— bacterial hypersensitivity.

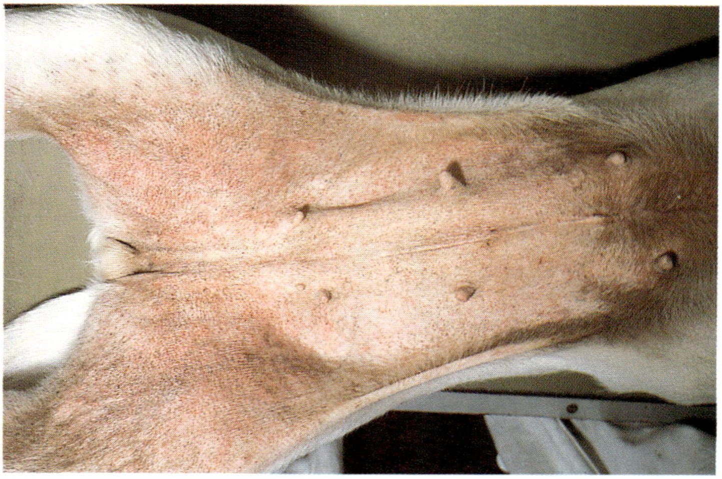

Fig. 5.14. Ventral pyoderma.

— atopy.

2 Nutrition. Other than allergy.

3 Functional skin disorder. Concurrent disease leading to seborrhoea.

CLINICAL SIGNS

These comprise a ventral papular–pustular rash extending from glabrous areas to dense-coated body and limbs.

There is intense pruritus with scratch reflex response on the posterior aspect of the forelimb just distal to the elbow, suggesting sarcoptic scabies. Lesions are not found on the fringe of the pinna.

In many patients the pustules are very small and there may not be an obvious pustular condition. Many dogs, particularly those having close coats, are found to be hyperhidrotic.

Persistent self-trauma causes chronic skin change with acanthosis, hyperpigmentation and hypertrophy of the nipples with excoriation.

Extension of lesions to the skin of the perineum, ventral tail base and anterior aspect of the elbow may also occur.

Animals with extensive lesions have a significant mal odour due to the accumulation of sebaceous and apocrine secretions on the surface of the skin.

DIFFERENTIAL DIAGNOSIS

1 Ectoparasitism.

2 Allergy.
3 Bacterial hypersensitivity.
4 Seborrhoea.

DIAGNOSIS

1 Clinically on the distribution of the ventral rash.
2 Biopsy. Histology may eliminate other causes for the changes seen but does not always demonstrate the pustules.
3 Skin scrapings. Negative for parasites.
4 Skin test. Eliminates allergic disease.

TREATMENT

1 Dietary investigation with implementation of a restricted diet routine.
2 Antibacterial therapy using potentiated amoxycillin, cephalexin or trimethoprim/sulphadiazine in extended dosage.
3 Shampoo using 2.5% benzoyl peroxide. Some patients will benefit from courses of *Staphylococcus intermedius* vaccine.

Deep pyodermas (Fig. 5.15)

As in other bacterial infections of the skin, deep pyodermas are secondary to a wide variety of predisposing factors.

The penetration of the dermal and subcuticular layers by bacteria may follow damage by parasites (Fig. 5.16), penetrating foreign bodies, physical agents or physical pressure. In addition, certain individuals are predisposed to bacterial infection by virtue of concurrent endocrine disease. This may be iatrogenic in its relationship to corticosteroid therapy, or naturally spontaneous as in Cushing's disease, hypothyroidism or diseases associated with immunosuppression or immunodeficiency.

Lesions of deep pyoderma may be localized or generalized.

Nasal pyoderma

The dorsum of the nose is the more commonly affected area (nasal pyoderma). Those breeds having a particularly pointed facial and nasal conformation, e.g. German shepherd, collie and Doberman, are prone to this condition.

Lesions in the early stage of the disease are papular and pustular, these develop to form tracts from which pus and

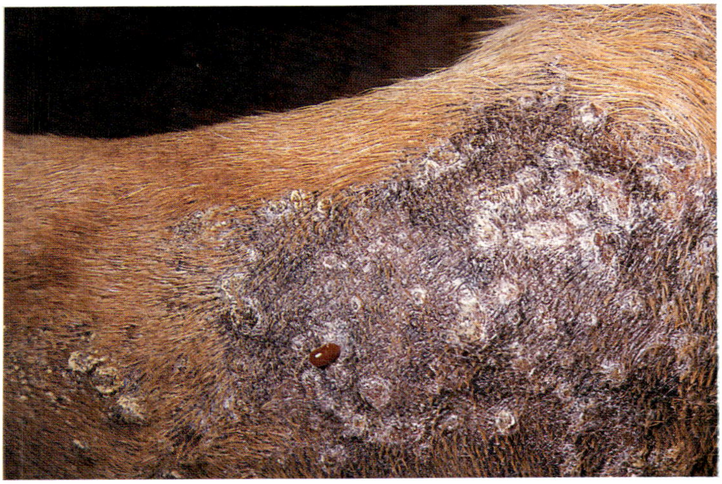

Fig. 5.15. Furunculosis on the dorsal skin of boxer.

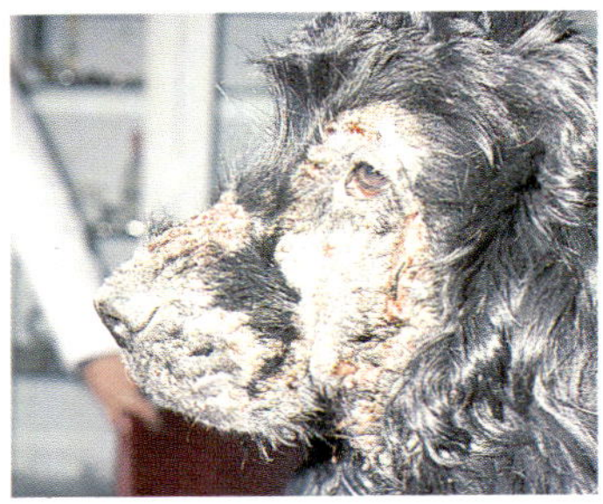

Fig. 5.16. Furunculosis secondary to demodicosis.

exudate can be expressed.

There is swelling at the site, erythema and hair loss due to follicular damage, and self-trauma from pruritus or inflammatory pain.

DIFFERENTIAL DIAGNOSIS

1 Parasitism — demodicosis. Since predilection sites for this infection are the muzzle, face and temporal region, scrapings to eliminate *Demodex* should always be examined.
2 Fungal infection. Infection of the skin of the bridge of the nose with ringworm fungi occurs in dogs having opportunities to root in woods and gardens as well as to encounter wild mammals infected with dermatophytes.

Lesions caused by *Trichophyton mentagrophytes* (Fig. 5.17), *T. erinacei* and *Microsporum persicolor* are often similar to those of pyoderma and arise from contact with hedgehogs and voles. In the UK the Jack Russell terrier appears more commonly affected than other breeds.
3 Autoimmune disease. Although rare, certain well-defined autoimmune disorders are recognized in dogs. Lesions, particularly on the nose and face, may resemble some stages in the development of nasal pyoderma; they are scaling, erosive and persistent.

Autoimmune conditions may well present with lesions at other sites, e.g. periorbital, mucocutaneous junctions and nail beds, and be less localized than pyoderma.

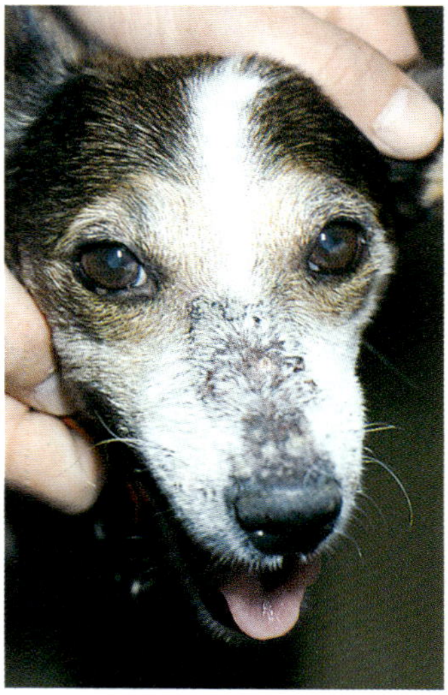

Fig. 5.17. *Trichophyton mentagrophytes.*

So-called 'collie nose', in most cases thought to be a solar-stimulated autoimmune response, should also be considered in the differential diagnosis.

DIAGNOSIS

The primary cause of nasal pyoderma may be behavioural – e.g. trauma from rooting.

TREATMENT

Extended therapy with antibiotics.

Callus pyoderma

Heavy, giant breeds show localized lesions of pyoderma at the sites of callus formation over bony prominences coming into contact with hard surfaces.

Pressure-induced lesions occur over the elbows, hocks and lateral toes. Some of the smaller breeds, e.g. short-haired pointer and shorthaired dachshund, become infected on the sternum.

CLINICAL SIGNS

These comprise chronic thickening at the site, accompanied by hair loss; infection with pyogenic organisms produces multiple tracts from which pus, serosanguinous exudate and blood can be expressed.

Pressure between thumb and finger shows the area to be of the consistency of a pus-filled sponge.

TREATMENT

A basic requirement is attention to management in order to reduce pressure damage. Some benefit is said to accrue from the application of protective clothing over the pressure areas.

Immediate treatment using hot hypertonic saline soaks followed by extended antibiotic therapy can be helpful.

Surgical ablation of the lesion has, in selected cases, been found to be beneficial.

Pedal pyoderma (Figs 5.18 and 5.19)

This is usually seen as deep pyoderma lesions affecting the

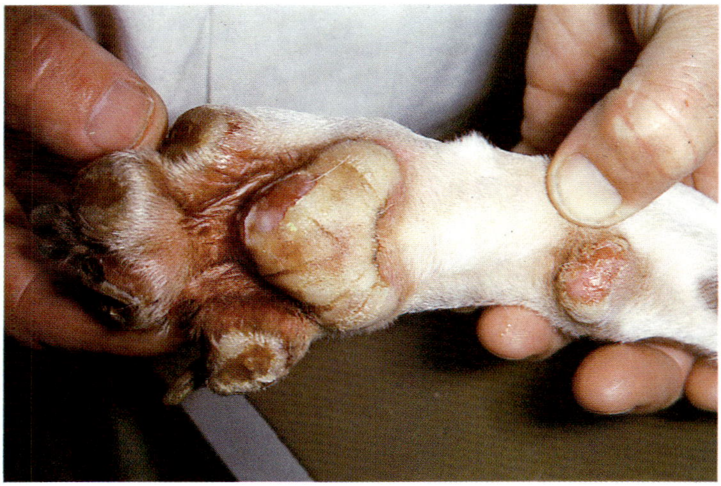

Fig. 5.19. Pedal dermatosis.

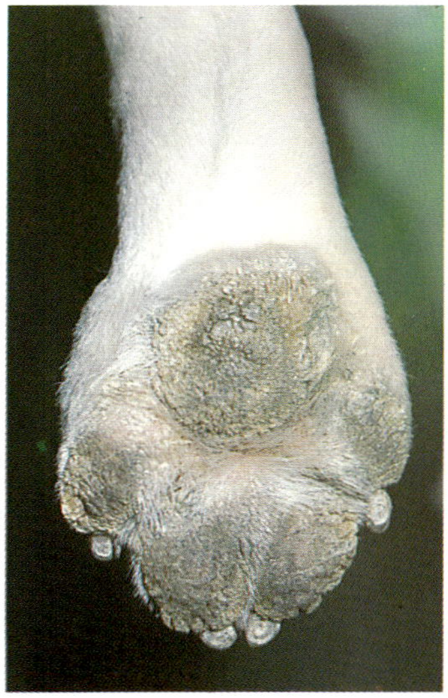

Fig. 5.18. Bull terrier with pedal dermatosis causing hyperkeratosis.

skin of the interdigital spaces or between the pads. It is sometimes referred to as pododermatitis.

Pedal pyoderma is an infective condition often of obscure aetiology and occurring in many breeds of dog of any age or either sex. It is rarely seen in the cat.

A higher incidence is recorded in the bulldog and bull terrier breeds although Muller *et al.* (1983) suggest that a number of the larger hound breeds are more commonly affected.

Many contributory factors of foot conformation can be considered to play a significant role.

1 Poorly ventilating interdigital spaces and webs of the feet give rise to a persistent moist situation with the accumulation of sebum and sweat with surface keratin debris, which is an ideal medium for the multiplication of micro-organisms (Fig 5.20).

2 Irritants (both physical and chemical, penetrating foreign bodies, e.g. grass awns) initiate primary skin damage with consequent infection and secondary self-trauma.

3 Parasites, notably demodectic mites, trombiculid larvae and hookworm larvae as well as some fungal organisms, may also initiate pododermatitis (Fig. 5.21).

4 Plugging of the follicles of the interdigital space to form comedones or hair abnormalities resulting in curling of the hair within its follicle, subsequent rupture and are also contributory causes of the condition.

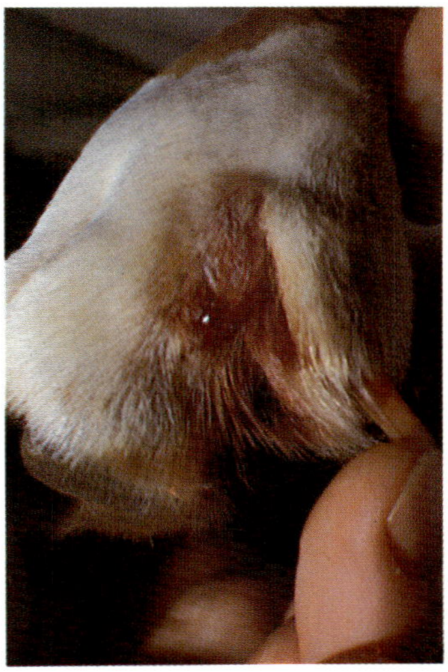

Fig. 5.20. Interdigital sepsis, well-developed cyst with rupture revealing purulent contents.

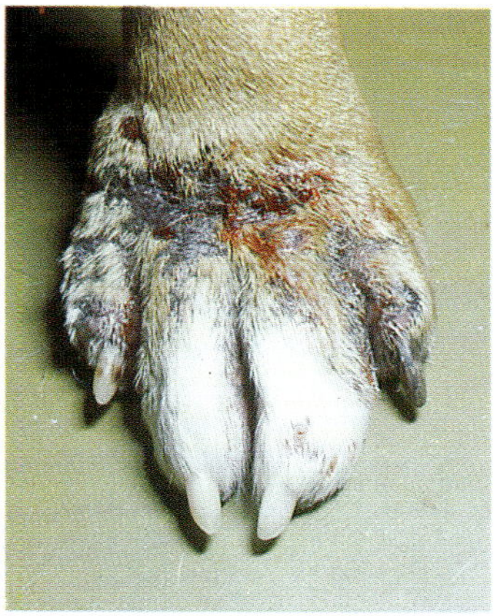

Fig. 5.21. Pedal pyoderma secondary to demodicosis.

CLINICAL SIGNS

Erythema of the interdigital skin and that of the web between the pads is often all that is found in the early stages, accompanied by evidence of discomfort; foot nibbling, etc.

The forefeet are more commonly affected. More obvious lesions take the form of bright-red, cyst-like swellings, which on rupture exude serosanguinous fluid, blood or pus. Alternatively the lesions may present as obvious abscesses or penetrating tracts. There may be a varying degree of lameness as well as associated regional lymphadenopathy.

DIFFERENTIAL DIAGNOSIS

1 Demodicosis.
2 Foreign body.
3 Autoimmune disease.

TREATMENT

This entails specific treatment of parasitism and fungal infections. Hot hypertonic saline soaks using magnesium sulphate or sodium chloride are administered at least three times daily for 10–15 minutes on each occasion.

A full therapeutic regime of antibiotics is administered for 3 weeks in the first instance. A double therapeutic dose may be required.

Generalized deep pyoderma

This condition is characterized by multiple, deep-tracking, furuncular lesions of the skin of the body and limbs, the underlying cause of which is often obscure. In some patients chronic parasitism or immunosuppression appear to play a part.

The disease is more prevalent in larger breeds, particularly the German shepherd.

CLINICAL SIGNS

These comprise extensive areas of furunculosis and total destruction of epidermis and some upper dermal tissue often involving the skin of the hindquarters, lateral thorax and lateral and dorsal abdomen extending to the upper limbs.

Lesions are present below masses of matted coat which when removed reveals their extent, often 5 cm or more in diameter.

In some dogs, fever, loss of appetite and lethargy may accompany the skin signs.

DIFFERENTIAL DIAGNOSIS

1 Demodicosis.
2 Diabetes mellitus.
3 Iatrogenic immunosuppression.
4 Hyperadrenocorticism with calcinosis cutis.

TREATMENT

1 Investigate and treat known precipitating cause as detailed in differential diagnosis.
2 Lesion hygiene.
3 Clipping away hair around the necrotic areas. The removal of matted hair, exudate and pus overlying lesions is paramount.
4 Cleansing with a hot hypertonic saline soak, solution of hydrogen peroxide or a preparation such as Dermisol solution.
5 Antibiotic therapy for an extended period.

Prognosis in these cases is poor, the outcome often being a recommendation for euthanasia.

Juvenile pyoderma (Fig. 5.22)

A condition of obscure aetiology but thought to be associated with infection by pyogenic staphylococci. The authors have seen outbreaks of the disease in weaning puppies, suggesting an allergic aetiology.

The disease affects young puppies under 4 months of age. Hound breeds are more commonly affected, particularly beagles. Wilkinson (1985) includes Labradors and Bassett hounds as also being susceptible.

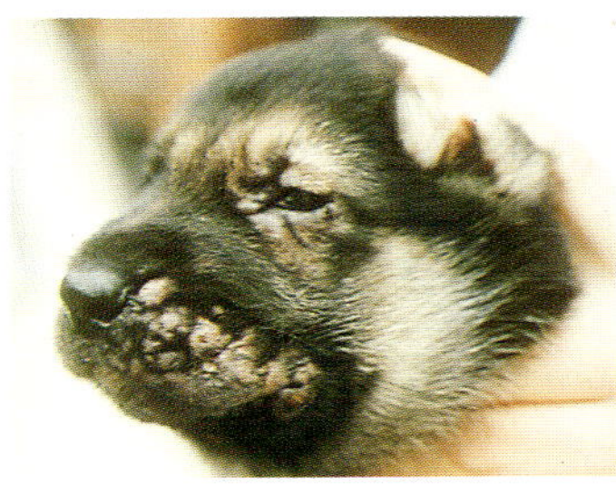

Fig. 5.22. A juvenile pyoderma with muzzle and head lesions.

CLINICAL SIGNS

These consist of oedema with pyoderma-like lesions, particularly involving the head. There is marked lymphadenopathy of the regional nodes around the head with impaired lymph drainage and consequent oedema; hence the term 'puppy-head gland disease' or 'strangles'. The disease progresses to the point where oedema is extensive and sinus tracts drain from the affected lymph nodes. Scarring of the muzzle is a common sequel.

Not all littermates are equally affected. Whilst it has been generally believed that the condition is bacterial in origin, few organisms of significance have been isolated from affected puppies — either survivors or at postmortem.

TREATMENT

The disease is usually treated by combined antibiotic and corticosteroid therapy with limited success.

Anal sepsis/anal furunculosis

This is a predisposition of larger breeds of dog and in particular of the German shepherd.

AETIOLOGY

The aetiology is obscure but is considered to be multifactorial; poor ventilation of the skin of the area due to conformation and tail carriage, accumulation of skin secretion and anal sacculitis are thought to play significant roles.

CLINICAL SIGNS

In the early stage of the disease, the only observation that may be noted is excessive moistness of perianal skin and the skin of the ventral tail base.

Erythema, sepsis, furunculosis with fissuring of the anus and surrounding tissue follow, often accompanied by mal odour.

Necrosis and tracking of infection into the deeper perianal tissues result in varying degrees of pain and self-trauma.

TREATMENT

1 Radical surgery.
2 Cryosurgery to remove necrotic tissue by debridement.
3 Supportive antibiotic therapy.

Chin/muzzle acne

Dogs (Fig. 5.23). Young dogs, particularly short-haired breeds and those having a conformation which leads to a tendency to persistent salivary wetting of the skin of the chin and muzzle (great Dane, Doberman, boxer) are predisposed to acne. The underlying cause is obscure but is considered similar to that in humans and results in colonization of the hair follicles of the chin and muzzle by pyogenic bacteria.

The differential diagnosis is demodicosis.

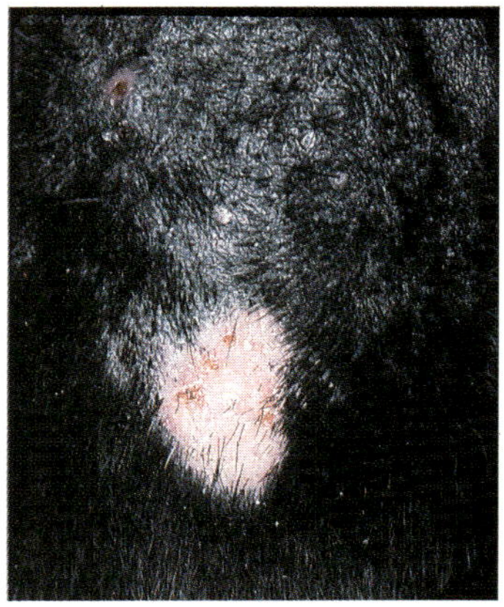

Fig. 5.23. Chin acne of a dog.

CLINICAL SIGNS

These include muzzle rubbing and recurrent abscessation of the large hair follicles of the chin in particular, leaving areas of erosion and ulceration of the skin following rupture, with exudation of pus or serosanguinous exudate.

The condition is chronic with recurrent episodes of swelling of the hair follicles, accompanied by self-trauma resulting from rubbing the chin and muzzle.

DIAGNOSIS

This is made on the basis of clinical signs and demonstration of micro-organisms in impression smears or cultures.

TREATMENT

1 Extended antibiotic therapy.
2 Cleansing with saline soaks or 2.5% benzoyl peroxide wash.
3 Antibiotic therapy.
4 Ablation of hair follicles by cryoprobe.
5 *Staphylococcus intermedius* vaccine.

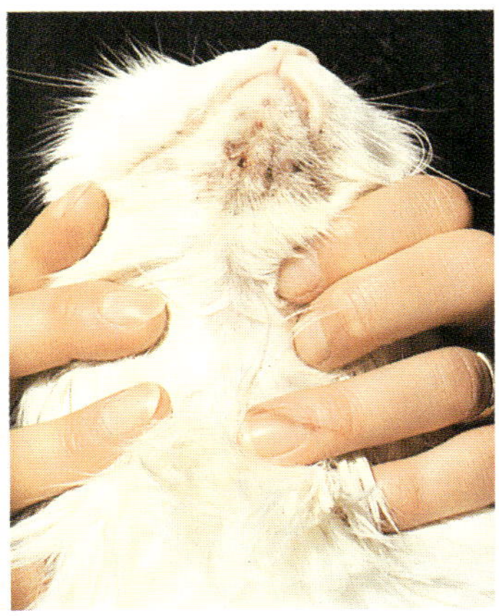

Fig. 5.24. Chin acne of a cat.

Cats (Fig. 5.24). The chin is used for territorial marking, and plugging of the hair follicles with black comedones composed of keratinous debris and skin-gland secretion is common; in some this may lead on to pustule formation.

Crust, exudate and comedone debris accumulate on the hair of the chin and may be accompanied by erythema and local oedema.

Cats of any age and either sex can be affected with this, often very chronic, condition.

TREATMENT

Since the underlying cause is essentially physiological and the lesions are very mild, no treatment may be justified.

Where lesions are infected and cause discomfort then antibiotic therapy should be instituted.

Mild cases may respond to daily cleansing with warm soap solutions and expression of the comedones.

Feline pyoderma

As a species, the cat is less commonly affected with bacterial skin disease than the dog, differing also in the species of infecting organisms; pasteurellae, haemolytic streptococci and fusiforms being predominant.

Superficial pyodermas are less common and lesions are usually deeper and focal rather than widespread on the skin surface as in dogs.

Many lesions arise as the result of bite and scratch wounds from fighting, being more commonly found around the head, extremities and dorsum near the tail base.

CLINICAL SIGNS

Pain, lameness, anorexia, fever and lethargy in established sepsis are accompanied by an area of swelling of the skin which is hot to touch and later becomes a fluctuating swelling.

Puncture wounds from claws or teeth may be visible at the site.

TREATMENT

1 Allow the abscess to point.
2 Provide drainage.
3 Cleanse with hot soaks.
4 Antibiotic therapy for 7 days.

Miscellaneous pyodermas

These consist of mycobacterial infections of the skin of dogs and cats.

Tuberculosis

Skin lesions due to infection with tubercle bacilli are now fortunately rare.

Mycobacterium tuberculosis has been isolated from chronic ulcerating skin lesions and nodules of the head, neck and limbs.

Systemic illness with fever, loss of appetite and weight loss or inexplicable lymphadenopathy should arouse suspicion of tuberculous infection.

DIAGNOSIS

This is based on demonstration of tubercle bacilli in smears and cultures.

TREATMENT

Because of danger of transmission to humans and other susceptible species only euthanasia should be considered.

Cat leprosy (Fig. 5.25)

Cases of infection of the skin with a variety of mycobacterial organisms have been reported from various parts of the world.

The most commonly isolated organism has been *Mycobacterium lepraemurium*.

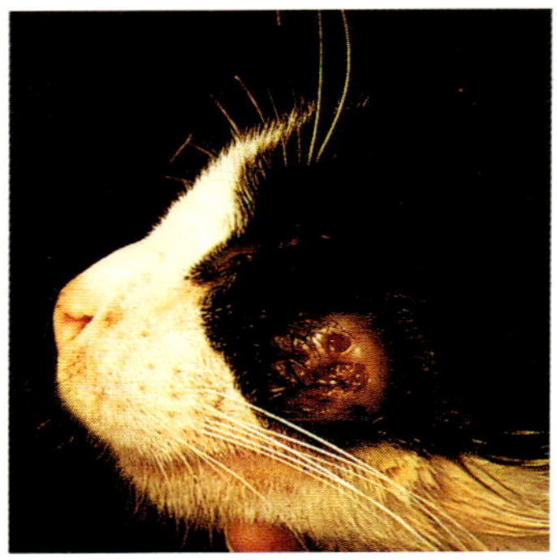

Fig. 5.25. Cat leprosy. (Courtesy of G.T. Wilkinson and Wolfe Medical Publications.)

CLINICAL SIGNS

These include chronic granulomata of the skin of the head and limbs, abscesses and indolent ulcers with regional lymphadenopathy but without systemic illness.

The feature differentiating these infections from that of *M. tuberculosis* is the absence of systemic illness.

TREATMENT

Where lesions are localized to a nodule or skin granuloma then surgical excision may be justified, although in a proportion of cases natural resolution may take place.

Wilkinson (1978), Wilkinson *et al.* (1982), Kunkle (1982) and Wilkinson (1985) have described cases of atypical mycobacterial infection of the skin of small animals where organisms such as *M. smegmatis* and *M. fortuitum* have been incriminated.

The course of the disease in such cases has been several months after which, in some infections, spontaneous remission has taken place.

Because of the chronic and unpredictable course of the

condition and lack of specific therapy, the likely outcome is a request for euthanasia for an affected animal.

Nocardiosis

Chronic infection of the skin and subcutaneous tissues may be caused by the weakly acid-fast soil saprophytic organism in the dog and cat of the genus *Nocardias*.

Infection is by contamination of wounds or the introduction of organisms by penetrating vegetable foreign bodies, e.g. grass awns. Occasional extension to the skin can occur from discharging sinuses draining a deep infected cavity.

TREATMENT

1 Surgical drainage of lesions.
2 Antibiotic therapy — penicillin, trimethoprim/sulphadiazine.

General considerations in the diagnosis and prognosis of pyodermas

Since nearly all bacterial infection of skin is secondary, the initial consideration in the investigation of pyodermas is to establish the underlying primary cause. This depends in the first instance on a detailed history and meticulous clinical examination.

The following predisposing causes should therefore be considered:
1 Management — housing, behaviour, diet.
2 Conformation — genetic predisposition.
3 Allergy.
4 Endocrine disease.
5 Immunodeficiency.
6 Infestation and infection with parasitic and fungal organisms.

The specific bacterial infecting organism may then be determined by:
1 Direct smear.
2 Culture and establishment of antibiotic sensitivity.

Pyoderma therapy

SUPERFICIAL PYODERMAS

Once the primary factor in the causation of the disease has been determined and corrected or eliminated, many patients will not require antibiotic therapy. The antibiotics of choice, if required, are lincomycin, cephalexin or trimethoprim/sulphadiazine.

DEEP PYODERMA

Comment has already been made in relation to the individual manifestations of deep pyoderma.

1 In general, the first consideration is lesion hygiene.
2 Clip away hair.
3 Provide drainage.
4 Assist with hot soaks — this line of treatment is of particular value where the lesions are on the extremities or are focal.
5 Repeated hot bathing (fomentation) using hypertonic magnesium sulphate or sodium chloride solution has been shown to be highly beneficial even when other treatments have failed.

ANTIBIOTIC THERAPY

Before commencing any treatment which is sustained for a long period, is expensive and requires owner participation, there should be discussion with the owner on these points.

The minimum duration of antibiotic therapy should be 3 weeks, and in many cases considerably longer; in excess of 6–8 weeks may well be required to ensure the infection will not recur.

Dosage of antibiotic

The guiding principle is 'maximum dose for maximum effect'. The dose of some preparations, e.g. trimethoprim/sulphadiazine, can justifiably be doubled. For other antibiotics, Grant (1986) recommends that antibiotic therapy be continued for a period of 10 days beyond the point of clinical cure in superficial pyodermas and for 3 weeks in cases of deep pyodermas. Dosage and duration of therapy have been reviewed by Ihrke (1986).

5.3 Fungi

Many diseases of animals are caused either directly or indirectly by fungi.

This may be by direct invasion of the host by a single invading species or in conjunction with other organisms or pathological processes.

Fungi may also initiate allergic reactions, produce mycotoxins which when ingested cause disease, or cause spoilage of feeding stuffs with consequent unpalatability.

In dermatological practice, the keratinophilic fungi — the dermatophytes — are responsible for the greater number of disease problems, although the incidence among small animals (dog and cat) is not high.

Fungal skin disease may be:

1 Superficial. Due mainly to dermatophytes of the genera *Microsporum* and *Trichophyton* and occasionally other species of surface-living pathogens, e.g. yeasts such as *Candida, Pityrosporon*.

2 Deep. Subcutaneous mycoses due to infection with non-keratinophilic organisms, e.g. *Sporotrichum, Aspergillus*, with the formation of mycetomata.

3 Systemic mycoses. Infection is due to organisms such as *Blastomyces* and *Cryptococcus* species.

Dermatophyte infections (ringworm)

A wide variety of fungal species have been incriminated in the aetiology of small-animal dermatophytosis.

Wright (pers. comm.), in a laboratory survey of samples submitted from cats and dogs in Britain, isolated *Microsporum canis, M. gypseum, M. persicolor, Trichophyton mentagrophytes, T. erinacei, T. verrucosum* and *T. terrestre* from dogs. Samples from cats showed *Microsporum canis, M. persicolor, Trichophyton mentagrophytes, T. terrestre* and *T. ajelloi* as the infecting organisms.

Microsporum canis was responsible for 94% of infection in the cat and 66% in the dog, a ratio of 1.4:1; this had been previously recorded in Germany (Weiss & Weber, 1982).

Considerable similarity exists between lesions of dermatophytosis in small animals and other infective and non-infective skin disorders of those species. Because of the difficulty of differential diagnosis which this situation presents and the infectivity of certain species of animal ringworm for humans, an appreciation of the clinical manifestation of dermatophyte infection in animal hosts and their differential diagnosis is essential.

Infection occurs when viable spores, transmitted by contact with infected animals, contaminated environment, fomites or airborne transmission, invade the keratin of hairs in the anagen growth phase.

Hyphal invasion of the hair keratin takes place, extending downwards to the level of Adamson's fringe, where active keratinization of the hair shaft takes place (Fig. 5.26).

The hair shaft, through destruction of keratin by the fungus, becomes weakened and breaks with resulting alopecia.

Depending on the species of fungus responsible and the host response, there is considerable variation in the inflammatory reaction to be seen in ringworm infection.

Many *M. canis* infections in the cat, and a significant number in the dog, stimulate a negligible inflammatory response. This contributes greatly to the difficulty of diagnosis as well as to the establishment of the carrier state in long-haired, fine-coated breeds, where detection of lesions at physical examination of the patient may be virtually impossible.

Trichophyton infection more commonly evokes a marked inflammatory response giving rise to lesions characterized by erythema, swelling, exudation and crusting with consequent hair loss. Extension to involve nails or claws occurs and in severe cases the skin lesions resemble those of a deep pyoderma.

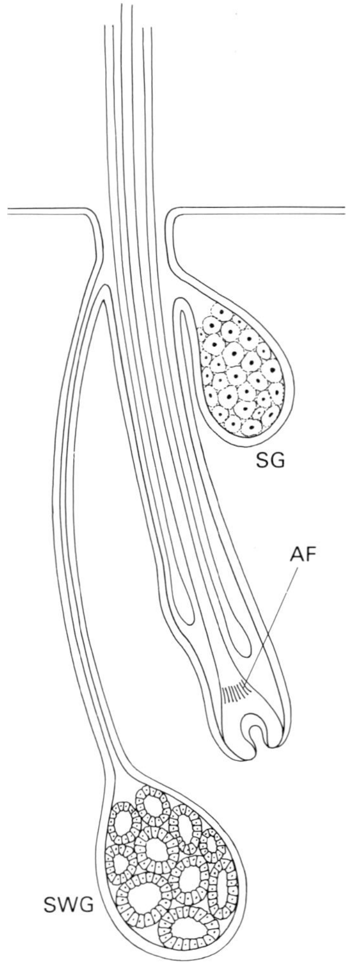

Fig. 5.26. Diagram to illustrate mode of infection of hair by dermatophytes. SG= sebaceous gland, AF= Adamson's fringe, SWG= sweat gland.

Microsporum canis infection

In both the cat and dog, the inflammatory response to this organism is commonly mild, the lesion being no more than a scaly area of alopecia.

Cats. A number of clinical signs may be seen:

1 Small, discrete, scaly or slightly crusted areas with little or no hair loss, possibly involving a small number of pilosebaceous units. Palpably and visually these may simulate small lesions of miliary dermatitis. (Figs 5.27 and 5.28.)

2 Extensive, slightly elevated irregular or circumscribed patches of alopecia with some mild hyperpigmentation and superficial scaling. (Fig. 5.29.)

3 No obvious lesion, slight hair thinning. The presence of infection is only confirmed by laboratory means.

Lesions may persist for 2–4 weeks or as long as months to years. Where discrete lesions are found, their distribution about the body has been shown to be associated with certain predilection sites. One author (Thomsett, 1962), in a study of

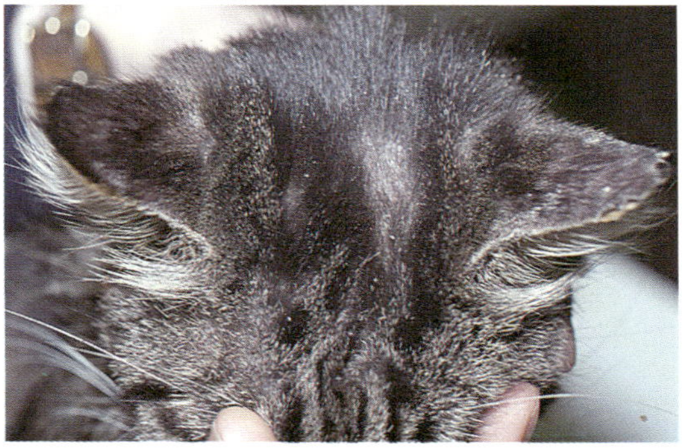

Fig. 5.27. Cat with *Microsporum canis* infection. Scaly and partially alopecic area on head.

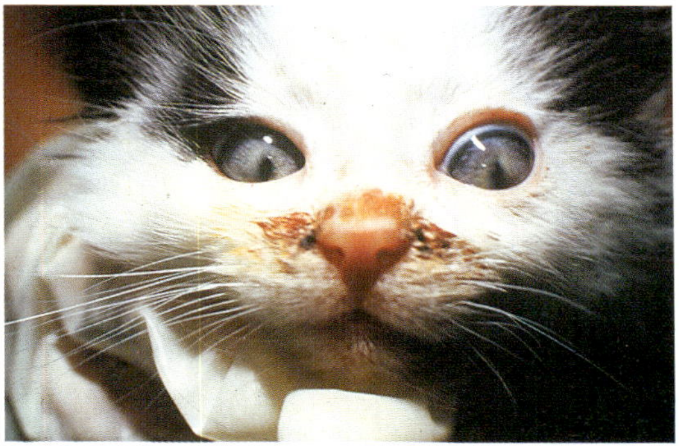

Fig. 5.28. Kitten with crusted lesion of *M. canis* around the nose.

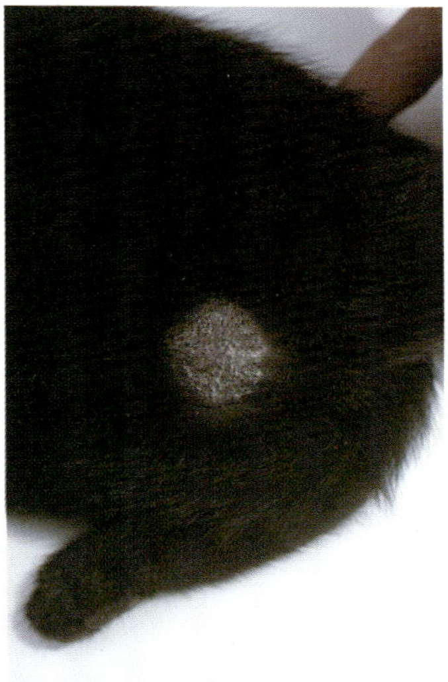

Fig. 5.29. Cat with *M. canis*. There is a crusted, scaling hairless lesion on left hind limb.

colony cats, found 66% of affected animals to have lesions on the head and ears, 25% on the limbs and 16% on the body.

Severely affected cats, particularly young kittens, may show total skin-surface infection.

Many *M. canis* infections in cats remain low grade and chronic, particularly in long-haired and very close-coated breeds. This hazard is potentiated in the boarding and breeding cattery environment.

Pepin and Oxenham (1987) studied the 'carrier state' in respect of *M. canis* infection of cats in a town practice in the South of England and demonstrated the presence of asymptomatic carriers, particularly in long-haired breeds. In the same study there was evidence to show that persistence of environmental contamination was minimal once infected cats were removed and that maintenance of infection within the environment was of less importance than had previously been believed. For this reason these workers considered it necessary to leave infected premises free of animals for at least 4 weeks before restocking, provided the premises were thoroughly disinfected.

Dog. Lesions in the dog are often discrete circular patches of scaliness with partial to total hair loss at the site of infection (Fig. 5.30).

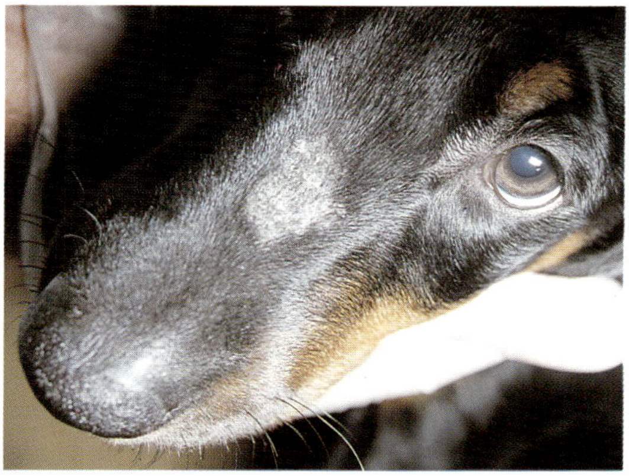

Fig. 5.30. Doberman with *M. canis* infection. There is a hairless, scaling lesion on the nose.

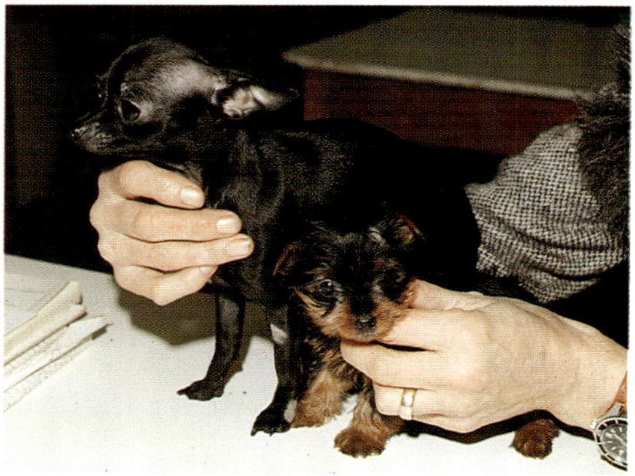

Fig. 5.31. Chihuahua and Yorkshire terrier both with *M. canis*. The Chihuahua has circumscribed lesions on left foreleg.

The affected areas increase in size until spontaneous limitation in size takes place.

As in the cat, some dogs will show involvement of extensive areas of the body and limbs.

Breeds having a long, fine coat, e.g. Yorkshire terrier, may show an almost asymptomatic infection and minimal skin response as in long-haired breeds of cat (Fig. 5.31). However, the same breeds may have extensive lesions.

Trichophyton infection

The most common species of the genus *Trichophyton* responsible for skin disease in the dog and cat is *T. mentagrophytes*, other species listed are responsible for a small percentage of the total incidence.

The clinical appearance of lesions produced by *Trichophyton* is usually more marked than that due to *M. canis*.

Host response to *T. mentagrophytes* is often an intense inflammatory reaction, particularly at the periphery of the lesion, with severe erythema, swelling, pyoderma-like suppurative change (Fig. 5.32) accompanied by hair loss and crusting, often extending to nail beds with consequent paronychia (Fig. 5.33).

Although some lesions are discrete and circular in outline, these may become confluent to involve large areas of the skin surface.

In some breeds, notably the smooth-coated Jack Russell

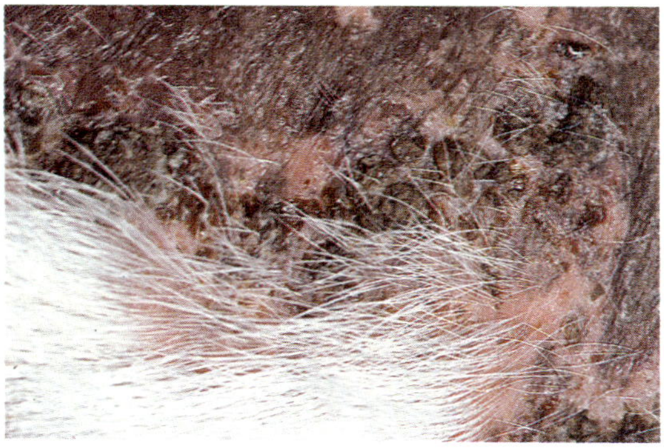

Fig. 5.32. *Trichophyton mentagrophytes* infection with a pyoderma-like inflammatory response.

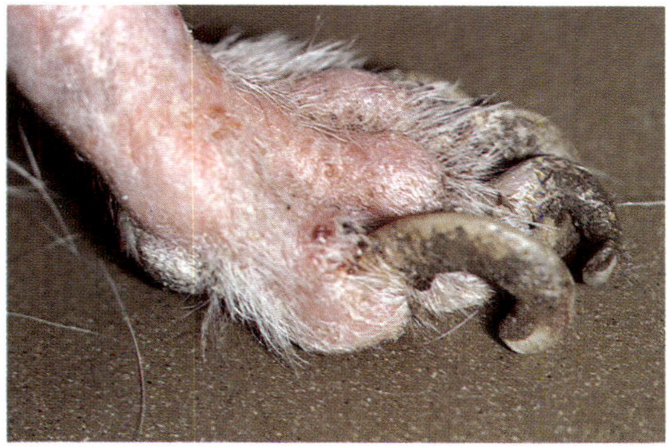

Fig. 5.33. *T. mentagrophytes* with paronychia.

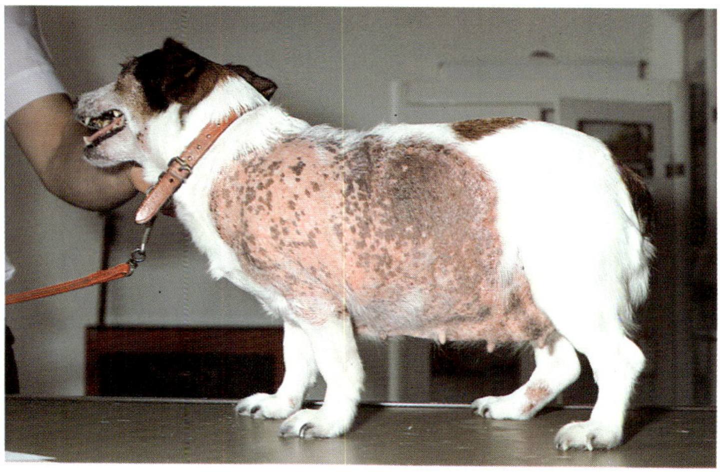

Fig. 5.34. Jack Russell terrier with *Trichophyton mentagrophytes* infection.

terrier, *Trichophyton* infections are more commonly seen (Fig. 5.34). As well as being responsible for generalized infection, *Trichophyton* species may be responsible for kerion-like lesions on the dorsal surface of the nose. This site is a predilection for *T. erinacei* infection (Fig. 5.35) since it is associated with trauma from hedgehog spines penetrating the skin when the dog plays with the curled up animal.

Burrowing into earth runs of other small wild mammals may lead to infection of this site with other zoophilic or geophilic species of fungus.

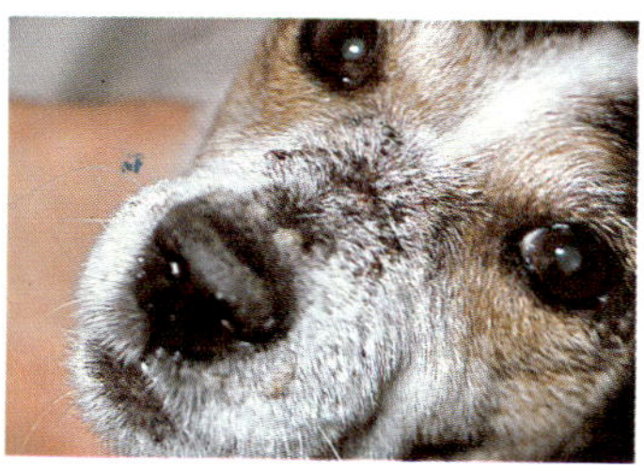

Fig. 5.35. *Trichophyton erinacei*, lesion on nose.

Mycotic granuloma

Deep follicular infection with granuloma formation has been recorded in association with dermatophyte infection.

DIFFERENTIAL DIAGNOSIS OF DERMATOPHYTE INFECTIONS

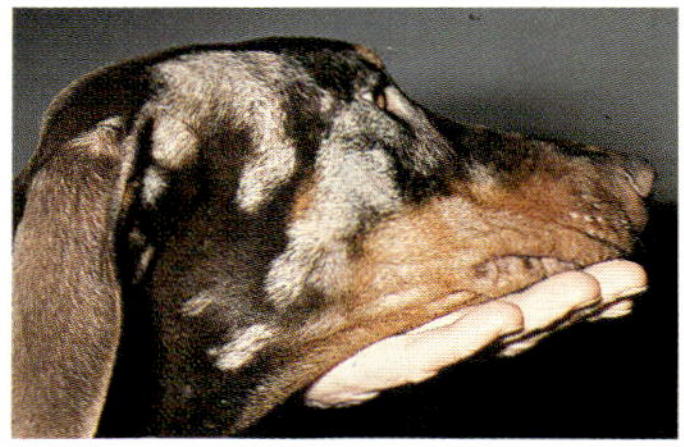

Fig. 5.36. Doberman with squamous demodicosis.

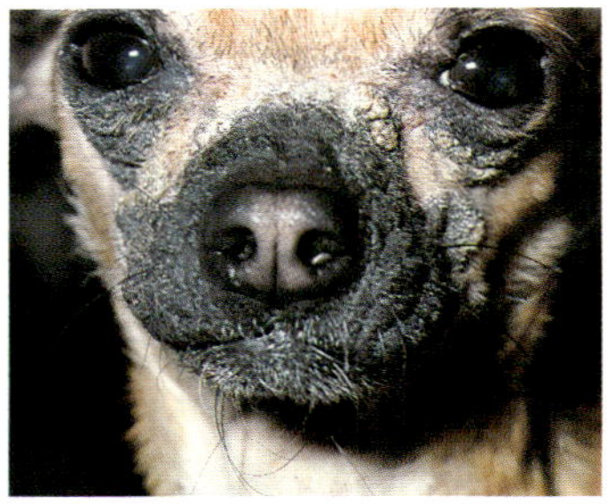

Fig. 5.37. Chihuahua with pustular demodicosis.

Demodicosis

Squamous demodicosis of both the dog and cat clinically simulates *M. canis* infection (Fig. 5.36).

Pustular demodicosis can resemble some more inflammatory fungal infections, particularly those due to *Trichophyton* species (Fig. 5.37).

Pyoderma

Severe infections with *Trichophyton* organisms can resemble pyoderma particularly where collarettes are present. The lesions seen in the end stages of superficial pyoderma where excess epidermal flaking occurs are often erroneously said to be those of fungal infection.

Seborrhoea

Excess scale formation with accumulations of any keratinous debris in diffuse or annular patches resembles mycotic lesions.

Autoimmune skin disease

Diffuse scaling, annular patches of scale and serpiginous or annular patterns of erythema with a covering of scale can arise due to autoimmune disease.

Nail bed lesions may suggest fungal paronychia.

Alopecia

Thinning of the coat accompanies most cases of dermatophyte infection although the extent of this is variable.

In cats, *M. canis* infection and in dogs *T. mentagrophytes* infection may cause extensive hair loss simulating endocrine disturbance or pyoderma respectively.

DIAGNOSIS OF DERMATOPHYTE INFECTIONS

The firm diagnosis of a dermatophyte infection is based on the positive demonstration of arthrosporic fungal elements with hyphal invasion of hair, stratum corneum or nail/claw

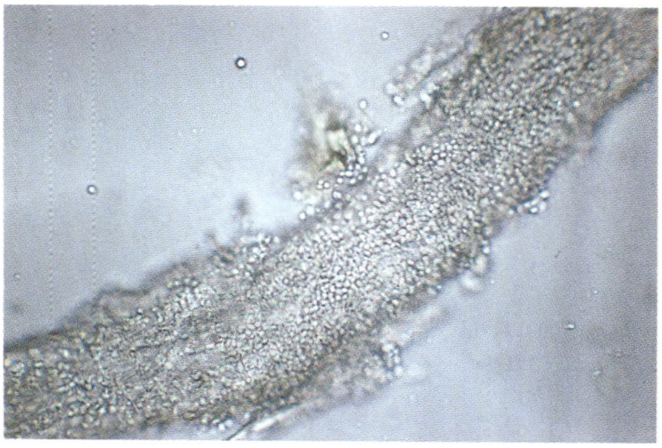

Fig. 5.38. *M. canis* arthrospore sheath around hair.

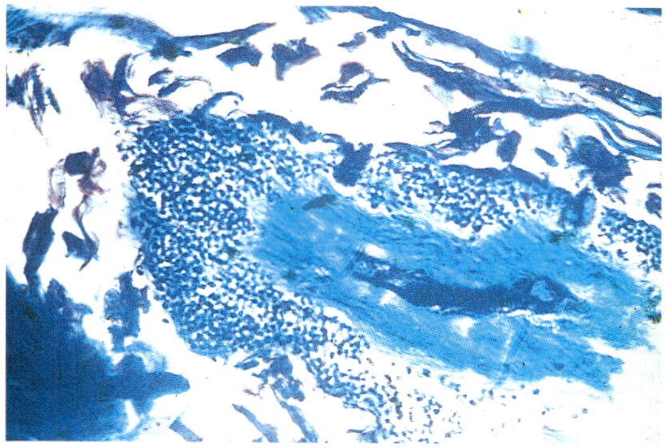

Fig. 5.39. Histological preparation showing *M. canis* spore sheath.

keratin.

This can be achieved by taking dry scrapings from the area of active fungal growth, usually the periphery of the lesion, by epilating infected hair or collecting nail or claw parings or clippings and submitting this material for microscopic examination. Wet preparations of such material, warmed in 20% potassium hydroxide (KOH) solution, lactophenol or other suitable solution on a microscope slide under a coverslip, give very satisfactory results (Fig. 5.38). Fungal material may also be stained by using a mixture of KOH solution and permanent black super Quink.

Similarly, the use of the Wood's lamp aids the collection of hair infected with *M. canis* by showing the positive material to have an apple-green fluorescence.

More definitive diagnosis may be achieved by culture of scrapings, clippings or MacKenzie's brush technique.

Histological techniques may be required where folliculitis and granuloma formation is present and where other diagnostic procedures have proved negative (Fig. 5.39).

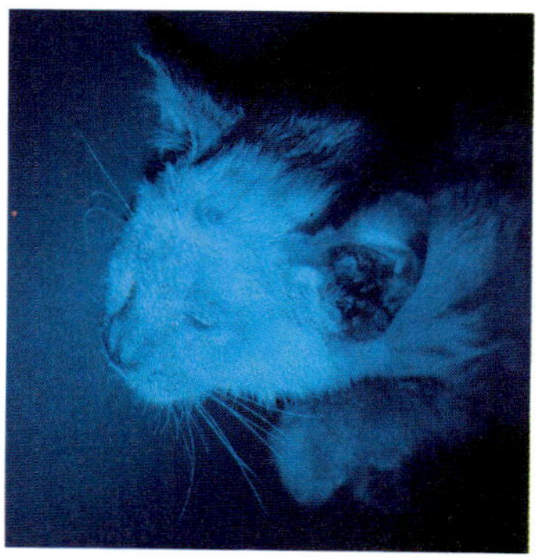

Fig. 5.40. Cat with *M. canis* infection revealed by Wood's lamp fluorescence.

Wood's lamp

The demonstration of fluorescence of hairs infected with species of the genus *Microsporum*, in particular *M. canis*, is an important aid to diagnosis. Where this infection is present a high proportion of animals will show positive diagnostic fluorescence (Fig. 5.40).

In a summary of 127 cases, Pepin and Oxenham (1987) showed that 89.8% of proven positive infections in cats fluoresced, confirming the earlier findings of Marples (1956) of 98.2% of 171 cases, and of Kushida (1978) of 83% of 87 cases.

The belief that Wood's-lamp screening for *M. canis* was unreliable and that a significant number of strains of that fungus do not show fluorescence in filtered ultraviolet light appears to be unfounded.

Carrier animals

The screening of cats, particularly long-haired breeds, as well as dogs for active infection, contamination or the identification of carrier animals often presents difficulty. Recent investigation by Pepin and Oxenham (1987) has shown that the use of a modification of the brush technique devised by MacKenzie (1961) is an effective way of detecting carrier cats.

Animals for investigation are brushed all over with a sterile, 9 cm diameter, plastic scalp-massage brush.

The teeth of the brush are then pressed into the surface of fungal culture medium in a Petri dish and incubated at 27 °C.

Culture

The diagnosis of fungal infection may also be confirmed by culturing hair, claw and nail clippings or scrapings from suspected or active lesions. Material is placed on Sabouraud's mycobiotic medium for incubation at 27 °C for the identification of the colonial characteristics and macroaeleuriospores (macroconidia), which may be seen after approximately 7–21 days.

Identification of the macroconidia is by lactophenol cotton blue stained, wet preparations examined under a light microscope.

TREATMENT AND CONTROL

Many treatment regimes have been devised for the management of both canine and feline ringworm and many substances are claimed to be therapeutically effective (Thomsett, 1962).

A combination of systemic antibiotic and topical imidazole therapy coupled with regular screening appears to give the most satisfactory approach. Close clipping of the area surrounding small lesions is desirable; if lesions are extensive the whole coat should be clipped off.

Griseofulvin administered in tablet form at 25–50 mg/kg daily with a fatty meal (vegetable oil) for 4–6 weeks is effective.

In *T. mentagrophytes* infection and refractory *M. canis*

infections, higher doses of griseofulvin may be required, e.g. 60–125 mg/kg daily, but these may give rise to toxicity (Muller *et al.*, 1983). It should also be borne in mind that griseofulvin is teratogenic and should not be used during pregnancy.

Supplementation of the antibiotic therapy using 0.2% enilconazole wash or local application of miconazole nitrate 1% lotion, or 2% miconazole nitrate cream or Surolan (miconazole nitrate, polymixin B, prednisolone acetate) is also recommended.

CONTROL OF *M. CANIS* INFECTION IN STUD AND SHOW CATS

All animals coming onto clean premises should be screened with the Wood's lamp and brush cultured. All positives should be isolated, clipped out, treated with griseofulvin and bathed with an antifungal, e.g. Captan. Animals are considered free of infection when two brush cultures are negative at 8-week intervals. Bedding should be destroyed and grooming utensils put into sealed plastic bags for safe disposal. Steel combs may be sterilized by placing in 5% formalin or boiling water for 5 minutes.

TREATMENT OF REFRACTORY CASES OF RINGWORM

In cases of ringworm responding poorly to griseofulvin therapy, ketoconazole has been shown to be an effective alternative, given at 5–30 mg/kg in divided doses daily.

This preparation does not have a product licence for dogs and cats and there should be discussion with the owner prior to use to establish their agreement in view of possible toxicity.

The use of antifungal agents in small-animal dermatology has been reviewed by Foil (1986) to which reference should be made.

Candidiasis (yeast infection)

Skin lesions due to infection with *Candida* species are rare. Experimental infection of canine skin with candidal organisms and the production of 'hot-spot' lesions was recorded by Schwartzmann *et al.* (1965). Naturally occurring skin disease of candidal origin does not appear to have been confirmed although mucocutaneous candidiasis should be suspected in cases of cheilitis.

CONFIRMATION OF DIAGNOSIS

This is based on cultural identification of the organism and differentiation from other infective and non-infective causes.

TREATMENT

This should be directed to eliminating the predisposing cause for the yeast infection:

1 Avoidance of excess wetting of the area.

2 Imidazoles topically and systematically, in particular ketoconazole orally.

Pityrosporum canis (malassezia pachydermatis)

This is a yeast, commonly found in the ears of small animals and possibly associated with situations of excess wax and moisture.

It is believed to play a role in the pathogenesis of otitis externa but it may be present as a commensal. Dufait (1983) considered *P. canis* to be the agent responsible for chronic dermatitis of the abdomen, feet, tail and skin folds in dogs and reported that the disease was responsive to topical imidazole therapy. Its presence may be revealed in smears made from swabs of the site stained with 1% methylene blue. It may be eliminated by therapy with a topical fungicide (Auroto ear drops contain thiabendazole which has fungicidal as well as miticidal properties). Thereafter, the site should be kept dry and free from debris.

Mycetoma

This is infection of deep structures with fungal organisms causing abscessation and erosions of the skin surface with discharge of purulent material containing granules of varying colour dependent on the species of fungus involved.

Mycetomata are very rare in temperate climates and uncommon even in tropical and subtropical regions. Van den Broek and Thoday (1987) described a case of eumycetoma in the cat due to a member of the genus *Torula* and reviewed the reports of the condition in animals.

DIAGNOSIS

This is based on fungal culture, bearing in mind that the organism may be classified as a 'contaminant' and require culture on media free of contaminant 'inhibitors', e.g. cyclohexamide.

HISTOLOGY

Histological preparations of biopsy material are stained by haematoxylin and eosin (H & E), periodic acid–Schiff stain (PAS) and silver techniques to demonstrate fungal elements in the granulomatous tissue.

Subcutaneous mycotic infection

This may arise as the direct result of traumatic implantation of infective fungal organisms from the environment.

Depending on the species of organism, a lesion of mycetoma, phaeohyphomycosis or sporotrichosis may arise.

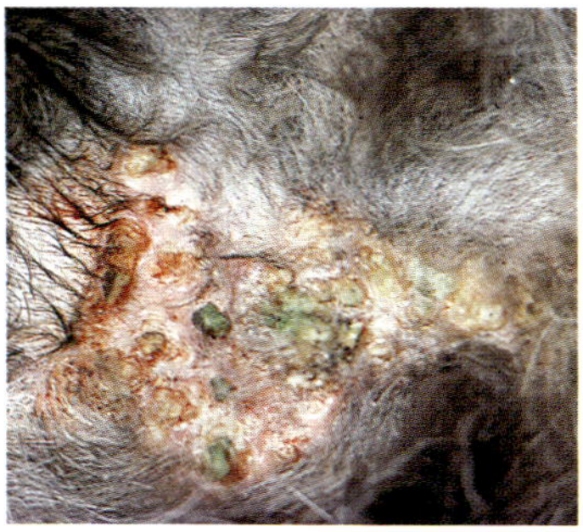

Fig. 5.41. Cat with mycetoma and sinus tracts. (The green stain is a topical dressing applied by the owner to the lesion.)

Mycetoma. Characterized by the formation of nodules and fistulae discharging granules (Fig. 5.41).

Phaeohyphomycosis. Subcutaneous or systemic infection with certain pigmented septate hyphae causing nodules and fistulae exuding purulent material.

Sporotrichosis. Localized or generalized infection with nodules and fistulation with exudation of brown pus due to *Sporothrix schenckii*.

Systemic mycosis. Deep infection with organisms classified as yeasts, moulds or actinomycetales, e.g. blastomycosis, aspergillosis, cryptococcosis, histoplasmosis, nocardiosis, coccidioidomycosis.

Deep mycoses

Deep mycotic infections of the skin of the cat or dog are rare in Europe. Those recorded are more likely to be found in warmer climatic areas of the world or are opportunistic in their occurrence. In humans, immunosuppressed or immunocompromised patients are more susceptible to deep mycotic infections. The role of long-term corticosteroid therapy or immunosuppressive viral infection as predisposing factors for the disease in animals is worthy of consideration.

CLINICAL SIGNS

Since the disease is characterized by its chronicity, the persistent intradermal or subcutaneous nodules and fistulous tracts make differential diagnosis difficult. The diagnosis of systemic mycosis can rarely be made on clinical grounds alone and the most reliable diagnostic aid is histology of biopsy specimens.

HISTOPATHOLOGY

This shows diffuse or nodular suppurative pyogranulomatous or granulomatous histiocytic inflammation. There may be pigmented or non-pigmented fungal elements present as 'grains' in the tissue, and fungal elements may be free in the tissue or within macrophages.

DIFFERENTIAL DIAGNOSIS

Deep pyodermas or follicular granulomata due to deep dermatophyte infection of the hair follicle.

THERAPY

Many deep mycoses require surgery. In the review of medical therapy for both superficial and deep mycotic infections made by Foil (1986) the value of the following drugs was discussed: sodium and potassium iodide, amphotericin B, 5-flucytosine and the imidazoles.

Dosage regimes are as indicated below.

Sporotrichosis. Sodium or potassium iodide (20% solution). Dogs 1 ml/5 kg daily for 6 weeks. Cats 0.5 ml/kg daily for 6 weeks.

Blastomycosis. Amphotericin B. 0.5 mg/kg three times a week to a total dose of 6 mg/kg.

Ketoconazole. 10 to 20 mg/kg in divided dose daily for 3–6 months respectively.

Cryptococcosis. Amphotericin B. 0.5 mg/kg three times a week to a total of 4 mg/kg.

5-Flucytosine. 100–200 mg/kg per day divided into three doses.

Nocardiosis/actinomycosis may be treated with penicillin 100 000 i.u./kg daily for 4 weeks or alternative antibiotics are tetracycline, chloramphenicol or erythromycin (Keep, 1981, 1982).

5.4 Parasites

The skin is an organ system that is exposed to a teeming multitude of potential parasites. It is therefore not surprising that during evolution numerous widely different species have adapted themselves to a parasitic mode of life both on the skin and within it.

The ideal parasite attempts to provoke a minimal reaction so that its host is not stimulated to respond in a way that results in the rejection of the parasite (Fig. 5.42). However, the body of a parasite or its products may be an irritant and provoke a foreign-body or allergic reaction. In both of these cases the resulting pruritus will cause scratching and thus aid the transfer of obligate parasites like *Sarcoptes scabiei* to new hosts. It is difficult to assess the value of the hypersensitive response to flea bites to the survival of the flea itself. This response only occurs in a small percentage of parasitized hosts so it is perhaps an aberrant reaction which neither aids nor hinders the survival of the fleas themselves.

A clinical understanding of ectoparasitic dermatology rests upon an understanding of the nature of the hosts' responses to the parasite, and of the life cycle of the parasite (Fig. 5.43).

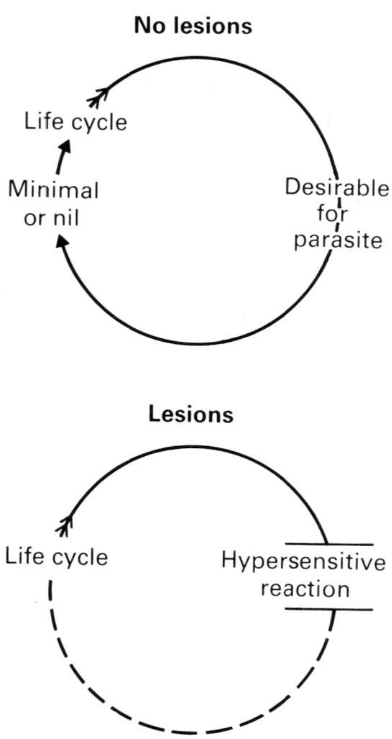

Fig. 5.42. Ectoparasite–host relationship. The ideal ectoparasite produces a minimal response in its host, e.g. the cat fur mite *Lynxacarus radovsky*.

Leishmaniasis

This is a geographically widespread chronic granulomatous disease caused by flagellate intracellular protozoan parasites belonging to the genus *Leishmania*. It is most usually reported in dogs and rarely in cats. The vector is the sandfly *Phlebotomus*, although spread by direct contact with infected material may occur. In northern Europe occasional cases are seen in imported dogs from endemic areas (the Mediterranean, Middle East, central America and parts of central Africa). Clinical signs may not develop for many months after importation (Longstaffe *et al.*, 1983).

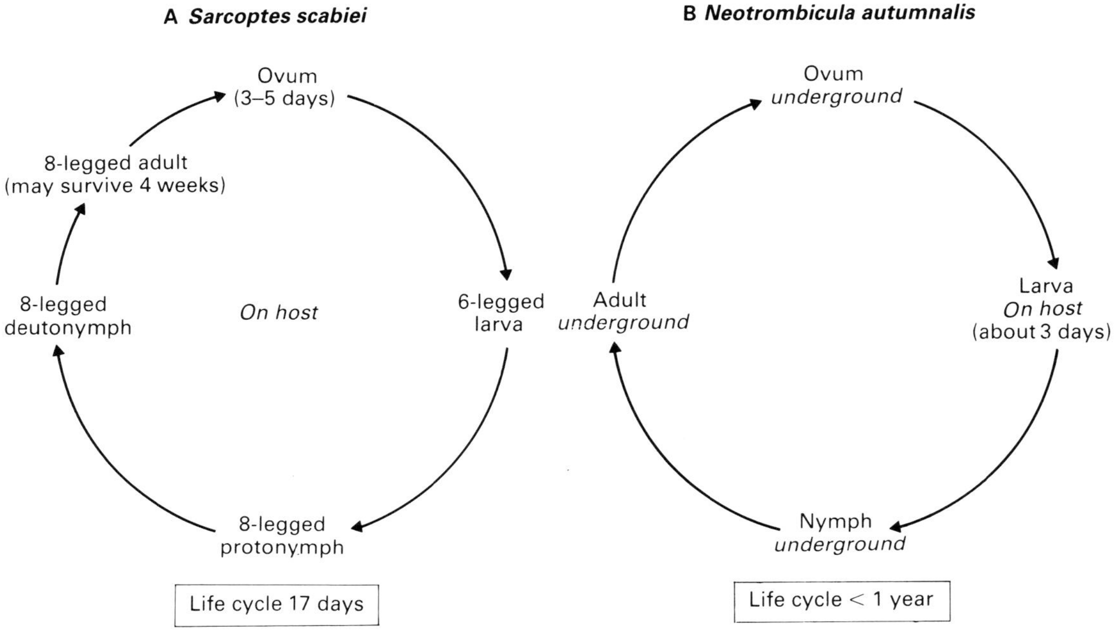

Fig. 5.43. A Sarcoptic mange is a relatively easy disease to treat and control as the life cycle of the parasite is spent entirely on the host.
B Harvest mite infestation is difficult to control as only the larva is parasitic and then only for a short time.

CLINICAL SIGNS

There is lymphadenopathy, hepatomegaly and splenomegaly with wasting. The skin lesions may be pruritic with exfoliative dermatitis and alopecia, particularly periorbital (spectacles or lunettes) and seborrhoea. Keratoconjunctivitis is seen. The coat is thin and lack-lustre with areas of alopecia.

DIAGNOSIS

Diagnosis is by the demonstration of intracytoplasmic bodies in smears from the lymph nodes or abscesses stained by the colophonium Giemsa staining method (Levine, 1985), or using Romanowsky stains. Von Schwalder (1977) states that there is a characteristic hyperproteinaemia electrophoresis and pathognomonic paper electrophoresis pattern.

THERAPY

Therapy is often unsatisfactory and relapses are common — the wide range of drugs prescribed indicates this. Metronidazole, amphotericin and the schistosomicides (sodium antimony-gluconate) have been used for humans. There is a real risk to those in contact with the animal of possible direct transmission and, since therapy is unsatisfactory, euthanasia should be advised.

Hookworm dermatitis

This is an erythematous pruritic dermatitis with a particular distribution involving the ventral pedal area, interdigital region and thinner skin on the ventral aspects of the body. It is caused by percutaneous entry of the infective third-stage (L3) larvae of *Uncinaria stenocephala* and *Ancylostoma caninum*. Infective larvae penetrate the skin with proteolytic enzymes.

In the UK both species parasitize dogs; *U. stenocephala* is far more common, *A. caninum* being reported in imported dogs only (Sloan, 1961). In Ireland only *U. stenocephala* is found whilst in North America *A. caninum* is the common species. Hookworm is mostly found in large sporting kennels.

Uncinaria stenocephala is well adapted for survival in temperate and subarctic regions and infective L3 larvae can survive on pasture throughout the year in England. Perinatal transmission is not important. Young animals become quickly infected after weaning; Jacobs (1982) found that faecal egg counts tended to reach a peak between 25 and 35 weeks of age.

CLINICAL SIGNS

Hookworms most usually enter the body by the oral route, but percutaneous penetration by the infective L3 stage can occur. This route is unusual because a marked inflammatory response occurs at the site of entry which is parasitologically undersirable. Signs of hookworm dermatitis are first recognized as red papular eruptions which are seen especially clearly upon the normally pale and thin skin of greyhounds and similar breeds. Later the affected area becomes uniformly erythematous and the focal lesions are more difficult to see. Finally, the skin becomes chronically thickened and discoloured with loss of hair although a complete alopecia is seldom seen.

The primary lesions are distributed in a quite characteristic manner (Fig. 5.44), occurring almost invariably on those parts of the body that touch the ground when the animal is standing, sitting or lying down. Dermatitis is recognized most commonly in the xiphoid and posterior sternal region but it also involves

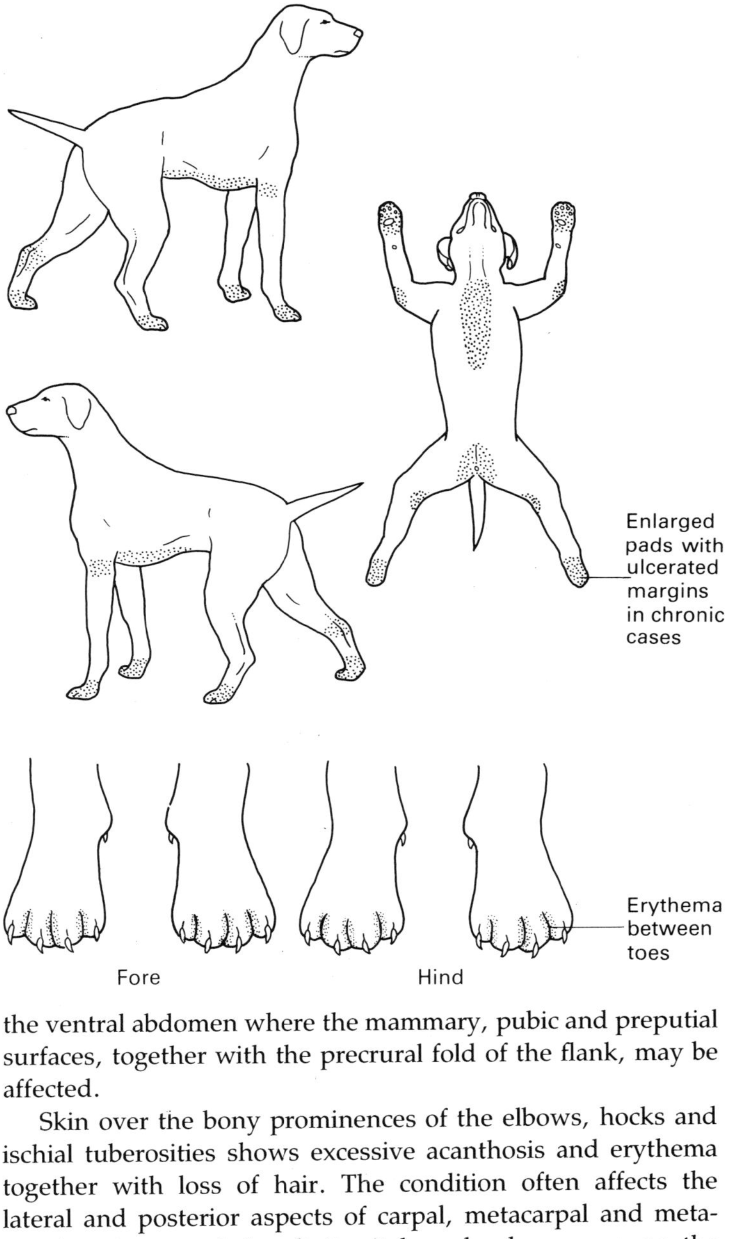

Fig. 5.44. Distribution of lesions in hookworm dermatitis.

the ventral abdomen where the mammary, pubic and preputial surfaces, together with the precrural fold of the flank, may be affected.

Skin over the bony prominences of the elbows, hocks and ischial tuberosities shows excessive acanthosis and erythema together with loss of hair. The condition often affects the lateral and posterior aspects of carpal, metacarpal and metatarsal regions, and the digits; it has also been seen on the outer aspect of the pinnae and on the ventral surface of the tail (Baker *et al.*, 1970; Baker, 1981).

A prominent and clinically recognizable feature of the feet of affected dogs is a change in the texture of the pads (Fig.

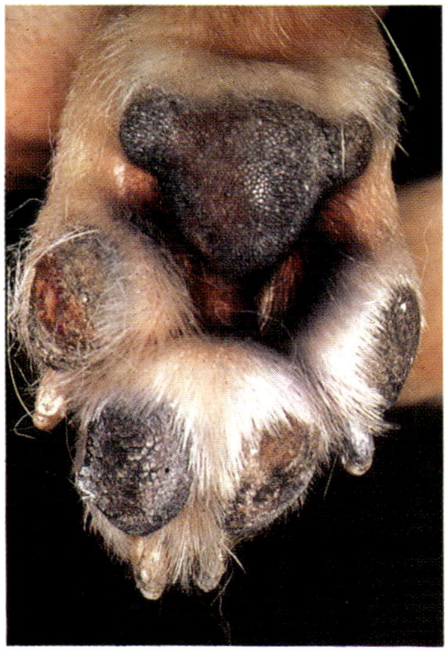

Fig. 5.45. Pedal lesions associated with migratory *Ancylostoma caninum*.

5.45). The skin of the foot pads is usually heavily pigmented and rough due to the presence of numerous heavily keratinized papillae which become smoother when the animal is exercised on concrete or other hard surfaces. In affected dogs this keratinized stratum becomes soft and spongy, especially around the pad margins, and it can be readily grooved and sometimes stripped from the underlying dermis by modest pressure with the examiner's fingernail. Partial and even complete spontaneous separation of the pad surface has been seen, exposing a pink and granular dermal surface.

The keratinized papillary nature of the pad becomes very obvious and the unworn surface may assume a frayed and crusty appearance. The interdigital web becomes rough, reddened and very thick, especially along its free border, a change which extends to the claw fold covering the ungual process of the third phalanx, which swells into a fleshy ring encircling the nail base. The feet may be grossly enlarged.

The nails themselves may be deformed. They become wider and thicker than normal at the base and more heavily ridged. The regular curved contour and surface gloss is lost and the nail may twist in its long axis or become friable and shear off below the ungual skeleton of the third phalanx to leave a thick and often sharply tapered stump. Paronychia may result in complete detachment and loss of the nail.

A coincidental severe arthritis of the distal interphalangeal joints has been encountered during examination of the feet of those hounds showing other signs of pedal involvement in a hookworm dermatitis. There is thickening of periarticular tissues and pain is obvious when the joint is squeezed or its manipulation is attempted. Almost invariably the affected digit shows some nail deformity.

Only rarely is an animal presented for examination because it is scratching or because a dermatitis is suspected, although in the advanced case the loss of hair is sufficient to stimulate the concern of the owner. Pruritus never appears to be very marked. The dog may nibble or lick transiently at the pedal and limb lesions or even scratch at chest or flank but the primary site rarely bears evidence of self-inflicted damage, and secondary infection is infrequent.

DIAGNOSIS

The history, type of management, isolation of hookworm eggs in the faeces and the typical signs and histopathology render the diagnosis straightforward. Pelodera dermatitis and contact dermatitis require to be differentiated. Sarcoptic mange is more pruritic and careful searching will reveal the mites and eggs in skin scrapes.

THERAPY

Hookworm may be eradicated by broad-spectrum anthelmintic therapy (thiabendazole, levamisole) and rigid control measures. The lesions will then quickly resolve. Where there is extensive associated pyoderma, determine the antibiotic sensitivity and prescribe the appropriate therapy.

CONTROL

Hookworm dermatitis is predominantly a problem in large kennels using grass exercising paddocks where infective L3 larvae may be present in large numbers. It is not possible to destroy larvae on grass runs but grass should be kept short. It is important to prevent the passage of ova by judicious use of broad-spectrum anthelmintics with frequent monitoring of faeces for evidence of infestation. Shedding of ova is irregular therefore counts should be made on a regular basis.

Faeces should be removed daily to diminish contamination. Resting the runs may not be an effective method of control because infective larvae are able to survive on grass pastures for prolonged periods. Replacement by concrete should be considered. Borax applied at a rate of $1\,kg/m^2$ of run may be used but this is expensive and destroys all vegetation.

The prevention of intradermal migration by effective control measures will permit resolution of lesions; cases complicated by secondary bacterial infection will require antibiotic therapy indicated by sensitivity tests.

Pelodera dermatitis

This is a rare but possibly under-reported disease caused by the entry of non-parasitic larval nematodes (*Pelodera strongyloides*) into the skin of dogs in contact with bedding material that is heavily contaminated by organic matter. The early literature is reviewed by Chitwood (1932). *Pelodera strongyloides* larvae are free-living nematodes occurring in damp soil rich in organic matter.

CLINICAL SIGNS

Lesions are found on the lateral aspect of the body and the ventral abdomen — those parts of the body which normally come into contact with bedding. Entry into the skin is more likely when the skin has already been excoriated as a result of ectoparasitism. The coat is dirty with the hair thinner or absent in the predilection sites, with erythema and papule formation. Subsequently, there may be pustules and crusts, severe pruritus and further self-excoriation.

DIAGNOSIS

Skin scrapings from the affected areas should be examined for larvae, which are motile, approximately 600 μm in length and 35 μm in diameter. Histopathologically, larvae are seen in the follicles with furunculosis. Many eosinophils are present.

TREATMENT

As the disease is associated with filthy bedding, owners must be aware that it is essential to remove contaminated bedding and to improve the living standards in which pets are kept. The environment must be thoroughly cleaned and sprayed with an insecticide and measures taken to avoid further contact with contaminated bedding; an alternative is paper or cotton sheeting. The patient should be gently washed with a mild soap then washed with an ectoparasiticide, e.g. Quellada (Stafford Miller), repeated 1 week later. If there is furunculosis, antibiotic sensitivity should be determined and the appropriate treatment prescribed.

Dracunculosis

Two species of this genus are important parasites: *Dracunculus insignis* attacks dogs in North America, whilst *D. medinensis* parasitizes dogs and cats in Africa and Asia. There are no reports of infection in Europe. The intermediate host is the small aquatic crustacean *Cyclops*, which is infected by the parasite larvae. The final hosts become infected by drinking water contaminated with the crustaceans. The larvae then develop over a long period in subcutaneous tissue of the host's limbs and abdomen, becoming large adult worms.

These form nodules which ulcerate and fail to heal. Before ulceration there may be local erythema and pruritus. The release of larvae from a female worm can be stimulated, lying beneath an open nodule, by application of a little cold water which can be collected for examination on a glass slide. The nodules may be surgically excised.

Neotrombicula autumnalis — the harvest mite

The harvest mite is commonly known as the harvest bug, berry bug or orange tawney. It is seldom seen but is extremely common: gardeners, soft fruit pickers and hikers will be aware of the extreme pruritus that it can cause. Birds and mammals are commonly parasitized, for the parasitic stage (larva) is not host specific. The season of activity in the UK extends from May to October, the mite being particularly active in warm, sunny weather.

Eggs are laid in the soil by the non-parasitic adult female mite (Fig. 5.46) and the larvae emerge to seek a host. The larva is an active six-legged mite about 250 μm in length. It is orange in colour and is capable of rapid purposeful movement. Mites are mostly to be found in open pastureland, whilst areas around soft fruit bushes and plants may be heavily infested. It is reported to be more common on limestone soils.

After emergence (Fig. 5.47) larvae climb to the tips of grass or low herbage and await a host, to which they attach themselves by extended hooked legs. Mites may congregate together to form small, visible, orange masses or on close inspection single mites may be seen. Mites tend to congregate on the edges of the pinnae in the ears and between the digits of cats, whilst in dogs they tend to congregate in skin folds and flexures of the limbs and between the digits. Once attached to the host, a feeding tube is quickly produced and the larva feeds on lymph and digested epidermal cells.

After several days, feeding is completed; the larva is now pale yellow in colour and about 550 μm in length (Fig. 5.48). When replete it leaves its host and returns to the soil where the non-parasitic nymphal and adult stages live. The life cycle is up to 1 year in length with successive broods being produced throughout the larval season (Jones, 1950, 1951, 1956). The larval stage is the only parasitic stage. This fact and non-dependence upon one host species is responsible for the large numbers of larvae which appear each year and for the difficulty in controlling the parasite.

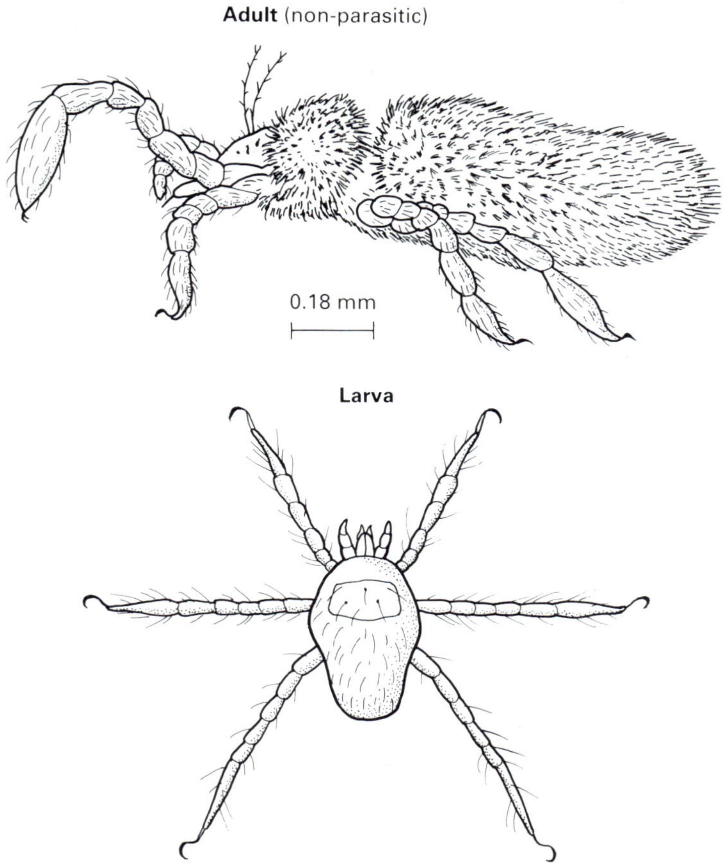

Fig. 5.46. Adult free-living *Neotrombicula autumnalis* in soil, and unfed larva at same scale.

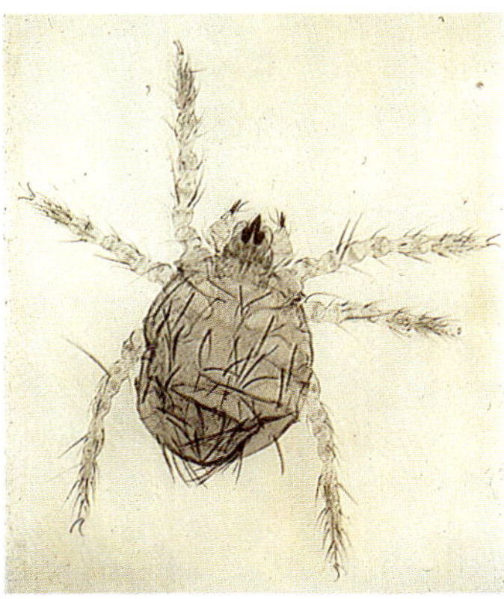

Fig. 5.47. Unfed larva *Neotrombicula autumnalis*.

CLINICAL SIGNS

The larva does not produce irritation when first attached. Subsequently there is pruritus, indicated by licking of the feet and limbs, flicking of the ears and shaking of the head. Small papules may develop which are quickly excoriated. Re-infestation may continue throughout the warmer months so that there may be continuous irritation.

DIAGNOSIS

Close inspection of the affected areas will reveal the mites. There will be orange blotches where present in large numbers (Fig. 5.49). Identification will be confirmed by microscopic

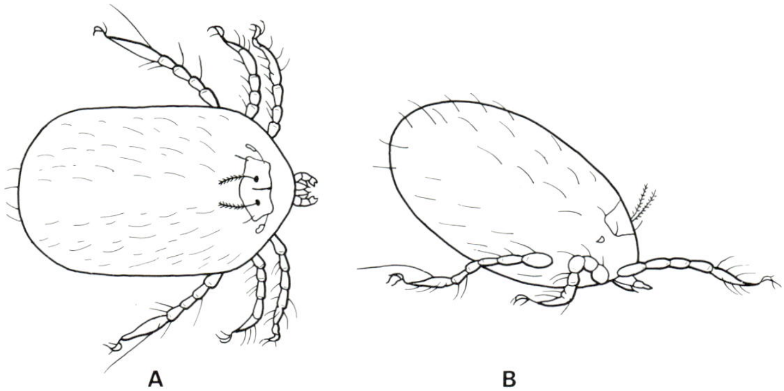

Fig. 5.48. Fully engorged larva of *Neotrombicula autumnalis*.
A Dorsal view. **B** Stance of settled larva. (From Jones, 1951)

examination of a skin scrape in 6% potassium hydroxide solution.

TREATMENT AND CONTROL

If reinfestation can be prevented the irritation is transient and is controllable with topical benzyl benzoate or caladryl lotion. Benzyl peroxide should not be used on cats. Ear drops containing thiabendazole may be used for treating cats by gently spreading the fluid on to the affected areas with a cotton bud.

Preparations applied to the skin as repellents are quickly licked off and are of little value.

Harvest mite infestation may be a very real problem in areas where numbers are high. Places to be avoided are pastureland in warm weather and the vicinity of soft fruit gardens and bramble patches: this may be possible with dogs but not cats. Exercising the latter at night may not necessarily be helpful, for the larvae are active during warm, still nights.

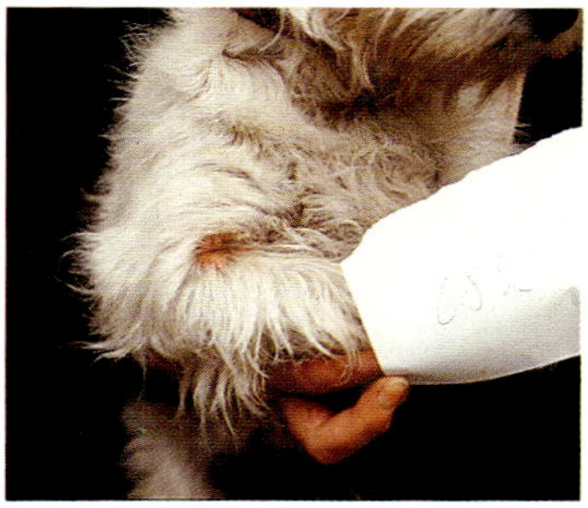

Fig. 5.49. Groups of harvest mite larvae shown as orange blotches particularly in skin folds; here the associated skin is discoloured brown by persistent licking.

Forage mites

A large number of mite species live in stored food products. Although not parasitic themselves, they are nevertheless important causes of prurigo in animals and humans. The increasing use of dry food for cat and dog feeding permits the exposure of pets to mites when such food has been stored in conditions which permit the development of mites.

CLINICAL SIGNS

Clinical signs are variable but usually long-standing; generalized pruritus, perioral pruritus, pododermatitis, seborrhoea and diarrhoea may be seen. Diagnosis may be difficult for the mites are transient passengers only; combings may reveal unusual mites, usually characterized by not being dorsoventrally flattened and having well developed legs and numerous long setae.

DIAGNOSIS

The report of Vollset *et al.* (1986) indicates that storage-mite allergy is common. Eighteen of 24 dogs with signs believed to be associated with allergy had positive skin reaction to intradermal challenge with *Acarus siro*, the most common storage mite, whilst only four of 29 dogs with no allergic signs developed skin reactions. The passive cutaneous test showed that an immediate type hypersensitivity was involved. Seven of 24 atopic dogs with positive skin reactions to house-dust mites had positive skin reactions when challenged with *A. siro* extract.

CONTROL

Forage mites will not survive on pets so that ectoparasitic dressing is unnecessary; however, it is essential that the environment be thoroughly vacuum-cleaned and dried food stored in cool, dry conditions. In confirmed cases existing food stocks should be destroyed.

House-dust mites

These mites, like storage mites, are not parasitic but are of considerable importance in atopy.

Two species are of greatest importance in the aetiology of atopic dermatitis: *Dermatophagoides pteronyssinus* and *D. farinae*, the former being of more significance in European countries. They are discussed in the section dealing with atopic dermatitis.

Sarcoptic mange

This is a non-seasonal, transmissible very pruritic skin disease of dogs resulting from infestation with the mite *Sarcoptes scabiei* var. *canis*. It is extremely rare in cats.

AETIOLOGY AND PATHOGENESIS

The mites are comparatively large and can just be seen with the naked eye (410 μm). The entire life cycle is spent on the host; the mite feeding on lymph collected through the epidermis (Fig. 5.43a).

The adult female lays 3–5 eggs daily in a burrow in the epidermis. Hatching occurs in 3–5 days with the emergence of a six-legged larva; these may remain in the burrow or emerge on the surface; many die but a few excavate feeding burrows. This stage is followed by two nymphal stages, both of which have eight legs, and the final moult into the adult. The period from egg laying to adult emergence is approximately 17 days, with adults surviving 4 weeks if conditions are optimum. All stages are susceptible to drying and will survive only a few days off the host. Transmission is by direct contact.

In animals not previously exposed to infestation, the presence of the mites does not provide a marked pruritic response. However, hypersensitivity develops accompanied by intense pruritus. In sarcoptic mange in pigs, infected adults may become non-reactive although harbouring mites. It is possible that this occurs in adult bitches who, although showing no clinical signs, transfer mites to their litters.

CLINICAL SIGNS

There is probably an incubation of several weeks before obvious signs of disease develop. These are most commonly seen in immature animals but older animals may occasionally develop a severe generalized reaction; this may also occur in animals on prolonged corticosteroid therapy.

There is intense pruritus with erythema, rapid self-excoriation and hair loss (Fig. 5.50): the contact surfaces of the body are most commonly affected. A marked scratch reflex is noticeable, particularly if the edge of the pinna is rolled between the fingers. Hyperkeratinization occurs with marked scaling; usually the edges of the pinnae are thickened, hairless and fissured (Fig. 5.51). In generalized cases all the body may be infected, with marked alopecia and hyperkeratinization (Fig. 5.52).

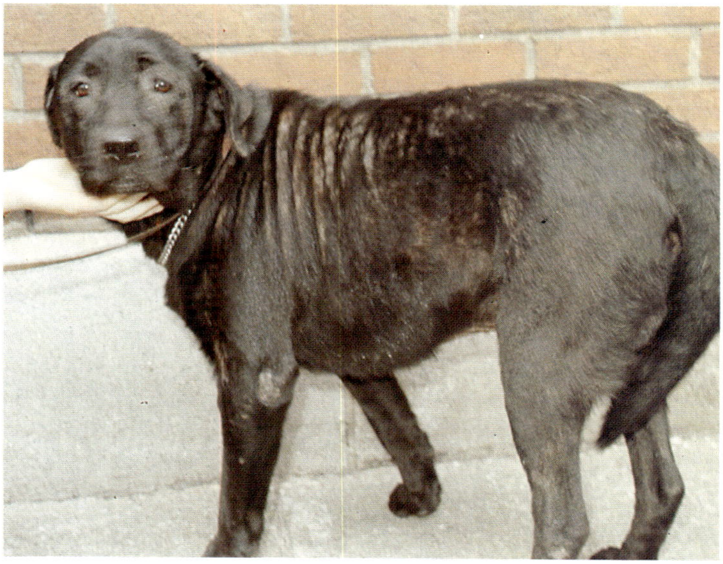

Fig. 5.50. 15-month-old Labrador with sarcoptic mange.

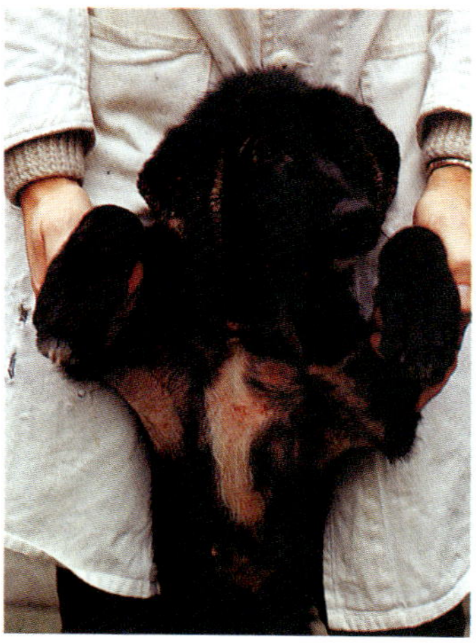

Fig. 5.51. 7-month-old mongrel, sarcoptic mange; the thickened encrusted margins of the pinna is a typical finding.

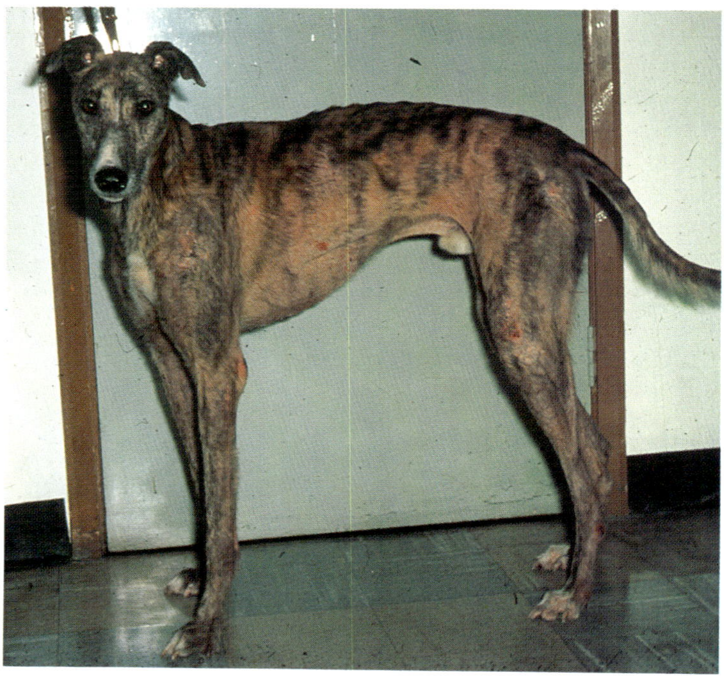

Fig. 5.52. Generalized sarcoptic mange in a greyhound.

The initial lesion is an irritant papule with erythema, but self-excoriation rapidly obliterates this. The skin becomes thickened, lichenified, scaly and excoriated. Spread to litter mates and other dogs in the vicinity is commonplace. The human contacts of the infested case will nearly always show a fine papular rash of the inner aspects of the forearms (Fig. 5.53) and/or of the chest and abdomen, with marked pruritus.

DIAGNOSIS

Sarcoptic mange is commonly misdiagnosed as an allergic disease; therefore, always examine carefully the clinical case history, the clinical signs and never neglect taking a skin scraping of all pruritic cases (Fig. 5.54). Several skin scrapings may need to be examined before the isolation of mites and/or the large oval eggs of *Sarcoptes* which have been laid in a row in a burrow in the epidermis (Fig. 5.55). Small foci of brown faecal pellets in skin scrapes are characteristic of *Sarcoptes scabiei* (Fig. 5.56).

THERAPY

Long-haired animals should be clipped short to allow penetration of the parasiticide used. If there is excessive scale a preliminary bath with a mild shampoo is advisable. Gammabenzene hexachloride, Sebacil, Alugan and Amitraz are effective but should be repeated at least once 5 days later. Bedding should be replaced and the animal's environment vacuumed, cleaned and sprayed with a parasiticide such as Nuvan.

Dogs in contact with the patient should be bathed at least twice in the ectoparasiticide.

Notoedric mange

Feline scabies is caused by the mite *Notoedres cati* which closely resembles *Sarcoptes scabiei*. It is very rarely seen now, but can infest dogs, whilst lesions can occur on humans in contact with infested animals.

The mite burrows into the skin, particularly of the head and neck. It is slightly smaller than *Sarcoptes scabiei* and although very similar it may be distinguished by a dorsal anus, *S. scabiei* having a terminal anus. The life cycle also is similar. In the UK the mite was very common in the 1940s and 1950s but has virtually disappeared since. Infested cats usually have

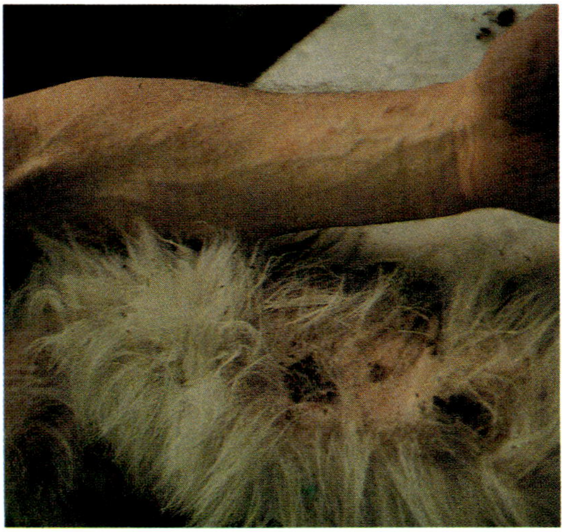

Fig. 5.53. Human sarcoptic lesions from infested dog.

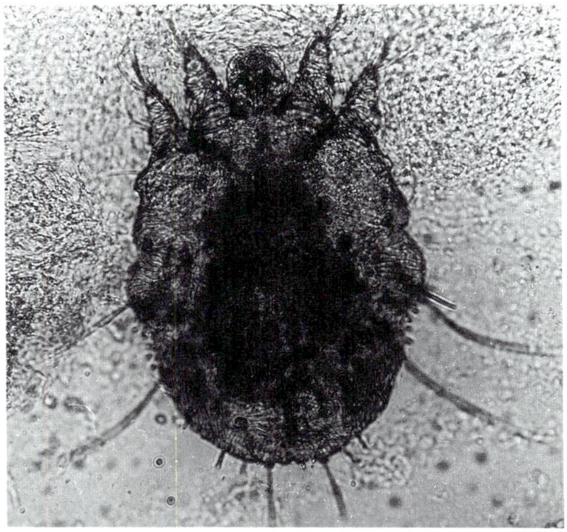

Fig. 5.54. *Sarcoptes scabiei* var. *canis*; typical appearance in skin scrape.

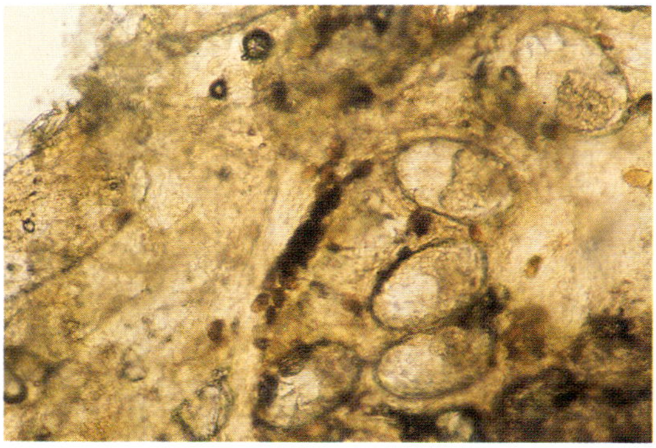

Fig. 5.55. Ova of *S. scabiei*, often seen in a row in skin scrapes.

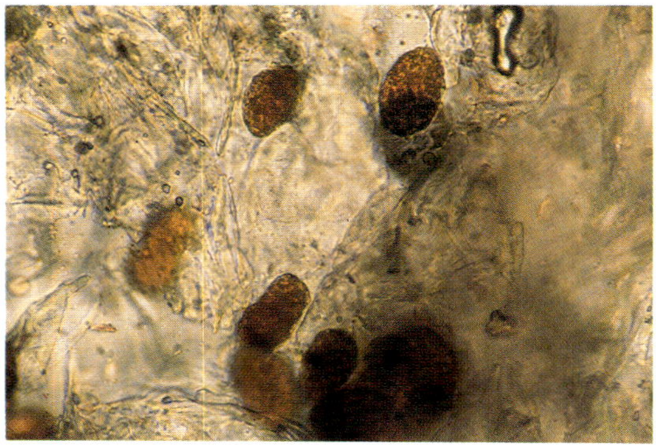

Fig. 5.56. Brown pellets are commonly seen in scrapes from the skin of cases of sarcoptic mange; these are mite faeces.

large numbers of mites present and they are easily found in skin scrapings.

CLINICAL SIGNS

The initial lesion is first seen on the edge of the pinna, but spread to the face and neck is rapid. Occasionally lesions are found on the feet and the perineum. Notoedric mange is characterized by intense pruritus; there is marked excoriation and thickening of the skin, whilst the ears, eyelids and face may be torn by frenzied scratching — a violent scratch reflex is easily initiated by gently rubbing the lesions. The skin becomes thickened, wrinkled and folded with much exudation and crust formation.

DIAGNOSIS

The intense pruritus, somewhat localized distribution, and isolation of the characteristic mite in scrapings determine the diagnosis. Affected animals resemble battle-scarred tom cats in appearance, therefore fight wounds should be eliminated in the differential diagnosis. Otodectic mange may also produce parotid and facial lesions but the otodectic mite is easily demonstrated and has a characteristic appearance.

Dermatophytosis is not as pruritic as notoedric mange, whilst pediculosis and cheyletiellosis affect other parts of the body as well. Pemphigus foliaceus may simulate this condition but may be eliminated by the history, failure to find mites and the histopathology.

The diagnosis rests upon the characteristic distribution, isolation of *Notoedres cati* and the response to therapy.

TREATMENT

The mites are sheltered by the encrusted inflammatory reaction they provoke: scale and crust must first be removed with mild soap and water. Gamma-benzene hexachloride as lotion or shampoo is effective and the diamide Amitraz is effective (0.025% reported by Wilkinson, 1983). Contact animals should also be treated with a parasiticide, the bedding should be changed and the immediate environment sprayed with an organophosphorus insecticide. Therapy should be repeated 5 days later.

Demodectic mange

Demodectic mange is relatively uncommon and may pose a diagnostic problem to the practitioner. Unlike sarcoptic mange, the clinical signs are very variable and may produce traps for the unwary: it is a great imitator of other skin diseases.

The genus *Demodex* is a ubiquitous one and has been recorded from 90 species. It is host specific and has been reported from all the major human races but the association with humans is probably an innocuous one. Hosts (e.g. humans) may harbour two species.

Several authors have reported that demodicosis is more common in short-haired dogs than in long-haired dogs. In Ireland the Doberman is statistically significantly over-represented in lists of clinical cases.

There are few references available for the prevalence of the disease in dogs: of all clinical cases presented the incidence was 0.99% in Scotland (Gregor, 1965) and 0.4% in the Republic of Ireland (Baker, 1969).

Demodex is an obligate parasite throughout its life cycle, which is spent in the hair follicle. Ova, 50 μm in length (about twice the size of keratinocytes, which they resemble) are produced; they quickly develop into six-legged larvae, followed by the eight-legged larval stage, the nymph, and finally the adult (Fig. 5.57). Spickett (1961) studied *Demodex* from human skin *in vitro* and stated that the life cycle is completed in 3 weeks. Transmission probably only occurs during suckling. It does not occur *in utero* (French, 1962; Sato *et al.*, 1965; Greve & Gaafar, 1966), or by close contact at other times; all stages of the life cycle are found in the hair follicle and sebaceous glands (Baker, 1969).

In generalized demodectic mange (GDM) all stages have been found in lymph nodes, bloodstream and alimentary system; however, this does not imply an extrafollicular life cycle, as forage mites have also been found in these tissues.

PATHOGENESIS

Demodectic mange is predominantly a disease of short-haired dogs that are less than 2 years old. It has a comparatively long incubation period. Initially in young animals, mites colonize the proximal third of the pilary canal and the root sheath is undamaged. With increasing numbers the pilary canal is distended, the root sheath is split and hair loss occurs. Distribution of lesions is shown in Fig. 5.58. From the time of initial infestation three possibilities of development may occur:

1 Resolution with extinction of the parasite.

2 Resolution with survival of the parasite; the carrier state. The follicular mite population is large. Unsworth (1946) reported an incidence of 10% of apparently normal dogs that he examined. Koutz *et al.* (1960) reported a percentage of 52.9 in the USA.

3 Clinically uncomplicated demodectic mange, with alopecia of the predilection sites sometimes with moderate furunculosis. This always occurs in dogs that are less than 2 years old; many cases are probably self-cured.

Approximately 16% of reported cases develop GDM. It occurs predominantly in young dogs but can occur in middle-aged and aged dogs. There is evidence that GDM is associated with depressed T-cell function, suppression rather than deficiency of T-cells, their function being restored when therapy

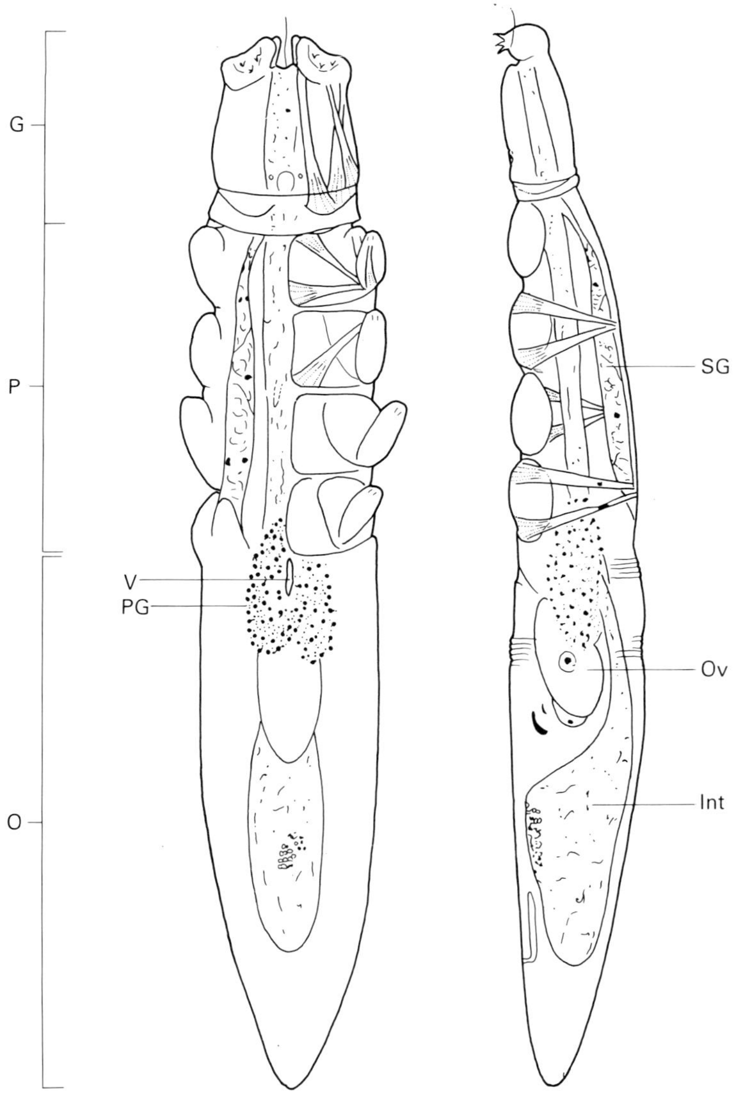

Fig. 5.57. *Demodex canis*: diagrammatic representation of adult female. G= gnathosoma, P= podosoma, V= vulva, PG= primary ganglion, O= opisthosoma, SG= salivary gland, Ov= ovary, Int= intestine.

results in the elimination of mites (Scott *et al.*, 1974; Scott, 1975; Scott *et al.*, 1976). If lymphocytes from normal dogs are cultured with serum from dogs with GDM having depressed *in vitro* lymphocyte blastogenesis (IVLB) responses, IVLB responses are suppressed in the normal cells — evidence of a humoral suppressive factor which is eliminated when mites are eradicated (Hirsch, 1975; Scott, 1975; Scott *et al.*, 1976).

Depressed T-cell function is not, however, seen in uncomplicated local demodicosis and early GDM. It is therefore secondary to GDM. Several authors have demonstrated immunodeficiency by the response of the skin of dogs with

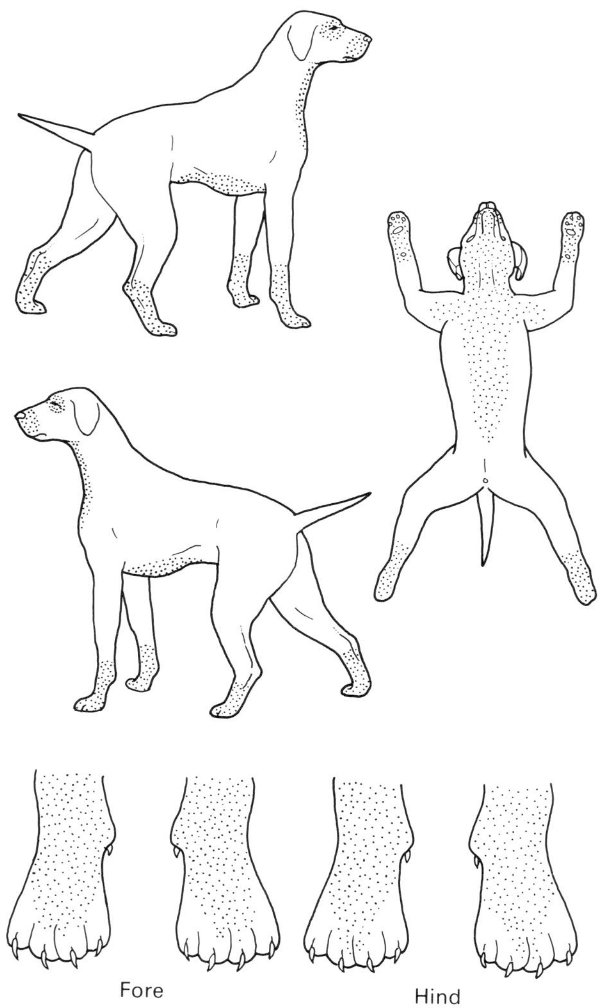

Fig. 5.58. Distribution of lesions in juvenile demodectic mange.

Table 5.2. Breed and prevalence of demodicosis of dogs in Ireland (n=100)

	No. of cases	Regional demodicosis	Generalized demodicosis
Doberman	26	6	20
Mongrel	25	21	4
Cavalier King Charles	6	4	2
Springer spaniel	5	4	1
Yorkshire terrier	4	2	2
Bull terrier	4	4	0
Labrador	4	2	2
Dachshund	4	4	0
Alsatian	4	4	0
Boxer	3	3	0
Jack Russell terrier	3	2	1
Pug	2	2	0
German pointer	2	1	1
Cocker spaniel	2	1	1
Greyhound	2	1	1
Bulldog	1	1	0
Corgi	1	1	0
West Highland terrier	1	0	1
Wire-haired terrier	1	1	0
Total	*100*	*64*	*36*

GDM to phytohaemagglutinin and concanavalin A (Scott *et al.*, 1974; Healy & Gaafar, 1977a, b), dinitrochlorobenzene (Corbett, 1975), and crude *Demodex canis* extract (Corbett, 1976). A possible genetic factor is indicated by the predisposition to GDM of pedigree dogs, particularly the Doberman pinscher (Table 5.2). Interestingly, Wilkie *et al.* (1979) identified Doberman puppies in a kennel with a high prevalence of demodectic mange by their response to intradermally injected phytohaemagglutinin.

CLINICAL SIGNS (Table 5.3)

These are extremely variable. Demodicosis may simulate many diseases. However, there are two distinct types. Firstly, a localized form, occurring in dogs usually 3–12 months of age; this involves alopecia and exfoliative dermatitis, which may be squamous and with a characteristic distribution — perioral, periorbital (Fig. 5.59), ventral cervical, anterior chest and on the lower limbs. In approximately 30% of such cases there is pruritus, and in approximately 14% pyoderma. Secondly, generalized demodectic mange, which is most commonly seen in dogs less than 2 years of age but may not become apparent until middle age. This is characterized by

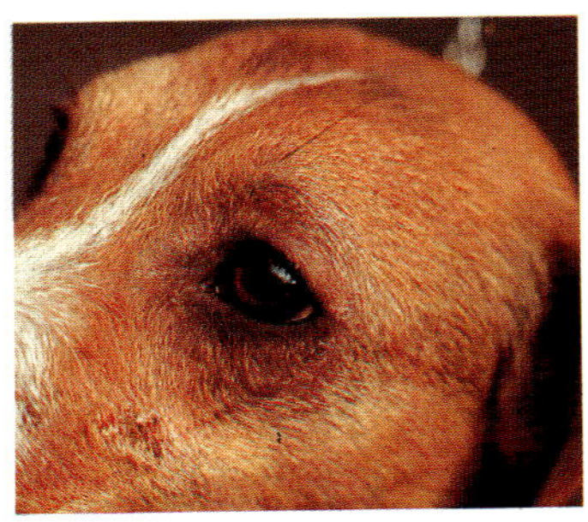

Fig. 5.59. Juvenile demodicosis in a 7-month-old mongrel. There is erythema and alopecia.

Table 5.3. Clinical signs of demodicosis

	Alopecia	Pruritus	Pustular	Hyperpigmentation
Localized (78 cases)				
No.	78	25	11	7
%	100	32.1	14.1	8.9
Generalized (22 cases)				
No.	22	16	22	11
%	100	72.8	100	50
Total	*100*	*41*	*33*	*18*

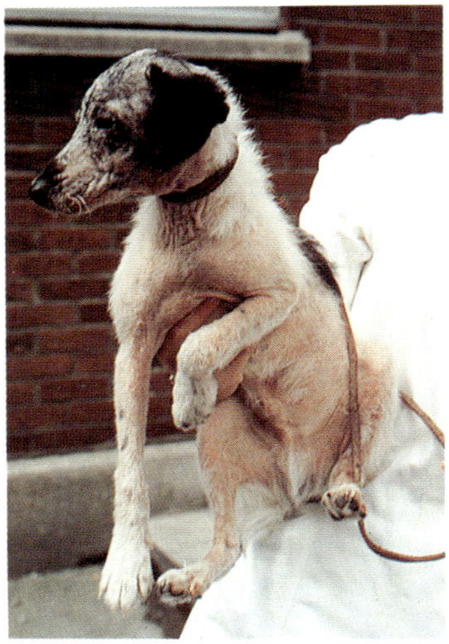

Fig. 5.60. Generalized demodicosis in a 6-month-old mongrel.

extensive alopecia, erythema, acanthosis and hyperkeratosis and seborrhoea, and is usually nodular, pruritic and pustular with oedema, particularly of the feet (Fig. 5.60). Occasionally there may be extensive squamous plaques without pyoderma. About 50% of generalized cases are markedly hyperpigmented (Fig. 5.61) (Baker, 1975) and about 75% are markedly pruritic. The skin in affected areas is fragile and bleeds easily, the dogs are depressed and there is lymphadenopathy; the skin has an offensive seborrhoeic odour.

In some cases in older dogs the affected areas may be quite localized, e.g. pododermatitis, ceruminous otitis externa, localized pyoderma.

HISTOPATHOLOGY

In juvenile demodicosis there is an infiltrate in the upper and middle dermis of histiocytes, fibroblasts, mast cells, neutrophils, plasma cells and lymphocytes. All stages of the mites are present in the hair follicle which becomes distended but does not rupture. In generalized demodicosis, the histopathology is dramatic, there is acanthosis and considerable sebaceous hyperplasia whilst rupture of follicles greatly distended by large numbers of mites results in a foreign-body reaction in the dermis with extensive cellulitis (Baker, 1969).

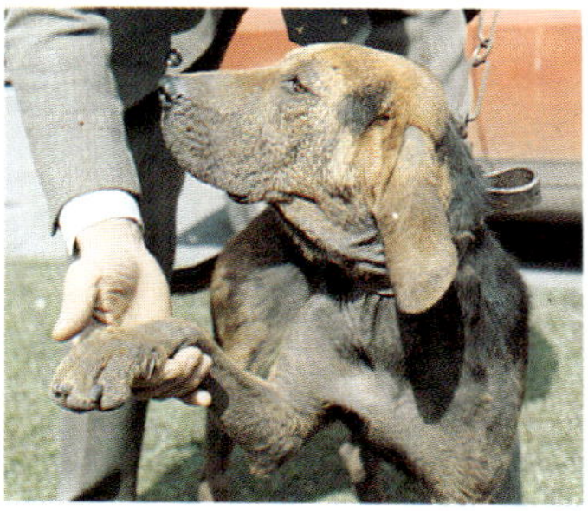

Fig. 5.61. Generalized demodicosis in a 10-month-old harrier hound; there is hyperpigmentation in 50% of the cases of generalized demodicosis.

DIAGNOSIS

Demodectic mange is often overlooked by the practitioner; the parasite is small and not easily discerned in scrapings. But diagnosis can only be confirmed by the demonstration of *Demodex* in the presence of typical lesions. In early infestation the distribution of lesions is characteristic; alopecia occurs with erythema initially; and pruritus is absent or, if present, is usually mild. In all other mite infestations pruritus is marked and self-excoriation occurs. Derwelis (1967) considers that examination of faecal samples concentrated by the flotation method is to be recommended in preference to the examination of skin scrapings. However, the mites are not always demonstrable by this method and for this reason a thorough examination of skin scrapings is essential. An active lesion should be chosen and a convex, curved scalpell blade is then used to produce capillary bleeding, over an area of 1 cm^2. The scrape may be made from a pinched area to slightly evert the follicles and so permit the sampling of their contents. The scraping is placed in 6% potassium hydroxide then examined diligently. Mineral oil may be used but does not clear the specimen. Too little time is spent examining skin scrapings. If the clinical history and signs are suggestive it is necessary to be patient and search until mites are found. It is to be regretted that students are too often introduced to the acarids as cleared specimens in the parasitological laboratory. They may not have been shown active mites in skin scrapings, nor have seen all stages in the life cycle — eggs and larvae may be overlooked. Finding *Demodex canis* in the skin of dogs without the characteristic signs of demodectic mange is not necessarily significant — many normal dogs harbour the parasite; Koutz *et al.* (1960) in the USA demonstrated the parasite in 52.9% of 204 clinically normal dogs, whilst Unsworth found a 10% incidence in England in 1946.

TREATMENT

Undoubtedly many dogs with uncomplicated juvenile demodectic mange resolve regardless of the treatment used; i.e. spontaneously. Nevertheless, the availability of the horticultural miticide Amitraz (a diamide, not an organophosphorus preparation) has been of great benefit. No case of GDM has been destroyed in the clinic of the Faculty of Veterinary Medicine, Dublin, since the compound has been routinely used there. Clinical trials in North America, Australia, France, England and the Republic of Ireland have indicated the efficacy of the preparation in both juvenile and generalized demodectic mange with excellent results (Bussieras & Chermette, 1986). Ancillary therapy for complicated secondary infections in GDM has usually been unnecessary with its use. It is used as a freshly prepared 1 : 250 part preparation with tepid water, which is applied to the lesions at 6-day intervals. Longhaired dogs should be clipped, examined regularly and skin scrapes taken. Treatment should continue until living mites cannot be demonstrated. At least 11 dressings are usually necessary. Occasional relapses in cases of GDM have occurred which quickly responded with topical therapy. There is no danger in using the product if the manufacturer's instructions are followed.

Avermectin has been used but is not licensed for use in dogs, and is definitely contraindicated for bearded collies, in which irreversible coma occurs following its use.

Rotenone in oil may be used by topical application at 3-day intervals. Long-haired dogs should be close-clipped and therapy is continued until no viable mites are found in skin scrapes; this may require dressings for 3 months.

Attempts to stimulate the immune response using levamisole have not been satisfactory. Corticosteroid therapy is definitely contraindicated. In some cases of GDM, pruritus may be severe, the skin being very erythematous and fragile. Urticaria (hives) occurs in such cases, and self-excoriation may be severe. It should be controlled by long-acting antihistamines like Phenergan. Affected bitches or carriers should not, of course, be bred. Transmission only occurs during lactation. No test is available to determine if a bitch previously producing infested puppies will pass on infestation to her next litter.

Feline demodectic mange

This is rarely reported. It is caused by *Demodex cati* which is host specific for cats. It resembles *Demodex canis* morphologically but is more slender: its life cycle is similar. An excellent description of this parasite is given by Desch and Nutting (1979) who also isolated it in normal cat skin. It is possible that it is usually a harmless common commensal (Hirst, 1919).

In cats, demodectic mange is a mild, localized exfoliative dermatitis of the periorbital regions which may spread to include parotid areas and the pinna. It has been isolated from the external auditory meatus (Desch & Nutting, 1979). Generalized demodicosis is very rare in the cat and then not as extreme as in the dog. Conroy *et al*. (1982) reported a second species from the cat; the subject was a 9-year-old Siamese cat. Their illustration shows a short mite resembling *Demodex criceti* of the golden hamster. It was isolated from areas of dermatitis involving the ventral abdomen and upper regions of the hindlegs. The lesions were reported to be mildly pruritic. The cat was bathed weekly for 3 weeks in a 1.6% lime sulphur suspension, after which scrapes were negative. Paramite was then applied weekly for 3 weeks and normal hair growth was restored. The habitat of this undescribed *Demodex* was within the stratum corneum and not in the hair follicles.

Many mammals commonly harbour two distinct species of the genus *Demodex*. Two cases treated in Ireland were in Siamese cats: Stogdale and Moore (1982) consider that feline demodicosis may be more common in pure-bred Siamese and Burmese cats.

Demodectic mange in cats may be treated successfully by the local application of 0.0025% Amitraz repeated at 6-day intervals using a hair dryer to prevent absorption by mouth during grooming. Rotenone may also be prescribed. A good prognosis can be given.

Dermanyssus gallinae (the poultry mite)

This is a parasite of birds but cats and dogs and other animals may become accidentally infested if in contact with poultry housing or infested bird nests. This is a large mite, red in colour when engorged and capable of rapid movement. The mite only visits the host to feed and spends most of its life off the host (Fig. 5.62). Isolation may therefore be difficult. The life cycle is completed in 7 days: eggs are laid in crevices of poultry houses and cages; they hatch quickly if conditions are favourable; six-legged larvae emerge, which moult to eight-legged protonymphs, and then to deutonymphs and finally to adults. Only the larvae do not feed.

CLINICAL SIGNS

The parasites are usually present in large numbers and are easily isolated with a fine-toothed comb. They cause intense pruritus, papulation and self-excoriation, with a ruffled coat along the dorsal midline. Repeated attacks produce anaemia.

TREATMENT

The mites may be destroyed using an organophosphorus insecticide like Alugan. It is most important that the environment be treated also, paying particular attention to cracks and crevices or other places where nocturnally active mites would hide during the day.

Otodectic mange

Otodectes cynotis is an obligate parasite throughout its life, primarily of the external auditory meatus of the cat, dog, fox and ferret. It is a non-burrowing mite and resembles *Chorioptes*,

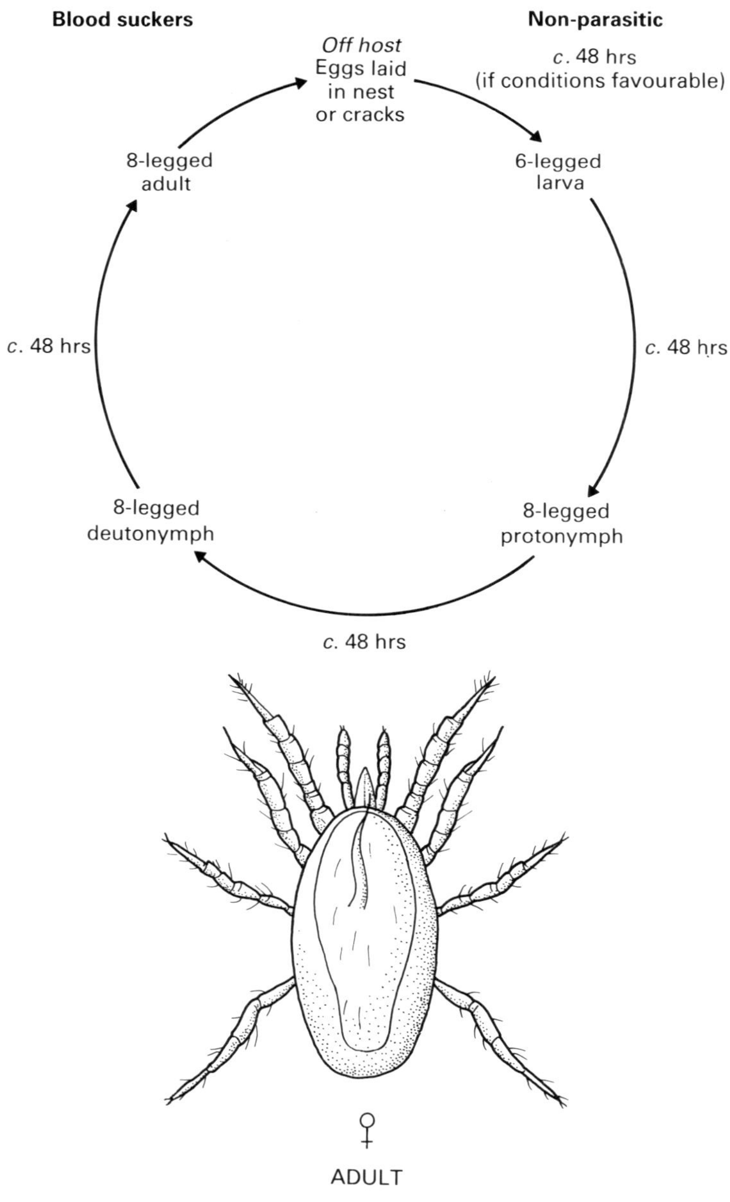

Fig. 5.62. Adult *Dermanyssus gallinae* and life cycle.

with prominent tarsal suckers but with less prominent male tubercles (Fig. 5.63). The life cycle is similar to that of *Sarcoptes scabiei* and lasts 3 weeks.

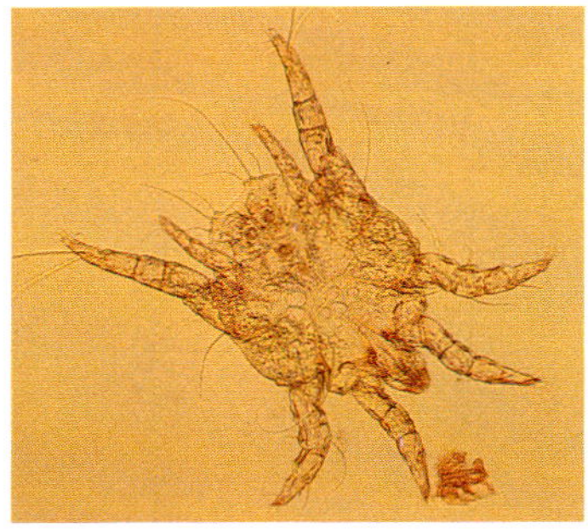

Fig. 5.63. *Otodectes cynotis.*

CLINICAL SIGNS

Whilst the mite may be tolerated in older cats it produces severe pruritus in dogs and some younger cats. There is much head shaking and scratching. Characteristically, brown crumbly wax occludes the orifice of the external auditory meatus.

Both ears are usually affected. Infestation may spread to the parotid area and, uncommonly, up to the tail tip. In severe cases there may be associated pyotraumatic dermatitis of the parotid area with a secondary bacterial otitis externa. A complication is rupture of the tympanum with the development of otitis media. Haematoma of the pinna is relatively common. Weisbroth *et al.* (1974) demonstrated a type of hypersensitivity to whole mite extracts in cats with otoacariasis: pathogen-free cats were non-reactive to intradermal injections of allergen and did not have precipitating antibodies.

DIAGNOSIS

Examination by auriscope will reveal the grey–white mites moving over the crumbly wax in the meatus. Alternatively a little wax may be removed and examined microscopically in 6% potassium hydroxide. Uncomplicated cases with excessive cerumen should have the auditory meatus gently syringed with a mild antiseptic detergent like Leo ear cleanser to remove debris. Preparations containing gammexane should be instilled into both canals on three occasions, at 5-day intervals. Several proprietary aural preparations are available which contain gammexane. If there are lesions elsewhere these should be treated.

Contact cats and dogs should also be treated, as the carrier state is common.

Where there is secondary infection, the pathogens should be isolated and their sensitivity determined. Direct smears stained with 1% methylene blue are useful to determine the presence or absence of the yeast *Pityrosporum*, which should be treated accordingly. Auroto drops contain thiabendazole which has fungicidal properties.

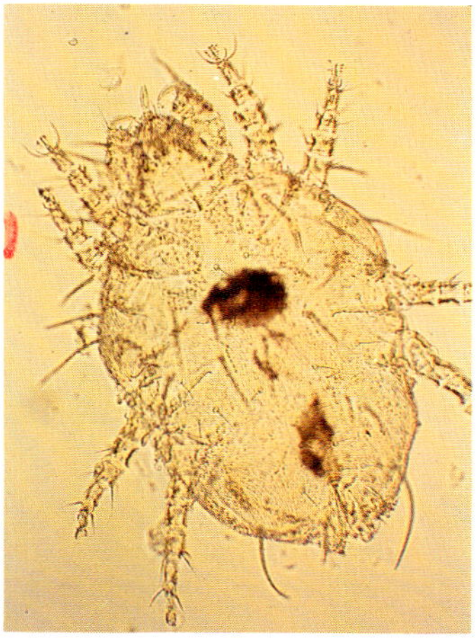

Fig. 5.64. Adult *Cheyletiella yasguri*.

Cheyletiella infestation

There are five members of the genus *Cheyletiella*, of which one species, *C. yasguri*, parasitizes dogs and one, *C. blakei*, affects cats. However, *C. parasitovorax* has also been identified on adult female cats (Fox & Ewing, 1969). The mites are comparatively large (Fig. 5.64) (500 μm) and visible to the naked eye. They are obligate parasites throughout their life cycle and actively move over the skin. The term 'walking dandruff' has been used to describe the appearance of infested skin debris.

There is no authoritative record of the period of the relative stadia. Humphreys (1958) gives a total lifespan of 35 days but reveals no experimental methodology. The eggs are non-operculate and are attached to a single hair by fine threads (Fig. 5.65). They are thus easily distinguishable from louse eggs, which are larger, operculate and are attached to the supporting hair by cement at their base. Active six-legged larvae soon emerge with development to the first and second nymphal stages and finally to adult males and females. Whilst the mites may survive short periods off the host, the mites are very susceptible to temperature changes and die rapidly.

Human contacts may develop a papular urticaria. Variable reactivity may indicate that some hosts develop hypersensitivity and show overt clinical signs.

CLINICAL SIGNS

These vary considerably; some animals, particularly cats, show no reaction to the presence of mites, even when present in large numbers.

Lesions in cats are characterized by mild exfoliation; discrete papules may be seen but erythema and excoriation do not occur.

In contrast, canine infestation is usually markedly pruritic, with mild to severe scale, particularly along the dorsal trunk, though the entire body may be affected.

'Walking dandruff' (Fig. 5.66) describes the effect of large numbers of mites moving over the skin in heavy infestation with associated scaling. There may be a mild papular rash present. Young cats and dogs will show severe signs of infestation. Most cases in the literature and in the author's experience occurred in dogs less than 6 months old. This suggests that older animals become non-reactive. The reaction in humans is not an exfoliative dermatitis but a papular rash.

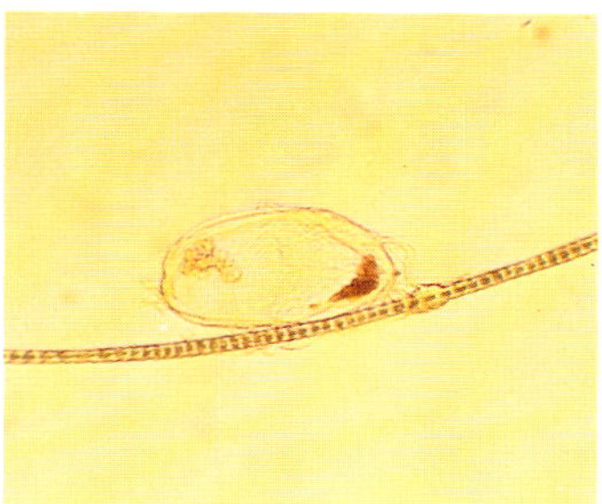

Fig. 5.65. The ovum of *Cheyletiella* is smaller than a typical louse egg; it is non-operculate with threads binding it to the hair.

Hewitt *et al.* (1971) report that one-third of affected people show small yellow macules developing to yellow crusted lesions with marked pruritus. Others may exhibit papules and wheals (Fig. 5.67). In some households, not all the contacts will develop a clinical response. However, the constancy with which clinical signs are shown in human contacts indicates that a thorough clinical history and investigation is always of value in diagnosis. Undoubtedly cheyletiellosis in humans is often undiagnosed by the medical profession.

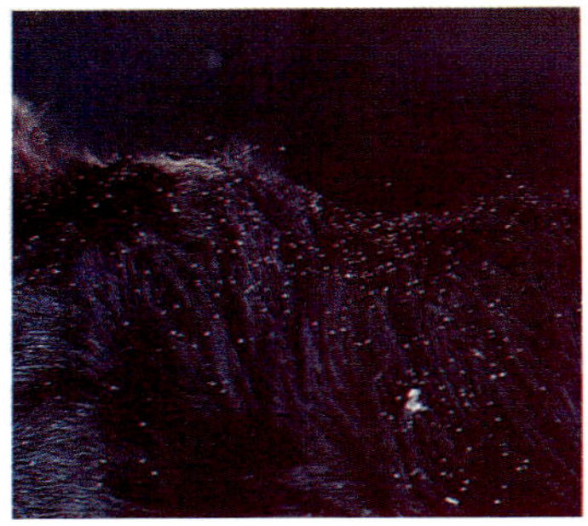

Fig. 5.66. Large numbers of *Cheyletiella yasguri* clinging to tips of hairs of dead miniature Yorkshire terrier, 3 months old.

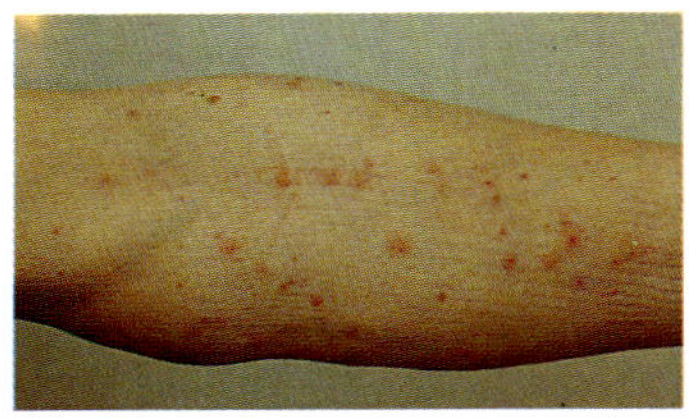

Fig. 5.67. Lesions on forearm of owner of an Irish wolfhound infested with *Cheyletiella yasguri*.

DIAGNOSIS

Close examination using a magnifying examination light will reveal the presence of the comparatively large, active mites. A fine-toothed comb and brushing and collection of debris for subsequent examination with a hand lens is advantageous. Microscopic examination is necessary to determine the species involved. Often the owner will admit to a pruritic papular rash on the arm and trunk.

Cheyletiella is dorsoventrally flattened, the nymphs and adults having eight well-developed legs which bear many setae and which have at their tips comb-shaped structures (Fig. 5.68); tarsal suckers are not present (Fig. 5.69). On either side of the chelicerae are the large hooked pedipalps. Specification is determined by the shape of the sensory organ on genu I (Fig. 5.70).

TREATMENT

Spread may be rapid, therefore all animals in the household should be examined. *Cheyletiella* may be killed by sulphur baths, selenium sulphide baths, organochlorines or organophosphorus preparations. All animals should be treated even if not showing clinical signs. Close vacuum cleaning of the animal's environs is advisable. *Cheyletiella* will not survive long on human skin so that human treatment should not be necessary if thorough measures are undertaken. The mite will quickly die off the host.

Ticks

The ticks are placed in the order Acarina in the families Ixodidae (hard ticks) and Argasidae (soft ticks). The latter are not found on domesticated animals in northern Europe.

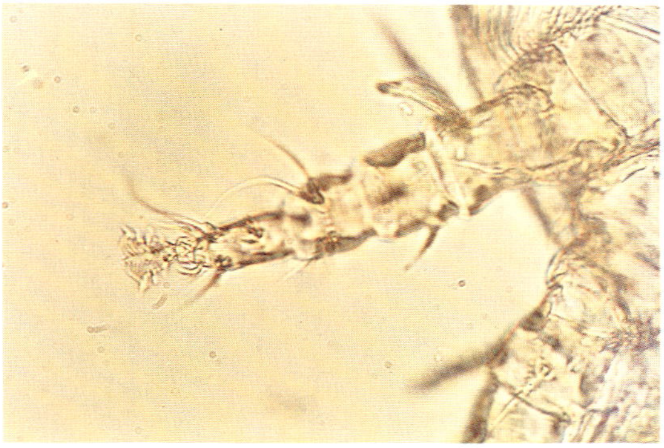

Fig. 5.68. *Cheyletiella yasguri* 'comb' at distal end of each coxa.

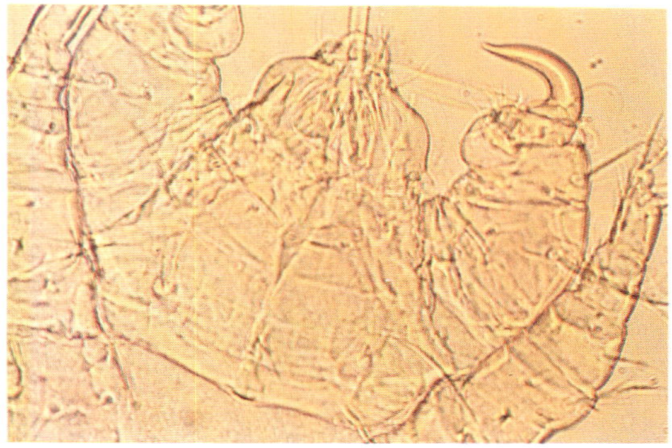

Fig. 5.69. Chelicerae and pedipalps.

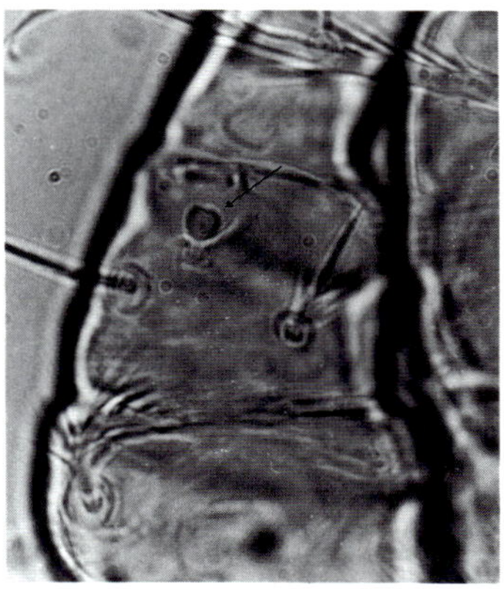

Fig. 5.70. *Cheyletiella yasguri* species-determining sensory organ (arrowed).

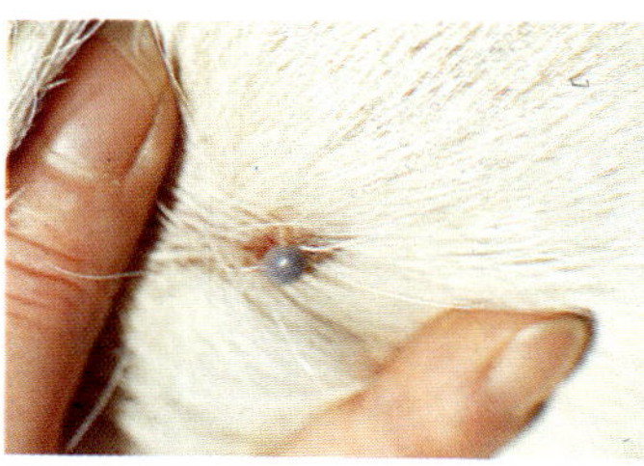

Fig. 5.71. Engorging tick in dog.

The Ixodidae have a rigid cuticle, on the dorsal side of which is a chitinous plate (scutum); in the male, this covers most of the dorsum, compared to only a small triangular anterior section in the female.

The mouth parts are well developed with a median denticulated structure, the hypostome, with a pair of chelicerae and a pair of pedipalps. The posterior curved teeth on the hypostome prevent dislodgement by force. Three species of the Ixodidae occur on cats and dogs: *Ixodes canisuga*, the dog tick; *Ixodes ricinus*, the sheep and cattle tick; *Ixodes hexagonus*, the hedgehog tick.

Ticks spend most of their life off the hosts. In some parts of the world ticks are important vectors of parasitic, bacterial and viral diseases, while some species may cause paralysis by their salivary secretions. In Europe only single or small numbers of ticks are found on the host, from which they suck blood for up to 2 weeks. They may be removed by enclosing them within a pledget of cotton wool soaked in surgical spirit or ether for a minute; firm traction at the site of attachment with the fingers or artery forceps will detach them. Removed ticks should be preserved in alcohol for identification and then burned. If an attempt is made to detach embedded ticks without first relaxing them, the hypostome will detach and remain in the skin where it may cause local inflammation (Fig. 5.71).

Ixodes canisuga

This is difficult to eradicate in kennels, where it may occur in large numbers. Feeding of this species is intermittent, the tick leaving the host to hide in crevices. In old premises these may be myriad. Leaving areas empty is not practical as the ticks can survive very long periods without feeding. In these cases, redesigning to eliminate crevices is advisable. Alternatively initial scrubbing with hot 5% washing soda to eliminate protective dirt is necessary following pressure hosing and finally cleansing with a synthetic pyrethroid.

Ixodes ricinus

The castor bean tick, so-called because of its superficial resemblance to the castor bean, is commonly found on farm animals except in the south east of England. In most parts of Britain it feeds from March to June; however, in western England, Wales, western Scotland and Ireland there is some feeding from August to November. Larvae, nymphs and adults are parasitic only once yearly during their 3 years of life.

Ixodes hexagonus

The hedgehog tick resembles the dog tick and is about the same size. It is found on hedgehogs and other wild mammals. Spring and autumn peaks of feeding activity are recorded on wild mammals.

Order Phthiraptera: the lice

The order Phthiraptera contains the lice which are parasites on the skin. Lice are usually host specific and are obligate parasites throughout their life cycle. Some feed on blood (the sucking lice or Anoplura), others feed on epithelial debris (the Mallophaga which, however, does contain more blood-sucking species).

All lice attach their operculate eggs to the hairs or feathers of their host, the life cycle is simple without metamorphosis and may be complete in 3 weeks (Fig. 5.72). Lice, unlike fleas, are host dependent throughout their life cycle; they survive for only a few days when separated from their hosts. Control is therefore relatively straightforward, as spread is by direct contact with an infested animal or by fomites.

SUBORDER MALLOPHAGA

Members of this suborder are more active than the Anoplura and consequently cause more irritation.

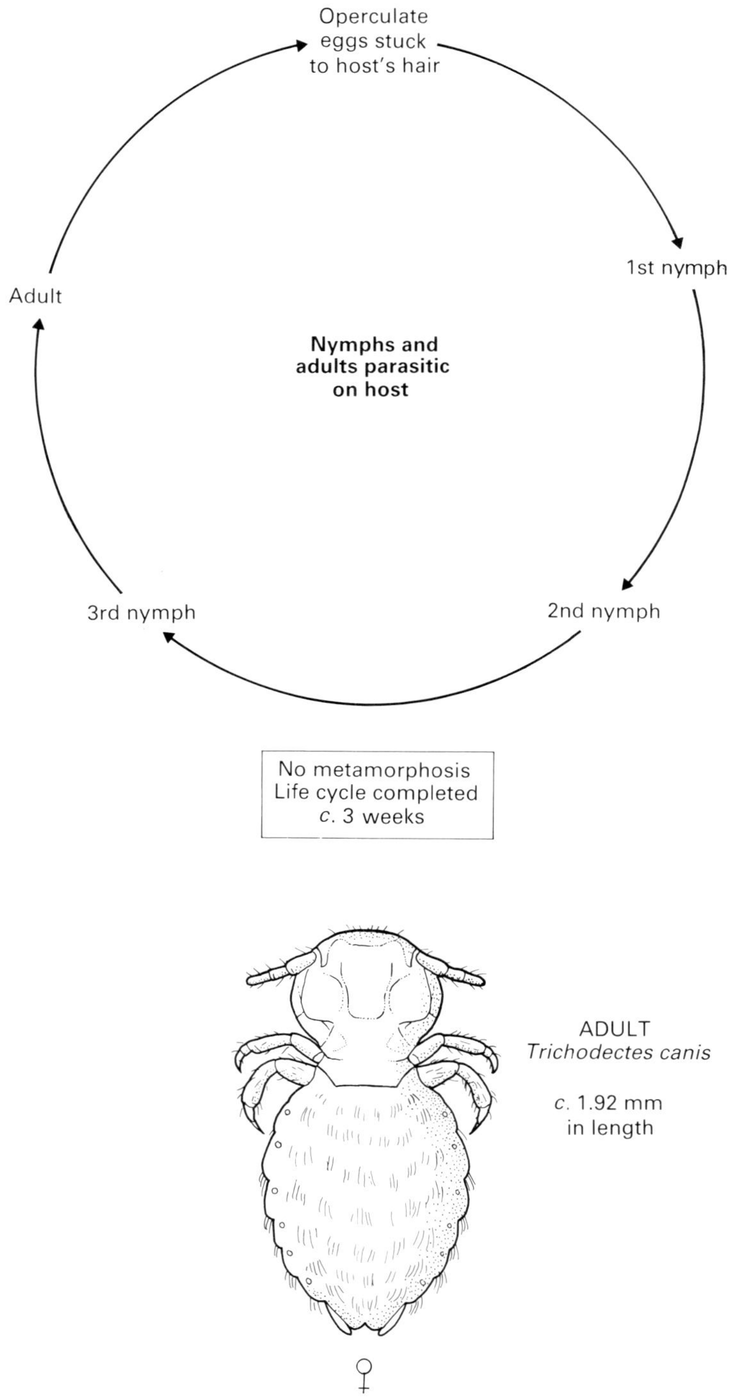

Fig. 5.72. Life cycle of typical louse and adult *Trichodectes canis*.

Trichodectes canis

This is the more common of the two species of louse parasitizing dogs in the UK. It is greyish yellow in colour and almost 2 mm in length when adult. It is a vector, acting as the intermediate host of the dog tapeworm *Dipylidium caninum*. It may also be found on cats.

Felicola subrostratus

This species parasitizes cats and is smaller than the above (adult females measure 0.29 mm in length) (Fig. 5.73).

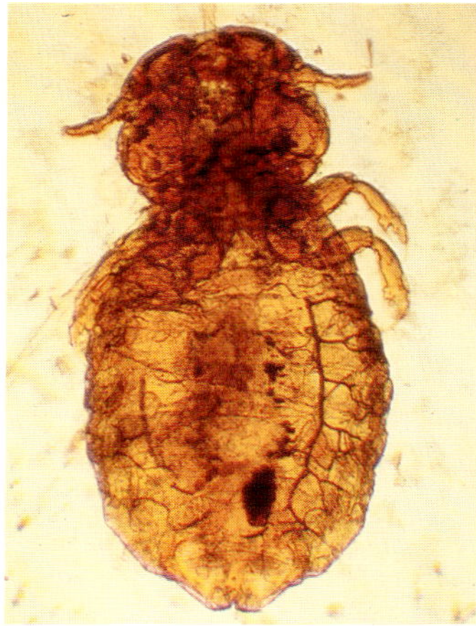

Fig. 5.73. Adult *Felicola subrostrata*.

SUBORDER ANOPLURA

The only sucking louse of dogs, *Linognathus setosus*, may be distinguished from the two biting lice by its somewhat larger size and smaller, more pointed head.

CLINICAL SIGNS OF INFESTATION

These are mostly seen in young animals; however, older, debilitated, neglected animals may be severely infested. There is irritation and consequent self-excoriation with patchy alopecia developing (Fig. 5.74). If large numbers of sucking lice are present, anaemia may develop. The parasites should be searched for diligently for they are small, comparatively slow moving and are easily overlooked, particularly if there is much skin scale present (Fig. 5.75). The eggs (nits), however, are more conspicuous. In light infestation, lice are most commonly found in the axilla, inguinal and perineal areas; when heavy, the entire body may be covered. A fine-toothed comb is a useful adjunct to isolate the lice. The pinna should also be examined for lice; these may provoke head shaking, and infestation has been known to be misdiagnosed as otitis externa.

The differential diagnosis should include diseases characterized by exfoliative dermatitis, such as other ectoparasites and seborrhoea sicca; it should be remembered that pruritus may not be a clinical sign.

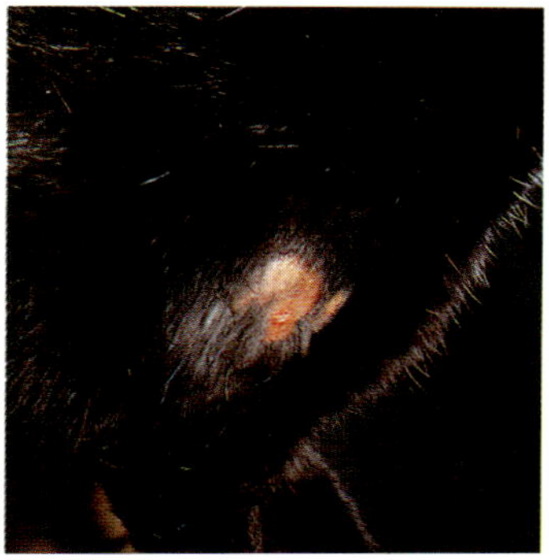

Fig. 5.74. Louse infestation, cat.

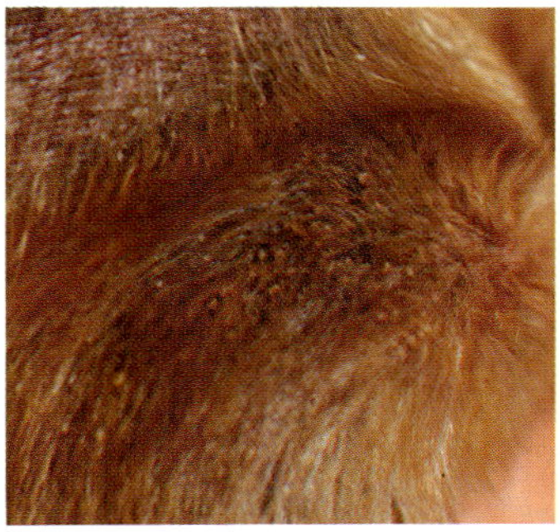

Fig. 5.75. Louse infestation, Basset hound.

TREATMENT

The knotted hair of long-haired, infested cats and dogs should be close clipped and burnt. All infected animals should be washed in a parasiticidal bath, rinsed and dried, taking care that the preparation is suitable for use on cats; this should be repeated 10 days later. All dogs and cats on infested premises should be so treated, for some adult animals may be carriers without showing clinical signs. Bedding should be removed and destroyed if it cannot be washed in a parasiticidal bath. Combs and brushes should be similarly treated.

Order Siphonaptera: fleas

Fleas are the most common cause of skin diseases in cats and dogs. The fleas differ from the lice in several ways: they are laterally compressed, obligate parasites for only part of their life cycle, not always host specific, and move rapidly as adults. These characteristics make control much more difficult. Also they are more likely to provoke severe allergic reactions. Unlike lice they undergo complete metamorphosis during their life cycle (Fig. 5.76).

Several species are found on cats and dogs, with some variation of species representation in different countries (Baker & Hatch, 1972; Amin, 1967). In the UK the most common parasite is *Ctenocephalides felis felis* followed by *Ctenocephalides canis* and *Pulex irritans* (Beresford-Jones, 1981). In Ireland *Ctenocephalides canis* is the most commonly found flea in dogs (Baker & Mulcahy, 1986). However, other species are also found, including the rat flea, *Xenopsylla cheopis*, the rabbit flea, *Spilopsyllus cuniculi*, and the hedgehog flea, *Archeopsylla erinacei erinacei*.

Females lay eggs at regular intervals and may produce over 600 during their adult life. These are comparatively large, white, non-sticky and visible to the naked eye.

The non-sticky eggs are laid on the host but fall to the ground where they develop. Because warmth and moisture are required for development, fleas have a restricted northern range; in Europe they are not found in central and northern Scandinavia. Adult fleas do not leave their host to lay eggs as is sometimes stated, in dogs they have a predilection for remaining on the dorsal midline of the body (Baker & El Harrem, in press). Egg production is variable, a blood meal being essential. Up to 400 eggs may be produced during a lifetime. The nesting sites of the host usually provide ideal conditions for development if the environmental temperature or relative humidity are favourable. Larvae feed on nest debris and dried blood: they resemble small caterpillars (Fig. 5.77).

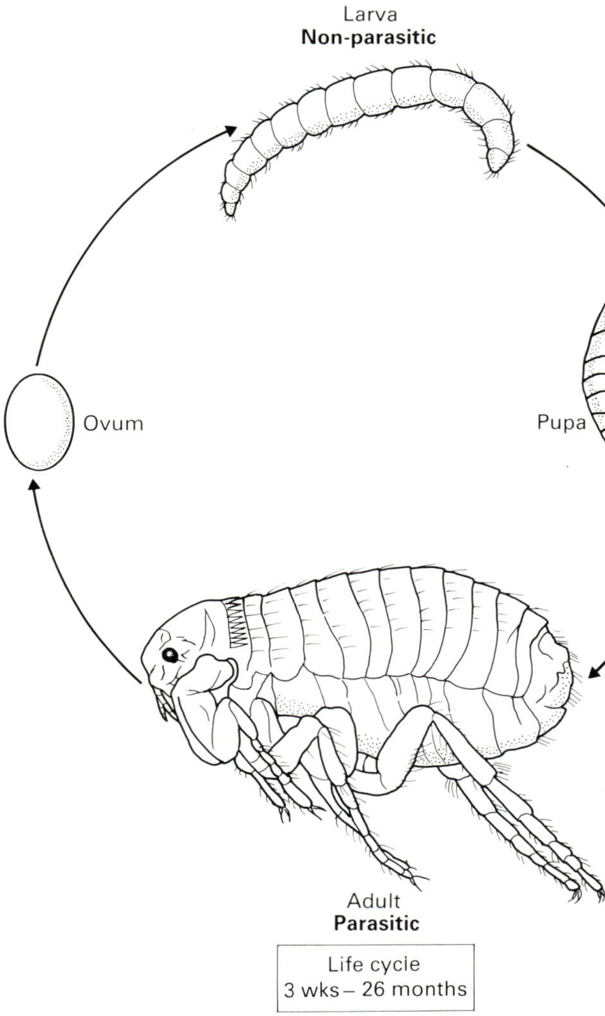

Fig. 5.76. Life cycle of *Ctenocephalides canis*.

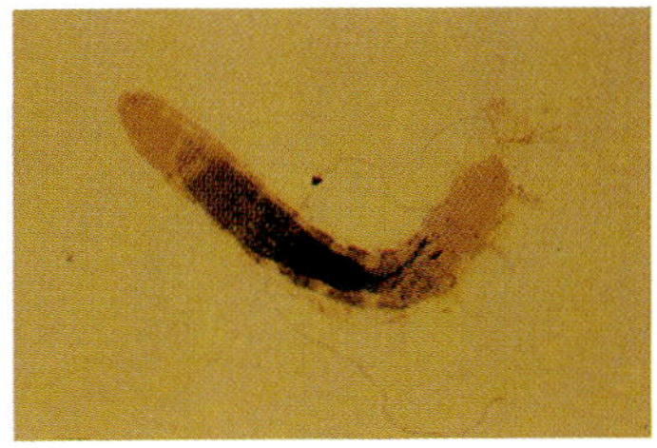

Fig. 5.77. First stage larva *Archeopsylla erinacei erinacei*.

There are three larval stages, the third of which, when mature, spins a coccoon and pupates. If conditions are favourable the larval period may be completed in 9 days, if unfavourable it may extend to 7 months. The inactive pupa develops to the adult stage in 7 days or remains dormant for up to a year if conditions of temperature and humidity are unfavourable.

Emergence is stimulated by vibrations, thus fleas may emerge after lying dormant in empty houses for months when so stimulated. Adult fleas are dark brown in colour, about 3 mm in length; males are smaller than females. A blood meal is required for normal egg development, but fed adults can survive for many months in the absence of hosts under laboratory conditions. Although the life cycle can extend beyond a year in length, under ideal conditions it may be completed in 3 weeks. Thus, with the great egg-laying capability of fleas and survival characteristics, large infestations may be produced. Once a host has been found, adult fleas remain on it, producing eggs and feeding regularly. Numbers of fleas on a particular host may be variable, from few to many; there tend to be few on hyposensitive dogs, less than 10. This has also been recorded in humans; Herms (1950) quotes McCoy who reported less than 12 *Pulex irritans* per human host. This probably reflects the skill of the host in removing them. However, debilitated or insensitive hosts may carry very large numbers; e.g. hedgehogs may be heavily infested. Mulcahy and Baker (1986) reported an average of 55.89 on hedgehogs in Ireland; however, Brinck and Löfqvist (1973) found an average of 129 *A.e. erinecei* on the hedgehogs they examined in Sweden.

The life cycle of fleas is favoured by civilization: central heating is common, homes with fitted carpets are shared by dogs and cats, the latter particularly being free to roam and so become infested. Fleas are to some extent host specific, thus *Ctenocephalides canis*, though feeding on cats, requires dog blood to complete its life cycle (Baker & El Harrem, in press). However, fleas share a common salivary hapten and therefore a hypersensitive dog will react if bitten by cat fleas.

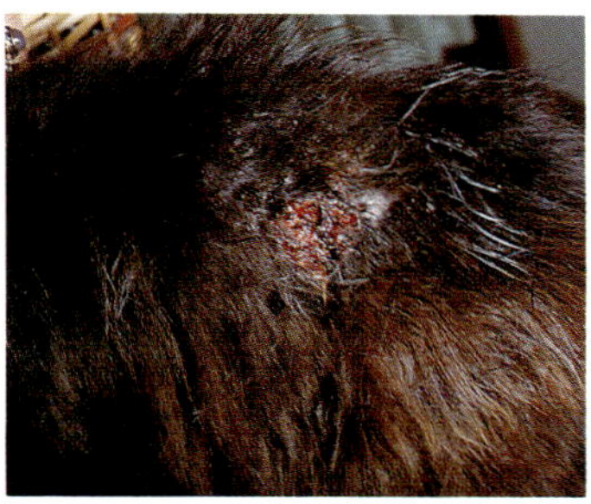

Fig. 5.78. Pyotraumatic dermatitis in feline flea hypersensitivity.

CLINICAL SIGNS

These are variable and range from mild pruritus with some self-excoriation and local alopecia to severe prolonged pruritus, marked excoriation, miliary eczema in cats and pyotraumatic dermatitis in dogs (Figs 5.78 and 5.79). The difference is explained by the fact that flea saliva contains a hapten (incomplete allergen) capable of producing a hypersensitive reaction which may be immediate and or delayed in the skin.

Hypersensitive reactions to fleas which constitute perhaps the most important disease numerically in small animal practice will be discussed in Chapter 8.

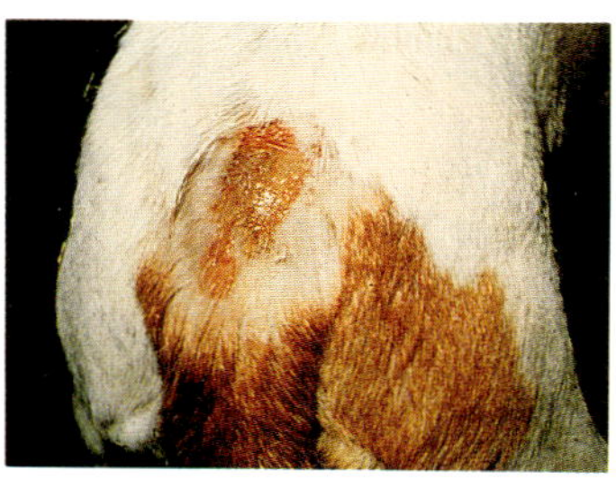

Fig. 5.79. Pyotraumatic dermatitis in flea hypersensitivity.

DIAGNOSIS

As ectoparasitism is easily the most important cause of pruritus the coat should always be diligently examined. This will be aided by a fine-toothed comb. Captured fleas should be immersed in a bowl of water to prevent escape and then placed on a slide under a coverslip for identification (Figs 5.80–82). Alternatively they may be captured on a Sellotape strip wrapped around a finger, its sticky face being applied to the flea which can then be transferred to a slide for microscopic identification. With experience flea faeces can be recognized; however, their true nature can be demonstrated by placing them on a piece of moist paper — a brown halo of digested blood will quickly develop. This is a helpful demonstration for pet owners who otherwise may be sceptical that their pet has fleas.

CONTROL

Where fleas are presenting problems the species involved should be identified to determine the source of infestation. Unfortunately it is not possible to completely eradicate fleas from most pets' environments. Careful counselling is important when discussing control measures with owners; e.g. a single flea may trigger a serious pruritic episode in hypersensitive hosts.

All dogs and cats in an infested household, kennel or cattery should be washed with a safe insecticide: gamma-BHC (not for cats), selenium sulphide, Derris or synthetic

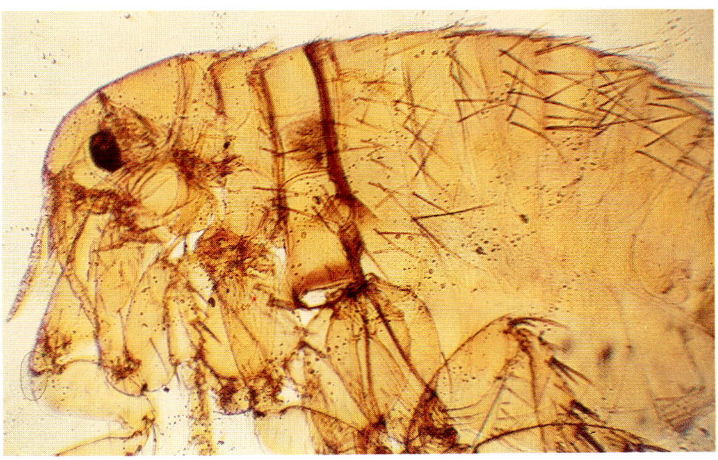

Fig. 5.80. *Pulex irritans*, adult.

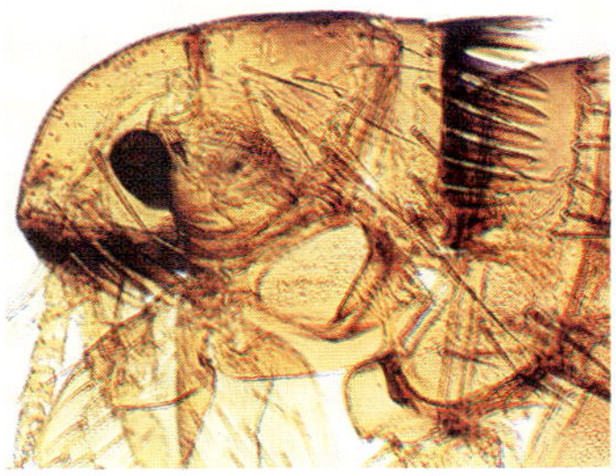

Fig. 5.81. *Ctenocephalides canis*, head of adult.

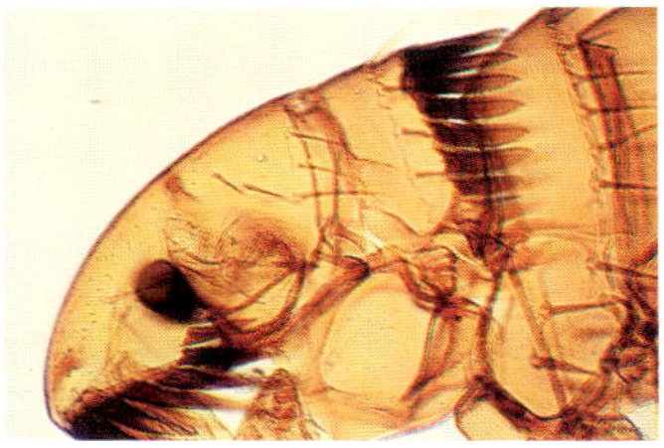

Fig. 5.82. *Ctenocephalides felis felis*, head of adult.

pyrethroids used as sprays, washes or dusting powders. Coopers' 'Head to Tail Shampoo' (Coopers Animal Health Ltd) will give a residual action for 2 weeks and prevent biting during this time (Baker & El Harrem, in press). Treatment should be repeated 7 days later. It is essential to treat bedding also: this should be washed or dusted with a parasiticide or destroyed if this cannot be satisfactorily done. Careful vacuuming of the sleeping area is essential. Places where stray dogs, cats and other animals are sleeping require attention too. A spray is available containing the juvenile insect hormone methoprene; this may be sprayed in the environment and is claimed to prevent metamorphosis to the adult stage for 6 months. The preparation should not be used outside the home because the life cycle of harmless insects may be damaged.

Flea collars give some control but should never be the only control measure implemented. They have a comparatively short active 'life' and may not prevent biting — a most important consideration in the hypersensitive animal. Occasionally pets develop contact allergic dermatitis to flea collars.

Fleas are the intermediate host of the tapeworm *Dipylidium caninum* and are vectors of several important infections of humans. In humans fleas cause utricaria (hives), which is an intensely pruritic condition, lesions are found particularly on the lower limbs, waist and lower neck but may occur anywhere on the body. Owners should be questioned regarding hives; if present it is an added indication of flea infestation of the pet's environment.

Diptera

GENUS *CULICOIDES*: MIDGES

There are about 50 different species of midge in the UK, of which the majority are haematophagous. The genus is implicated in the aetiology of summer seasonal recurrent dermatitis (sweet itch) of horses.

The larvae and pupae are aquatic and non-parasitic (Fig. 5.83). Only the adult females of the genus are haematophagous and are active from April to November particularly on warm, still, humid days, where they may be active throughout the day. At sunrise and nightfall, when conditions are favourable, large numbers may develop and individual dogs may become hypersensitive to bites. Small irritant papules may develop on the pinna and frontal area with head shaking and pawing.

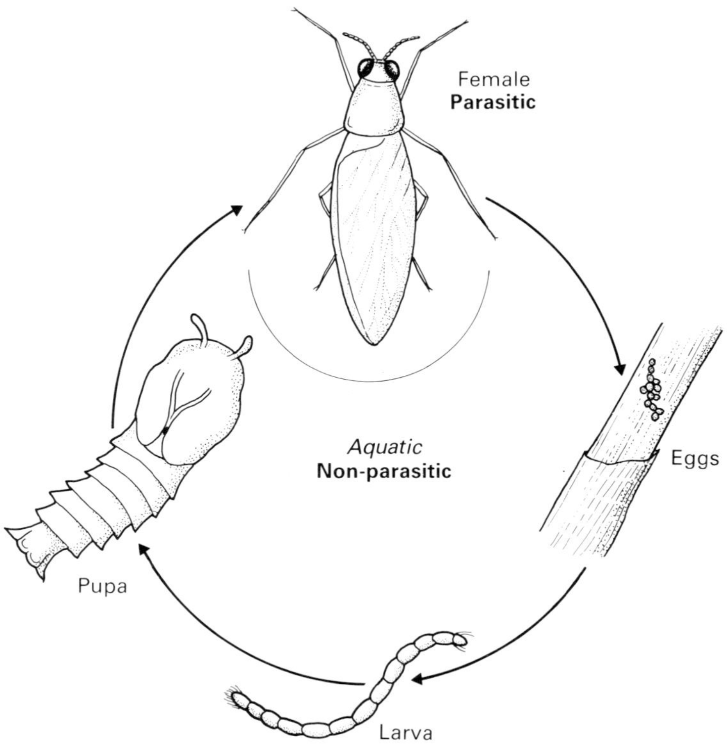

Fig. 5.83. Life cycle of the midge *Culicoides* spp.

Examination of the patient outside at home may indicate the presence of biting midges. Combings and scrapings taken in the consultation room will not reveal ectoparasites, although histopathological examination should indicate an immediate hypersensitivity reaction. *Culicoides* extracts are not available for skin testing.

Prednisolone by mouth (2 mg/kg) may be necessary to control intense pruritus. As biting activity occurs mainly at daybreak and nightfall, sensitive animals should be housed at this time. Topical synthetic pyrethroids (Barricade 1 : 50 dilution in water) will give protection for several days.

GENUS *LUCILIA*

The most important cause of myiasis is *Lucilia sericata*, the green-bottle fly.

Myiasis in cats and dogs only occurs in neglected or weak,

recumbent animals in warmer weather, when the egg-laying females are attracted by soiled bedding, skin and fur. The perineum is the most commonly affected area but pressure points may also be attacked.

With favourable conditions of moisture and warmth the eggs hatch quickly and the larvae may reach maturity within 2–7 days. Severely debilitated animals may not react to larval activity, others may show tail wagging or evidence of pruritus.

Eggs and developing larvae are easily seen by the naked eye.

The hair around lesions should be clipped short and the area and lesions washed with strong saline baths. A hair dryer will be effective in causing the larvae to leave the lesions rapidly; they should then be collected and destroyed. Thereafter the lesions should be kept clean and dry and inspected regularly to prevent further deposition of eggs until healing is complete.

References

Bacteria

Grant D.I. (1986) Skin diseases of the dog and cat. *Library of Veterinary Practice* pp. 21–22. Blackwell Scientific Publications, Oxford.

Ihrke P.J. (1983) The management of canine pyodermas. In *Current Veterinary Therapy VIII* (Ed. Kirk R.W.) pp. 505–517. W.B. Saunders, Philadelphia.

Ihrke P.J. (1986) Antibacterial therapy in dermatology. In *Current Veterinary Therapy XI. Small Animal Practice* (Ed. Kirk R.W.) pp. 566–571. W.B. Saunders, Philadelphia.

Krogh & Kristensen S. (1976) A study of skin diseases in dogs and cats. II. Microflora of the normal skin. *Nordisk Veterinaer Medicin* **28**, 459–63.

Kunkle G.A. (1982) Cutaneous atypical mycobacterial infections. *The 8th World Congress of World Small Animal Veterinary Association*, Las Vegas.

Medleau L., Long R.F., Brown J. & Muller W.H. (1986) Frequency and antimicrobial susceptibility of *Staphylococcus* species is dated from canine pyodermas. *American Journal of Veterinary Research* **47**, 229–231.

Muller G.H., Kirk R.W. & Scott D.W. (1983) *Small Animal Dermatology*, pp. 206, 222. W.B. Saunders, Philadelphia.

Ness E. (1984) Patterns of antibodies to staphylococcal DNases in dog sera. *Journal of Clinical Microbiology* **20**, 806–7.

Wilkinson G.T. (1978) Cat leprosy. *Veterinary Annual*, **18**, 270–275.

Wilkinson G.T. (1985) *A Colour Atlas of Small Animal Dermatology*, pp. 68–73, 89–94. Wolfe Medical Publications Ltd, London.

Wilkinson G.T., Kelly W.R. & O'Boyle D. (1982) Pyogranulomatous panniculitis of cats due to *Mycobacterium smegmatis*. *Australian Veterinary Journal* **58**, 77–78.

Fungi

Dufait R. (1983) *Pityrosporum canis* as the cause of canine chronic dermatitis. *Veterinary Medicine for the Small Animal Clinician* **78**, 1055–1057.

Foil C.S. (1986) Antifungal agents in dermatology. In *Current Veterinary Therapy XI. Small Animal Practice* (Ed. Kirk R.W.) pp. 560–565. W.B. Saunders, London.

Keep J.M. (1981) *Feline Dermatoses*. University of Sydney, Postgraduate Foundation in Veterinary Science. Veterinary Review No. 20.

Keep J.M. (1981) *Canine Dermatoses*. University of Sydney, Postgraduate Foundation in Veterinary Science. Veterinary Review No. 21.

Kushida T. (1978) A survey on canine and feline medicine. *Bulletin of the Nippon Veterinary and Zootechnical College* **27**, 33–46.

Mackenzie D.W.R. (1961) The extra-human occurrence of *T. tonsurans* var. *sulfureum* in a residential school. *Sabouraudia* **I**, 58.

Marples M.J. (1956) The ecology of *Microsporon canis* Bodin in New Zealand. *Journal of Hygiene* **54**, 378–387.

Muller G.H., Kirk R.W. & Scott D.W. (1983) Dermatophytosis. In *Small Animal Dermatology*, 3rd edn. pp. 275–284. W.B. Saunders, London.

Pepin G.A. & Oxenham M. (1987) Feline dermatophytosis. The diagnosis of subclinical infection and its relevance to control. *British Veterinary Dermatology Study Group Newsletter* **11**, 22.

Schwartzmann R.M., Deubler M.J. & Dice P.F. (1965) Experimentally induced monilia (*Candida albicans*) in the dog. *Journal of Small Animal Practice* **6**, 327.

Thomsett L.R. (1962) *Microsporum canis* infection in cats treated with griseofulvin. *British Journal of Dermatology* **74**, 66–71.

van den Broek A.H.M. & Thoday K.L. (1987) Eumycetoma in a British cat. *Journal of Small Animal Practice* **28**, 827–831.

Weiss R. & Weber A. (1982) Cultural demonstration of dermatophytes from 2865 pets having skin lesions. 28 Jahrestagung der Fachgruppe. *Kleintierkrankheiten*, Frankfurt, October 14–16 Deutsche Veterinarmedizinische Gesellschaft 342–348.

Parasites

Amin O.M. (1967) The fleas of Egypt, distribution and seasonal dynamics of fleas infesting dogs in the Nile Valley and Delta. *Journal of Medical Entomology* **3**, 293.

Baker K.P. (1969) Canine demodicosis. *Journal of Comparative Pathology* **79**, 321

Baker K.P. (1975) Hyperpigmentation of the skin in canine demodicosis. *Veterinary Parasitology* **1**, 193–197.

Baker K.P. (1981) Clinical aspects of hookworm dermatitis. *Veterinary Dermatology Newsletter* **6**, 69–74.

Baker K.P., Grimes T.D. & Winstanley E.W. (1970) Cutaneous lesions in dogs associated with hookworm infestation. *Veterinary Record* **87**, 376–379.

Baker K.P. & Hatch C. (1972) The species of fleas found in Dublin dogs. *Veterinary Record* **91**, 151–152.

Baker K.P. & Mulcahy R. (1986) Fleas on hedgehogs and dogs in the Dublin area. *Veterinary Record* **119**, 16–17.

Beresford-Jones W.P. (1981) Prevalence of fleas on dogs and cats in an area of London. *Journal of Small Animal Practice* **22**, 27–29.

Brinck & Löfqvist J. (1973) The hedgehog, *Erinaceous europaeus*, and its flea, *Archeopsylla erinecei*. (Suppl. 1), 97–103.

Bussieras J. & Chermette R. (1986) Amitraz and canine demodicosis. *Journal of the American Animal Hospital Association* **22**, 779–782.

Chitwood B.G. (1932) The association of *Rhabditis strongyloides* with dermatitis in dogs. *North American Veterinarian* **13**, 35–40.

Conroy J.D., Healy M.C. & Bane A.G. (1982) New *Demodex* sp. infesting a cat: a case report. *Journal of the American Animal Hospital Association* **18**, 405–407.

Corbett R. (1975) Cellular mediated immune responsiveness in dogs with demodectic mange. *Transplant Proceedings* **1**, 557.

Corbett R. (1976) The cell-mediated immune response: its inhibition and *in vitro* reversal in dogs with demodectic mange. *Federation Proceedings* **35**, 589.

Derwelis S.K. (1967) Presence of *Demodex canis* in dog skin and faeces. *Illinois Veterinarian* **10**, No. 3, 10–11.

Desch C. & Nutting W.B. (1979) *Demodex cuti* Hirst 1919: a redescription. *Cornell Veterinarian* **69**, 280–285.

Fox T.S. & Ewing S.A. (1969) Morphologic features, behaviour and life history of *Cheyletiella yasguri*. *American Journal of Veterinary Research* **30**, 269–285.

French F.E. (1962) Biology and morphology of *Demodex canis*. PhD Thesis, University of Iowa.

Greve J. & Gaafar S.M. (1966) Natural transmission of *Demodex canis* in dogs. *Journal of the American Veterinarian Association* **148**, 1043–1048.

Gregor W.W. (1965) The incidence of skin disease in small animal pruritus. In *Comparative Physiology and Pathology of the Skin* (Ed. Rook A.J.O. & Walson G.S.) pp. 33–36. Blackwell Scientific Publications, Oxford.

Healy M.C. & Gaafar S.M. (1977a) Demonstration of antibody (IgE) in canine demodectic mange, an immunofluorescent study. *Veterinary Parasitology* **3**, 107–119.

Healy M.C. & Gaafar S.M. (1977b) Immunodeficiency in canine demodectic mange II. Skin reaction to phytohaemagglutinin and concanavalin A. *Veterinary Parasitology* **3**, 122–141.

Herms W.B. (1950) *Medical Entomology with Special Reference to Health and Well-Being of Man and Animals*, 4th edn. Macmillan, New York.

Hewitt M., Walton G.S. & Waterhouse M. (1971) Pet animal infestation and human skin disease. *British Journal of Dermatology* **85**, 215–221.

Hirsch D.C. (1975) Suppression of *in vitro* lymphocyte transformation by serum from dogs with generalised demodicosis. *American Journal of Veterinary Research* **36**, 1591–1595.

Hirst S. (1919) *Studies on Acari No. 1. The genus Demodex*. British Museum (Natural History).

Humphreys M. (1958) *Cheyletiella parasitovorax* infestation of the dog. *Veterinary Record* **70**, 442.

Jacobs D.E. (1978) The epidemiology of hookworm infestation of dogs in the U.K. In *The Veterinary Annual*, 18th issue (Eds Grunsell C.S.G. & Hill F.W.G.) pp. 220–224. Scientechnica, Bristol.

Jones B.M. (1950) The penetration of the host tissue by the harvest mite *Trombicula autumnalis* shaw. *Parasitology* **40**, 247–260.

Jones B.M. (1951) The growth of the harvest mite *Trombicula autumnalis* shaw. *Parasitology* **41**, 229–248.

Jones B.M. (1956) The British harvest mite. *New Biology* **21**, 74–86.

Koutz F.R., Groves H.F. & Gee C.M. (1960) A survey of *Demodex canis* in the skin of clinically normal dogs. *Veterinary Medicine* **55**, 52–53.

Longstaffe J.A., Jeffries A.R., Kelly D.F., Bedford P.G.C., Herrtage M.E. & Darke P.G.C. (1983) Leishmaniasis in imported dogs in the United Kingdom; a potential health hazard. *Journal of Small Animal Practice* **24**, 23–30.

Levine N. (1985) *Veterinary Protozoology*. Iowa State University Press.

Mulcahy R. & Baker K.P. (1986) Fleas on hedgehogs and dogs in the Dublin area. *Veterinary Record* **119**, 16–17.

Osbrink W.L.A. & Rust M.K. (1984) Fecundity and longevity of the adult cat flea *Ctenocephalides felis felis* (Suphonaphlera: Pulicides). *Journal of Medical Entomology* **21**, 727–731.

Owen L.N. (1972) Demodectic mange in dogs immunosuppressed with antilymphocyte serum. *Transplantation* **13**, 616–617.

Powell M.B., Weisbroth J.H., Roth L. & Wilhelson C. (1980) Reaginic hypersensitivity in *Otodectes cynotis* infestation of cats and mode of mite feeding. *American Journal of Veterinary Research* **41**, 877–922.

Sato T., Higuchi H. & Saito J. (1965) *Japanese Journal Dermatology* **75**, 331–337.

Scott D.W. (1975) Further studies on the immunologic and therapeutic aspects of canine demodicosis. *Journal of the American Veterinary Medical Association* **167**, 855.

Scott D.W., Farrow B.R.H. & Schulz R.D. (1974) Studies on the therapeutics and immunologic aspects of generalized demodectic mange. *Journal of the American Animal Hospital Association* **10**, 233–244.

Scott D.W., Schulz R.D. & Baker E. (1976) Further studies on the therapeutic and immunologic aspects of generalized demodectic mange of the dog. *Journal of the American Animal Hospital Association* **12**, 203–213.

Spickett S.A. (1961) Studies on *Demodex folliculorum* Simon (1942) life history. *Parasitology* **51**, 181–192

Stogdale L. & Moore D.J. (1982) Feline demodicosis. *Journal of the American Animal Hospital Association* **18**, 427–432.

Unsworth K. (1946) Studies on the clinical and parasitological aspects of canine demodectic mange. *Journal of Comparative Pathology and Therapeutics* **56**, 114–127.

Vollsett I., Larsen H.J. & Mehl R. (1986) Immediate type hypersensitivity in dogs induced by storage mites. *Research in Veterinary Science* **40**, 123–127.

Von Schwalder P. (1977) Lesihmaniose bei Hund und Katze. *Kleinties Praxis* **22**, 237–246.

Walker M.T. & Jacobs D.E. (1981) Studies on the epidemiology of *Uncinaria stenocephala* in British greyhounds: development and persistence of larvae on herbage. *Research in Veterinary Science* **31**, 264–265.

Walker M.J. & Jacobs D.E. (1982) Epidemiology of *Uncinaria stenocephala* infections in greyhound breeding kennels. *Veterinary Parasitology* **10**, 317–321.

Weisbroth S.H., Powell M.P., Roth L. & Sches S. (1974) Immunopathology of naturally occurring otodectic otoacariasis in the domestic cat. *Journal of the American Veterinary Medical Association* **165**, 1088–1093.

Willers W.B. (1970) *Pelodera strongyloides* in association with canine dermatitis. *Journal of the American Veterinary Association* **156**, 319–320.
Willie B.N. & Markham R.J.F. (1979) Deficient cutaneous response to PHA-P in healthy puppies from a kennel with a high prevelence of demodicosis. *Canadian Journal of Comparative Medicine* **43**, 405.
Wilkinson G.T. (1985) Demodicosis in a cat due to a new mite species. *Feline Practice* **13**, No. 6, 32–36.

Further reading

Viruses

ORAL PAPILLOMATOSIS

Moulton J.E. (1978) *Tumours of Domestic Animals* 2nd edn. University of California Press, Berkeley.

CANINE DISTEMPER

Farrow B.R.H. & Love D.N. (1982) Bacteria viruses and other infectious problems. In *Textbook of Veterinary Clinical Medicine* Vol. I, 2nd edn. (Ed. Ettinger S.J.) pp. 269–273. W.B. Saunders, Philadelphia.

FELINE POXVIRUS (COWPOX) INFECTION

Baxby D., Ashton D.G., Jones D., Thomsett L.R. & Denham E.M. (1979) Cowpox virus infection in unusual hosts. *Veterinary Record* **104**, 175.

Fungi

Campbell M.C. & Stewart J.L. (1980) *The Medical Mycology Handbook*. John Wiley & Sons, New York.
Rebell G. & Taplin D. (1979) *Dermatophytes, their Recognition and Identification*. University of Miami Press, Florida.
Thomsett L.R. (1977) The diagnosis of ringworm infection in small animals. *Journal of Small Animal Practice* **18**, 803–814.
Thomsett L.R. (1986) Fungal diseases of the skin of small animals. *British Veterinary Journal* **142**, 317–325.

6 / Neoplasia and Cysts

The skin contains several different tissues and it may therefore give rise to many types of tumours. It is most important to diagnose accurately skin tumours; many are malignant and metastasis is common (Table 6.1). Skin tumours are usually observed at an early stage and veterinary advice is quickly sought. However, long hair in short-haired coats may hide early development of tumours which may not then be presented for examination until they are quite large.

The skin is the organ system most commonly affected by neoplasia (Cotchin, 1954). However, there are some differences in the literature. In a large survey of animal neoplasms in North America 67.6% of tumours of the dog and 44.8% of tumours of cats were in the skin and subcutis (Dorn *et al.*, 1968). Frese *et al.* (1982) reported 38% of 3492 canine tumours submitted for examination were skin tumours; however, these authors consider that the incidence of metastasis of skin tumour to internal organs is very low.

Dorn *et al.* (1968) considered the frequency of skin neoplasia in the USA to be about 450 new cases for 100 000 dogs yearly and 120 new cases per 100 000 cats; this represents one in three of all dog tumours and one in four of all cat tumours.

Middle-aged and older dogs are most at risk; however, viral papillomata are confined to dogs less than 2 years old, whilst histiocytomata predominantly occur in this age group. Dorn *et al.* (1968) reported a median tumour age of 10½ years in dogs and 12 years in cats.

Bostock (1986) reported close similarity of the various types of tumours in dogs in the USA and UK, the notable variations being anal adenomata, which are apparently twice as common in the USA, and histiocytomata, which are more common in the UK. In cats the most obvious difference is in the relative distribution of fibromata and fibrocarcinomata. In the USA these two tumours arise with the same frequency, whereas in the UK the malignant type is 10 times as common as the benign.

The tumour node metastasis (TNM) system of classification should be used when recording neoplasms to prevent ambivalence and confusion (Owen, 1980):

M0 no metastasis
M1 solitary isolated metastasis
M2 multiple metastases
M_s skin metastasis
M_p pulmonary
M_h hepatic, etc.

Table 6.1. Criteria for distinguishing between benign and malignant tumours. (From Schneider, 1978)

Criterion	Benign tumour	Malignant tumour
Growth rate	Slow	Rapid
Growth limits	Circumscribed, encapsulated	Unrestricted
Mode of growth	Expansive, pedunculated	Expansive, infiltration
Metastasis	None	Frequent
Recurrence after removal	Rare	Frequent
Anaplasia	No	Yes
Histology	Nearly normal	Abnormal (imperfect differentiation)
Stroma	Usually abundant	Usually scanty
Mitotic figures	Few	Usually numerous
Invasion of other structures	Rare	Frequent
Blood supply	Unlikely to be adequate	Adequate but tumour may outgrow it
Tissue destruction	Minimal	Frequent
Cell size	Uniform	Pleomorphic
Nuclear chromatin	Nearly normal amount	Hyperchromatic (may be polyploid)
Nucleoli	Normal	Large

An indication of the rate of growth of a tumour is the mitotic index. This is measured by counting the number of mitotic figures in 10 high-power fields randomly examined (magnification ×400).

For example, T4, N4, $M2_h$ is a massive invasive neoplasm with extensive lymph node involvement and multiple metastasis to the liver.

Bostock (1986) compared the relative proportions of different tumours in dogs and cats in surveys reported from the USA, the UK and Australia. Although the list is long, 10 tumour types in dogs and five in cats account for 80% of the total number. The mastocytoma is the most common tumour in dogs in each country.

Neoplasia of the skin and mammary glands in dogs and cats

The occurrence of metastasis of internal tumours of cats and dogs to the skin is apparently very low (Weiss & Frese, 1974). The occurrence of skin neoplasia in cats is roughly half that of dogs (Dorn *et al.*, 1968); however, feline tumours are more likely to be malignant (Moulton, 1965; Engle and Brodey, 1965; Bostock, 1977). Cotchin (1961) reported that there is less histological type variety of cat neoplasms. Most surveys indicate a relatively high incidence of adnexal tissue and fibrous tumours (Table 6.2) (Cotchin, 1961; Moulton, 1965; Whitehead, 1967; Engle & Brodey, 1969).

Some tumours show site predilection: basal-cell tumours and sweat-gland adenomata of dogs occur more commonly in facial skin, whilst canine mastocytomata are more often found in the skin of the hindquarters.

Lack of skin pigmentation in relatively hairless areas constitutes a genetic predisposition for solar keratosis (Macey & Reynolds, 1981). The chances of squamous carcinoma arising in the skin of the ears, eyelids and nose of white cats is 13 times that of cats with pigmented skin (Dorn *et al.*, 1968). Particoloured cats with white markings in these areas are also predisposed. Only one infectious agent, the feline sarcoma virus, has been shown capable of producing tumours in the skin of the cat. Viral papillomata have not been reported in the cat, in which the incidence of senile papillomata is low (Cotchin, 1961; Whitehead, 1967; Bostock, 1977).

In dogs, tumour occurrence shows breed variation. The boxer, West Highland terrier, bull mastiff, basset hound, Weimaraner, Kerry blue terrier and Norwegian elkhound have the highest incidence. In contrast, the Brittany spaniel, Chihuahua, Pekingese, Pomeranian and poodle have the lowest reported incidence (Dorn *et al.*, 1968; Moulton, 1978). Frese *et al.* (1982) reported that 37% of their tumour cases were in Schnauzers which, however, constitutes only 4% of the dog population. Two reports give no breed predilection for tumours in cats (Moulton, 1978; Scott, 1980).

Mast cell tumours, melanomata and squamous-cell carcinomata are potentially malignant. Basal-cell tumours uncommonly recur and only a few cases of metastasis have been reported.

Histiocytomata are entirely benign with spontaneous regression occurring in the majority of cases. Recurrence is common with circumanal adenomata because of difficulty of adequate removal whilst lipomata and sebaceous adenomata provide uncomplicated postsurgery recovery. Local recurrence is a recognized problem with fibrosarcoma and haemangiopericytomata but they rarely metastasize. Malignant haemangioendotheliomata have a grave prognosis with local recurrence and widespread metastasis.

DIAGNOSIS

Visual inspection alone is insufficient for the diagnosis of skin neoplasia. Inflammatory tissue and cysts may simulate

Table 6.2. Distribution of skin tumours in the dog and cat based on histological examination of surgically excised material. (From Bostock, 1977, 1986)

Tumour	Relative frequency of all tumours in dogs (%)		Relative frequency of all tumours in cats (%)	
	USA*	UK†	USA*	UK†
Mastocytoma	21.34	19.15	7.33	7.69
Circumanal hepatoid adenoma	18.29	9.82	–	–
Lipoma	8.64	8.49	6.02	2.34
Sebaceous adenoma	N/S	8.22	N/S	2.34
Fibrosarcoma	5.89	7.42	12.05	25.42
Melanoma	5.01	6.27	1.20	2.68
Squamous-cell carcinoma	3.86	5.39	16.28	17.39
Fibroma	3.15	2.29	12.05	2.68
Haemangiopericytoma	3.15	4.24	1.20	–
Haemangioma	3.00	2.44	2.27	0.33
Histiocytoma	2.54	6.04	–	–
Basal-cell tumour	N/S	4.13	N/S	14.72
Reticulum-cell sarcoma	N/S	3.33	N/S	2.68
Papilloma	2.54	2.26	–	–
Perineural fibroblastoma	N/S	1.64	N/S	0.33
Hepatoid adenocarcinoma	N/S	1.53	–	–
Malignant haemangioendothelioma	1.52	1.30	1.20	1.00
Sweat-gland adenocarcinoma	N/S	1.17	N/S	–
Myxosarcoma	N/S	0.99	N/S	0.67
Leiomyoma	N/S	0.88	N/S	0.33
Sweat-gland adenoma	N/S	0.73	N/S	0.33
Sebaceous adenocarcinoma	N/S	0.45	N/S	–
Trichoepithelioma	N/S	0.44	N/S	0.33
Liposarcoma	0.41	0.38	1.20	–
Calcifying epithelioma	N/S	0.34	–	–
Ceruminous gland adenocarcinoma	N/S	0.29	N/S	13.04
Lymphosarcoma	N/S	0.27	N/S	1.00
Leiomyosarcoma	N/S	0.15	N/S	0.67
Myxoma	N/S	0.15	N/S	–
Ceruminous gland adenoma	N/S	0.05	N/S	1.67

N/S = not separately specified.

* Figures for USA on a series of 984 canine and 83 feline tumours reported by Brodey.

† Figures for UK obtained from a study of 2616 canine and 288 feline neoplasms received from veterinarians for histology diagnosis at the Department of Clinical Veterinary Medicine, Cambridge, UK.

neoplasia, therefore in all cases skin biopsy is necessary for diagnosis. A thorough clinical examination should be undertaken; lesions which have been present for an extended period are likely to be benign and relatively asymptomatic unless the mass is large or (by means of its locality) is interfering with normal body functions. Malignant tumours are relatively fast-growing and may cause a wide range of clinical signs. Examination should therefore include haematology, enzymology and radiography of the thorax and abdomen for elucidating metastasis.

Tissue from the neoplasm itself should be examined, and interpretation undertaken by a competent veterinary histopathologist. However, the veterinarian by his training should be able to assess the nature of stained smears of ulcerating tumour, or aspirated tumour tissue.

Exfoliative cytology

Ulcerating neoplasms may be sampled directly by placing a glass slide on the ulcerating surface, air drying to fix, then staining with 1% toluidine blue or Papanicolau's stain for 1 minute. Surplus stain is washed off with tap water and, after drying, the slide is ready for examination under the microscope.

Needle aspiration

A 1-inch 22 standard wire gauge (s.w.g.) needle is fitted to a 2 ml syringe and inserted towards the centre of the suspected mass under sterile conditions (Fig. 6.1). The plunger is withdrawn and the needle and syringe contents are then discharged on to a glass slide, spread as for making a blood smear, air dried and stained for microscopic examination (Fig. 6.2). A second sample can be taken through a different region. The technique may be used to assess the nature of the tissue in an associated lymph node. The aspirated tissue is expressed on to a glass slide, air dried and stained with Wright's stain, Papanicolau's stain or with 1% toluidine blue for microscopic examination.

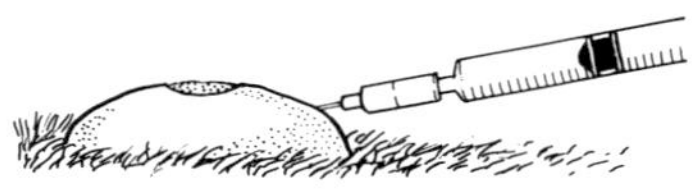

Fig. 6.1. Aspiration of cells from a suspect mass.

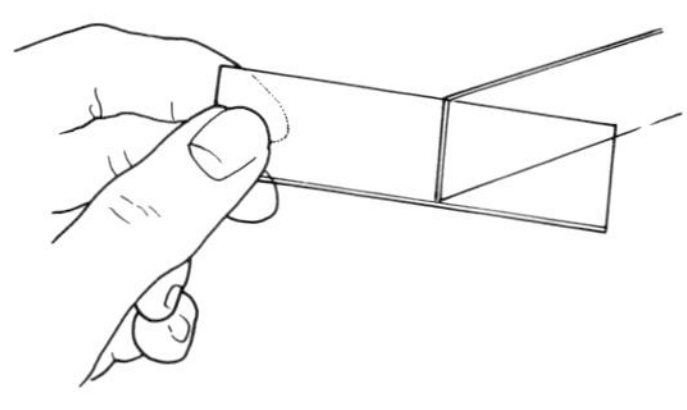

Fig. 6.2. The aspirated tissue is placed on a glass slide and a thin smear made for subsequent staining and microscopic examination.

The advantages of the technique are its simplicity, speed and rapid assessment; the disadvantages are those for exfoliative cytology — only a few, possibly unrepresentative, cells are made available for examination whilst only inflammatory cells may be withdrawn. Nevertheless, the procedure is to be highly recommended for rapid sampling of the interior of suspect masses. Griffiths *et al.* (1985) report the value of fine-needle aspiration cytology in diagnosis. Using this technique the cytological and histopathological interpretation agreed in 105 of 147 canine tumours examined (71.4%).

Biopsy

When a presenting mass is very large it is possible to remove a small representative piece of tissue; this should include a piece of apparently normal adjoining tissue and suspect tissue. However, surgical excision of the entire mass is preferable. Representative segments not more than 1 cm in thickness should then be submitted to the histopathologist in 10× volume of 10% formalin, the tissue being placed in the fixative before drying occurs. It is essential that sufficient detail is included with the specimen submitted for examination; this should include the following: the species, breed, sex, age and results of clinical examination, with a brief description of the tumour, and details of its position, size, whether pedunculated, nodular, ulcerating, umbilicate, mobile, solitary or multiple. Haematoxylin and eosin staining is satisfactory for most tumours and metachromatic stains like toluidine blue should be used to demonstrate mast-cell tumours. Bostock (1986) reported that of 5000 unselected but suspected canine skin tumours, 30% were found on histopathological examination to be potentially malignant, whilst 20% were non-malignant. Heavily pigmented melanomata will require bleaching before staining; the Mason Fontana stain is good for recognizing unpigmented or lightly pigmented melanomata. The cut surface of a pigmented melanoma will leave a black imprint when pressed onto paper.

Tumours are described in order of frequency in dogs.

Mastocytoma (mast-cell tumour) (Figs 6.3–6)

The mastocytoma is the most common tumour in the dog. Bostock (1986) reports that boxers, Labradors and terriers together account for 70% of all mastocytomata presented. No breed predilection has been reported in cats. There is considerable variation in the size, texture and location site in the skin. Manipulation of some masses may result in associated oedema formations, and blood coagulation defects, gastrict and duodenal ulceration may be associated clinical signs.

The TNM system for mastocytomata is shown in Table 6.3.

Patnaik *et al*. (1984) reported that mastocytomata of the skin make up 7–20% of canine skin neoplasms. Mastocytomata have twice the expected frequency in Chihuahuas and are usually seen in middle-aged or older dogs.

Mastocytomata may be graded according to their histopathology.

Grade I tumours are located in the dermis, the cells are well differentiated, in rows or in groups.

Grade II tumours are invasive extending into the subcutaneous and may invade other tissues. There is moderate pleomorphism but the cytoplasm is obvious. Oedema and necrosis is seen. A small number of mitotic cells are present.

Grade III tumours. The cells are more plasmorphic than those classified in Grade II, and other tissues are actually invaded. The cytoplasm, is indistinct multinucleated cells are common whilst more mitotic figures are seen than in Grade II tumours. There is associated oedema, haemorrhage and necrosis.

All mastocytomata should be regarded as potentially malignant and excised with a margin of non-tumorous tissue. The prognosis is closely related to tumour grade (Table 6.4). Bostock (1973) reported that 39% of dogs with mastocytomata were destroyed for tumour-related diseases within 6 months of surgery. More recently, Patnaik *et al*. (1984) reported a tumour-related death rate of 46% in the 4-year period following surgery. Bostock (1986) correlated his results with those of Patnaik *et al*. (1984).

Wilcock *et al*. (1986) examined mastocytomata of the skin removed from 85 cats in Canada and identified two histological types. The first type was observed in 65 cats which had severe, solitary tumours, the cells of which were only slightly atypical mast cells and were benign: seven solitary tumours showed marked anisocytosis and mitotic activity; these recurred after excision or had metastasized within 3 months. The tumours of 18 cats (17 Siamese) were categorized in the second type and in cats less than 4 years old these were discrete subcutaneous nodules (usually multiple), the predominant cell being histiocyte-like with equivocal cytoplasmic staining with toluidine blue, but identifiable as mast cells by electron microscopy. The subsequent history of four cases in the second group was reported; in these there was apparent spontaneous tumour regression within 2 years.

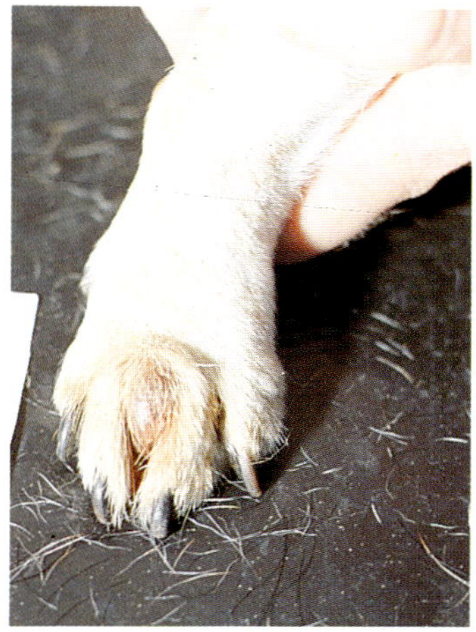

Fig. 6.3. Mastocytoma of a terrier, interdigital region.

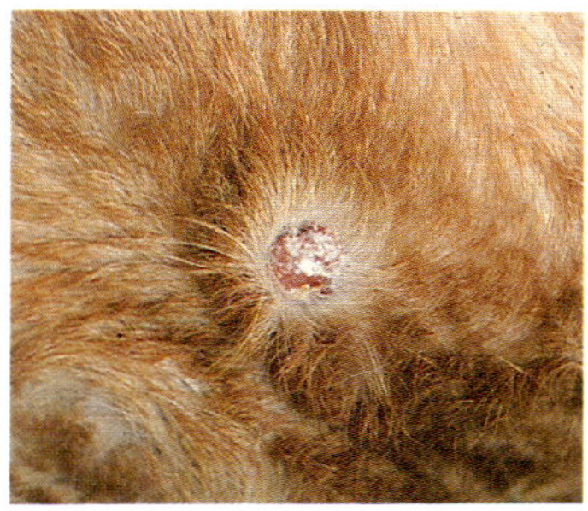

Fig. 6.4. Mastocytoma — a small, discrete tumour of a golden retriever.

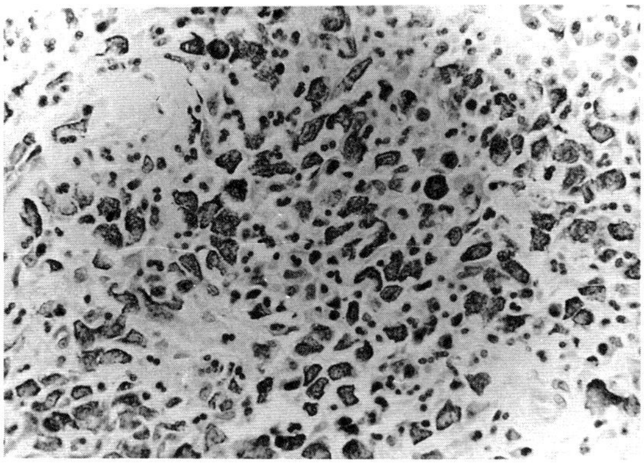

Fig. 6.5. Canine mastocytoma. Toluidine blue stain with characteristic mast-cell granules in this well-differentiated tumour.

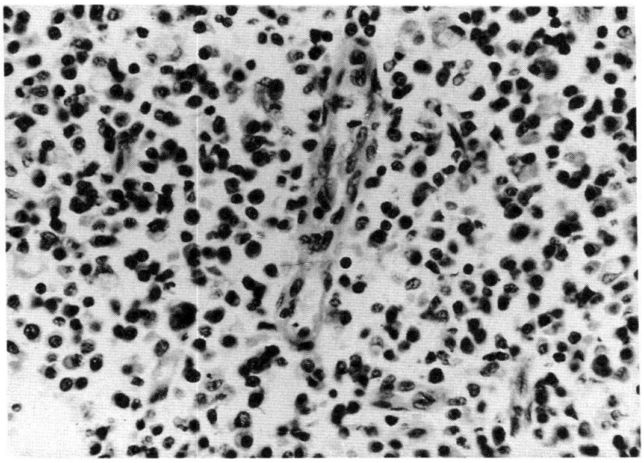

Fig. 6.6. Canine mastocytoma. The cells are poorly differentiated. Haematoxylin stain.

Table 6.3. TNM system for mastocytomata. (From Bostock, 1986)

Clinical stage	Description
I	One tumour only which is confined to the dermis. No regional lymph node involved
II	One tumour only confined to the dermis but *with* regional lymph node involvement
III	Multiple dermal tumours, *or*, large infiltrating tumour with or without regional lymph node involvement
IV	Any tumour with distant metastasis or recurrence with metastasis

Table 6.4. Histological classification and postsurgical survival rate of dogs with mastocytomata. (From Bostock, 1986)

Histological grade	Median survival times (weeks)	% dead from tumour in follow-up period
Well differentiated (Fig. 6.5)	>200	10
Intermediate	64	20–50
Poorly differentiated (Fig. 6.6)	14	80

Mastocytomata in boxers, although common, are usually well differentiated and relatively non-malignant so that a more optimistic prognosis may be given for this breed than others. In view of the potential danger of the poorly differentiated mastocytomata ideally radiotherapy should be initiated but this is rarely available. Therefore, after excision, chemotherapy should be commenced and continued for 6 months using prednisolone. Cytotoxic agents have also been used. However, any benefit is only temporary. Moreover, this is an expensive regime and the owner should be informed of this.

In cats there is insufficient information for detailed conclusions to be drawn but metastasis occurs in more than 50% of cases. Macey and Reynolds (1981), however, after examining 390 skin tumours in cats found a much greater prevalence of cutaneous mastocytomata (about 15%) than reported elsewhere: the results of Holzinger (1973) and Seawright and Grono (1964) agree with those of Macey and Reynolds.

The mean age of cats in Macey and Reynolds' (1981) series was 9.6 years, to be compared with the mean of 10.2 years reported by Cotchin (1961) in England. Tumours were mostly small (<2 cm), discrete, hairless or ulcerating with some predilection for the head, upper thigh and dorsal tail base.

A guarded prognosis must be given, and if the tumours are multiple the prognosis is poor.

Circumanal hepatoid adenoma (Fig. 6.7)

The circumanal hepatoid glands are modified sebaceous glands encircling the anus lateral to the prepuce. Circumanal hepatoid adenomata occur only in dogs, with a male to female ratio of 8 : 1. However in the USA both sexes of cocker spaniels show an extremely high risk. There is a predisposition in beagles, British bulldogs and cocker spaniels (Hayes & Wilson, 1977). It is the second most common canine skin tumour in the UK and the USA, and ranks third in frequency of diagnosis after those of the skin and testis (Hayes & Wilson, 1977).

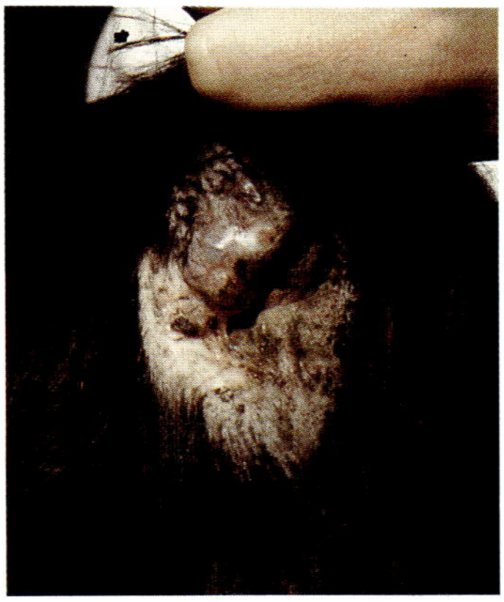

Fig. 6.7. Circumanal hepatoid gland tumour of a 12-year-old mongrel.

Whilst benign neoplasia is very common, malignancy is rare. In the former the cells are well differentiated and normally orientated. These tumours mostly occur in old male dogs and there is least occurrence in middle-aged to old, spayed females. Histopathologically, benign tumours are composed of well-differentiated hepatoid cells with occasional cystic ducts typical of the normal gland (Fig. 6.8).

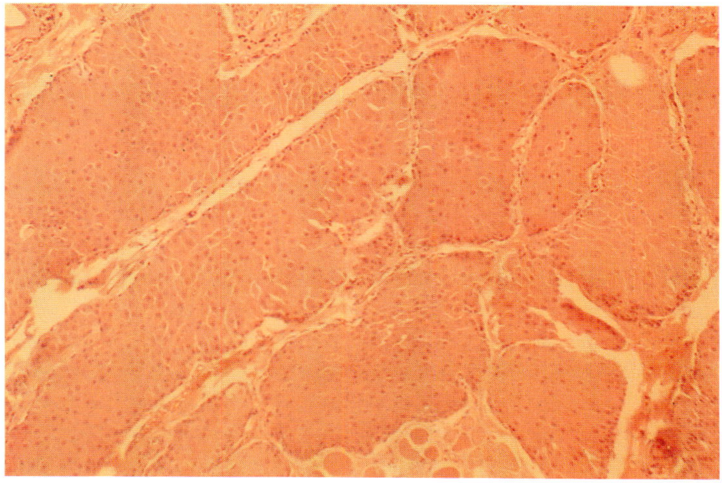

Fig. 6.8. Circumanal hepatoid gland tumour. Well-differentiated glandular acini.

When aspirated tissue or impression smears are examined, malignancy is indicated by pleomorphic cells with invasion of the surrounding tissue. Malignant tumours may be large but slow-growing and ulcerating. Satellite masses in the pelvic canal may produce tenesmus. Tumours of the hepatoid glands of the prepuce may also be large.

Tumours of the apocrine glands which surround the anal sac are usually malignant adenocarcinomata. Curiously, they may be associated with pseudohypoparathyroidism (Hause *et al.*, 1981).

THERAPY

Castration is the therapy of choice. If this does not produce the desired response, oestradiol may be considered (however, long-term therapy may result in bone-marrow depression and regrowth occurs once therapy is withdrawn). It may be given by a single intramuscular injection 0.5–2.0 mg or three weekly intralesional injections of 10–20 mg diethylstilboestrol, if available. Tardak and megestrol acetate are alternatives. Surgical excision is not advisable. A poor prognosis must be given for malignant tumours. These are invasive and metastasize readily to the local lymphatics, with narrowing of the pelvic canal, and distally to the liver and lungs. For malignant tumours, castration is not beneficial and oestradiol therapy is not satisfactory. If possible the tumour should be removed and systemic oestradiol therapy prescribed; however, the incidence of recurrence within 6 months of excision is very high. Gillette (1976) reported that radiotherapy for malignant tumours gave results no better than excision.

Lipoma

Bostock (1986) listed the lipoma as ranking third in order of occurrence in the dog but less common in cats (about 6% of total). They are tumours of fat cells located in the subcutaneous tissue and are more common in obese animals.

Lipomata occur most frequently in the thorax, abdomen and forelimbs. Often they are quite large, when presented (2 cm) and are spherical and somewhat rubbery in texture with a thin capsule, freely movable, and well delineated. They may become very large with associated haemorrhage and necrosis.

When lipomata are aspirated often only a few large cells are found in oily fluid. Lipomata float in 10% formalin and may be single or multiple. They do not ulcerate and are covered by hair.

In dogs lipomata are reported most commonly in cocker spaniels, dachshunds, Weimaraners, Labradors and smaller terriers (Brodey, 1970; Bostock, 1977). Lipomata are less common in cats and breed predilection is not reported.

Uncommonly, infiltrating fibromata are seen. These are ill-defined, are usually located in the upper limbs and may become large enough to hinder movement; they are non-encapsulated and may involve muscles, separating the fibres.

The adipose tissue in lipomata is similar histologically to normal adipose tissue there is a thin capsule and a uniform mass of large cells with small, dense nuclei.

Malignant lipomata (liposarcomata) are rare; however, they frequently metastasize but surgical excision will give a good prognosis in both dogs and cats (Strafuss & Bozarth, 1973; Scott, 1980). They are most common in dachshunds and Brittany spaniels (Strafuss & Bozarth, 1973). Liposarcomata are poorly delineated or firm. The cells are not uniform and are vacuolated, mitoses are common and the nuclei are larger and pale staining compared with lipomata cells.

THERAPY

The surgical excision of encapsulated tumours presents no problem. Careful and meticulous dissection of the infiltrating type will be necessary and it may not always be possible to remove all the infiltrating tissue. However, growth is slow and metastasis rare. The removal of a large infiltrating tumour may prolong life and permit greater activity.

Sebaceous adenoma

This is a very common canine neoplasm and is probably under reported in tumour series. Many old dogs show nodular evidence of sebaceous hyperplasia; sebaceous adenomata are often multiple, but because of their small size they are not reported.

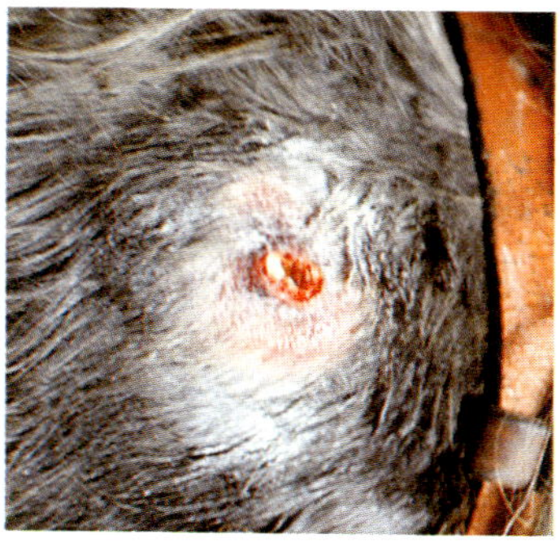

Fig. 6.9. Canine sebaceous adenoma on the shoulder.

Nodular hyperplasia is more common than true adenomata. The former may be multiple, small (≈ 1 cm), circumscribed, flat elevations which may be verrucose in appearance and often have a pedicle. They are usually hairless. They may be located all over the body and may break with pressure to reveal their creamy contents. In contrast true adenomata are usually large when presented (≈ 2 cm), domed and without a pedicle (Fig. 6.9).

Bostock (1986) reports no sex predisposition but states that cocker spaniels, poodles and terriers develop sebaceous adenomata more than other breeds. In contrast, they are relatively uncommon in cats.

Histological examination is necessary for differentiation. In sebaceous hyperplasia the normal glandular and well-differentiated architecture is apparent. Adenomata are well demarcated from the surrounding tissue but the cells do not form obvious acini — there are admixtures of mature sebaceous cells and germinating (reserve) cells with a few mitotic figures (Fig. 6.10).

In contrast, sebaceous adenocarcinomata infiltrate the surrounding tissue. Most cells are reserve cells and there will be numerous mitotic figures with little differentiation. Sebaceous adenocarcinomata are single, rapidly growing and often ulcerating.

THERAPY

Sebaceous-gland tumours are often multiple and there may be too many for complete surgical removal. However, regular clinical inspection is advisable and if ulceration occurs histopathological examination should be undertaken to determine the nature of the tumour. Surgical excision is the treatment of choice. Adenocarcinomata may recur at the site of excision therefore wide excision is advised.

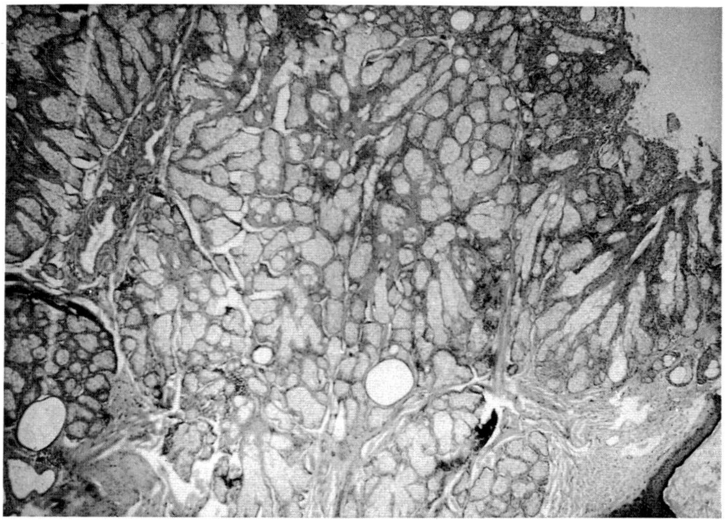

Fig. 6.10. Canine sebaceous adenoma.

Sebaceous hyperplasia may recur at other sites after excision and therefore owners should be advised of this possibility.

Melanoma

Melanomata are common in dogs and uncommon in cats. They are derived from melanocytes — dendritic cells in the basal layer of the epidermis which pass their pigment to epidermal cells. Phagocytic cells which have engulfed melanin are termed melanophages.

The aetiology is uncertain; however, in humans there is a definite association with increased solar radiation, with increasing incidence and higher death rate closer to the equator. Also the occurrence in Caucasian populations is six to seven times that in black populations in the same geographic localities. In humans there is no difference in incidence between the sexes (Sober *et al.*, 1979) but in dogs melanomata are more common in the male. Black-skinned dogs are more often affected, and the following breeds are definitely predisposed: Scottish terriers, Border terriers, Airedales, cocker spaniels, boxers, Irish setters, Irish terriers, chows and Chihuahuas (Cotchin, 1955; Head, 1965; Brodey, 1970). Tumours of melanocytes make up 9–20% of canine skin tumours in various nerves (Moulton, 1978). They are much less common in cats — 2% was reported by Cotchin (1954) and Moulton (1978) (Fig. 6.11).

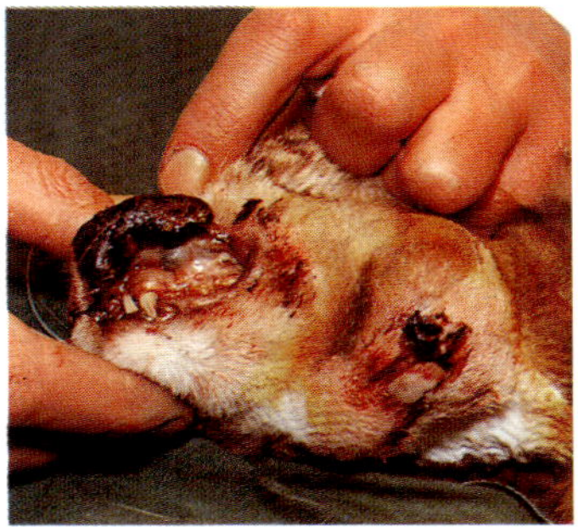

Fig. 6.11. Cat melanoma.

Melanomata may occur anywhere in the skin but more particularly on the face, trunk, the base of the tail, scrotum and hindquarters. The buccal cavity is the most common site in dogs, where 90% are malignant, although most skin melanomata are benign (Moulton, 1965). No predilection is reported in cats.

Benign melanomata are well-defined, very pigmented, dome shaped masses which are not moveable (Fig. 6.12). Malignant melanomata grow rapidly, ulcerate readily, infiltrate surrounding tissues, are less mobile and show variable pigmentation (Fig. 6.13). Melanomata are not encapsulated but benign tumours are well defined from the surrounding tissue. Rapidly growing, malignant tumours are composed of spindle shaped cells in bundles or whorls. To the naked eye, melanoma, haemangioma and haemangiosarcoma resemble each other; however, the melanoma if cut, blotted and then pressed on to white tissue, leaves a *black* imprint.

Weiss and Frese (1974) divide melanomata into seven types on the basis of their histological character. Table 6.5 gives the prognosis according to histological type. However, Bostock (1986) warns that approximately 10% of 'benign' tumours do metastasize with subsequent death, compared to about 50% of tumours described as malignant.

Macey and Reynolds (1981) warn that some feline non-melanocytic tumours may be heavily pigmented and so mistaken for melanomata.

Metastasis occurs by the lymphatic and vascular system. The regional lymph nodes are first affected, with the lungs being the most common visceral site.

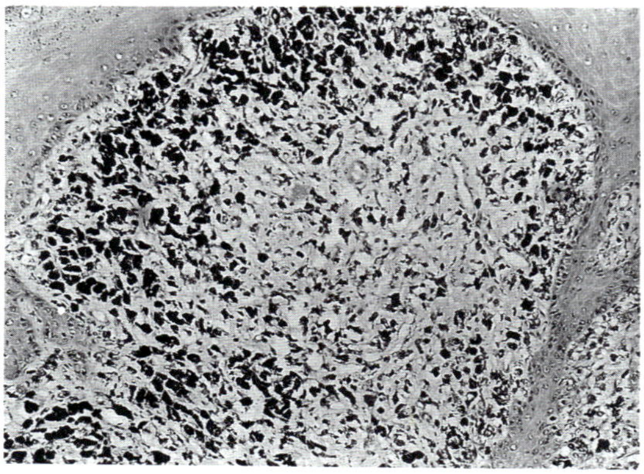

Fig. 6.12. Benign melanoma.

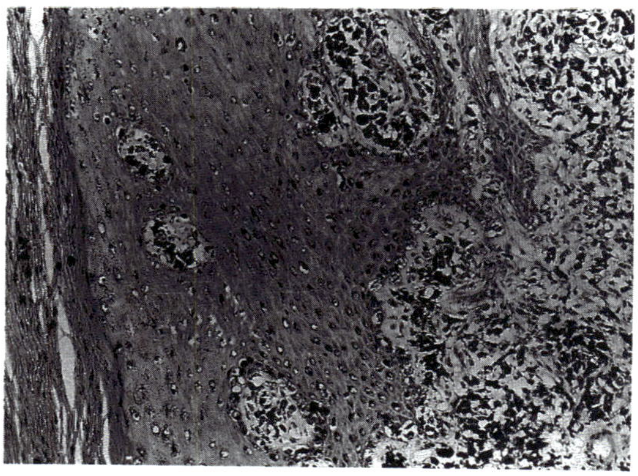

Fig. 6.13. Malignant melanoma.

Table 6.5. Histological classification and postsurgical survival rate of dogs with melanomata. (From Bostock, 1979)

Type of melanoma	Median survival time (weeks)	% dead from tumours after 2 years
Benign		
With junctional activity*	112	10
Cellular	120	10
Fibromatous type	98	11
Malignant		
Epithelioid	24	73
Spindle	75	40
Mixed	66	37
Dendritic and whorled	56	40

THERAPY

Melanomata should be completely excised and submitted for histopathological examination. A good prognosis can be given for benign tumours. Malignant tumours should be given a guarded prognosis; radical excision is essential. After excision bacille Calmette–Guérin (BCG) vaccine has been used by intradermal injection. No clinical trial results are available to assess its efficacy.

One in four melanomata will have metastasized to viscera within 6 months of surgical excision. If metastasis has not occurred after 1 year a good prognosis can be given.

Histiocytoma

Whilst these are relatively common tumours, they are benign and reported only in dogs. Some authorities consider them to be non-neoplastic inflammatory reactions but no infectious agents have been documented.

The histiocytoma is a tumour of mostly young dogs aged less than 2 years. Histologically histiocytomata have the features of rapid growth but they remain small and disappear spontaneously with age. They tend to be located on the extremities and are not more than 2 cm in diameter (usually ≈ 1 cm), firm and freely mobile, raised and hairless or comparatively hairless and sometimes ulcerated (Fig. 6.14).

Taylor *et al.* (1969) state that histiocytomata are more common in boxers and dachshunds.

Histologically, histiocytomata have a high mitotic index (less than 10), the cells are ovoid with large nuclei and abundant

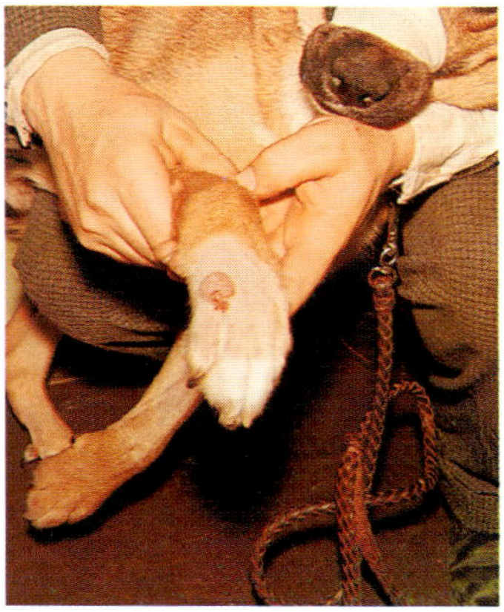

Fig. 6.14. Histiocytoma.

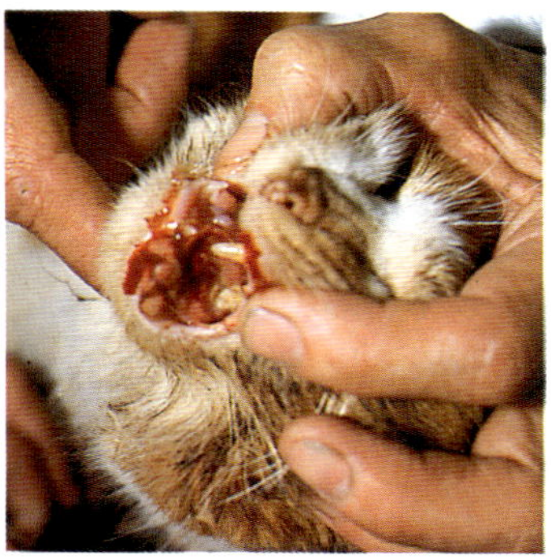

Fig. 6.15. Squamous-cell carcinoma of the lips.

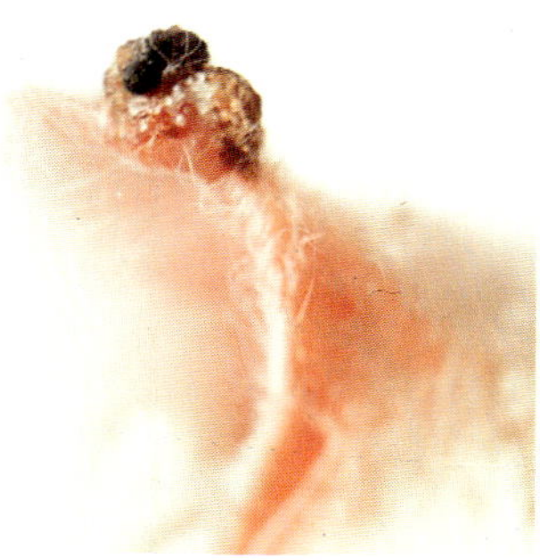

Fig. 6.16. Squamous-cell carcinoma of the ear.

cytoplasm. The evidence of ultrastructural characteristics and cytochemical staining indicates that they are histiocytes, while reticular aggregation within them may mean that the tumour is virally induced (Glick *et al.*, 1976). Although apparently malignant histologically, a very good prognosis can be given. After excision, they do not metastasize and they spontaneously regress.

Squamous-cell carcinoma

In the past, these have been overdiagnosed and are less common in dogs than is usually considered. In contrast, they are common in cats. The prevalence is greater in free-roaming white cats or cats with white extremities, particularly the ears. White cats are 13 times more susceptible than cats with pigmented skin (Dorn *et al.*, 1968). Approximately half of the cases in cats are on the tips of the pinnae, lips and nose. These tumours account for 2% of all feline tumours (Figs 6.15 and 6.16) (Cotchin, 1959; Engle & Brodey, 1965). Ceruminous gland tumours represent 1–2% of feline tumours (Cotchin, 1961; Schmidt & Langham, 1967). Older cats appear to be at a greater risk (Cotchin, 1961). Ear tumours appear more prevalent in cats than in dogs. The cell of origin is the keratinocyte of the epidermis. In dogs they are often located on the extremities (particularly if unpigmented). The reported breed predispositions are Scottish terrier, Pekingese and boxers (Bevier & Goldschmidt, 1984), poodles (Van den Ingh, 1973) and Norwegian elkhounds (Fig. 6.17). When located in the coronary band of the nail they are very invasive and commonly metastasize. They usually present as single tumours of variable size (1–5 cm), firm, often ulcerating without mobility, indicating extensive infiltration.

The neoplasm consists of columns of epidermal cells extending into the dermis with formation of keratin. If the neoplasm is well-differentiated concentric whorls of keratin are produced (horn pearls) (Fig. 6.18). If poorly differentiated these are absent; only a few keratinized cells are then seen. Desmosomes will be observed in all but the most anaplastic tumours.

In cats, squamous-cell carcinoma of the pinna is initially indicated by erythema of the tips and edges of the pinna. The hair is lost, the skin becomes scaly, the edge ragged, and there is crust formation and ulceration which may extend to involve the entire pinna but rarely metastasizes. Most feline

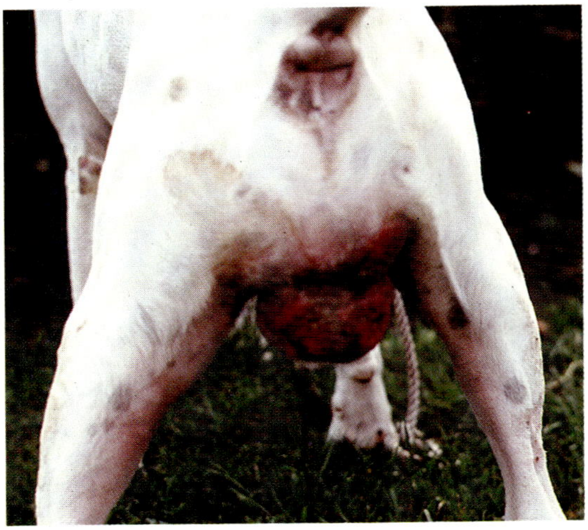

Fig. 6.17. Squamous-cell carcinoma of the prepuce and scrotum of a boxer dog.

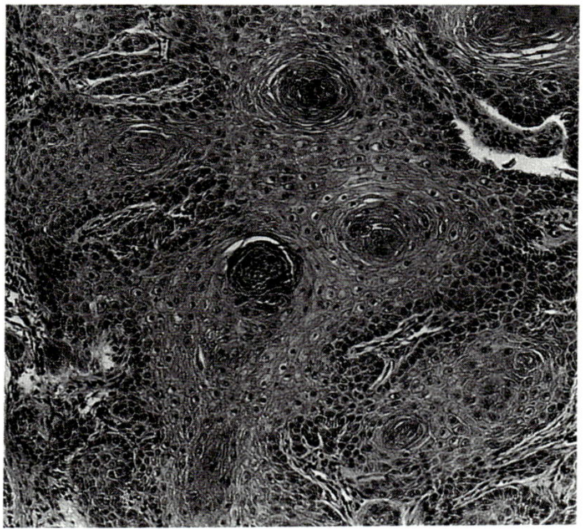

Fig. 6.18. Canine squamous-cell carcinoma, horn pearls.

squamous-cell carcinomata occur on the pinna, nose, eyelids or elsewhere on the face.

THERAPY

The tumours in dogs are slow-growing and well differentiated. Thus wide excision should permit a good prognosis except for digital tumours. These may invade bone, then phalangeal amputation is indicated. Wide excision of the pinnae is indicated in cats, with cryosurgery for lesions elsewhere on the head if total surgical excision is not possible.

A guarded prognosis should be given if the tissue is anaplastic. Bostock (1972) reported recurrence or metastasis in cats between 5 and 20 weeks after excision in nearly all cases (Table 6.6).

In cats, full-thickness excision therapy is advised to include 5 mm of normal marginal tissue. The skin incision is shaped

Table 6.6. Prognosis following surgical excision of feline squamous-cell carcinoma. (Biopsy for 21 cases.) (From Bostock, 1977)

Tumour type	Median survival time (weeks)	Six-month survival (%)
Well differentiated	42	100
Fairly well differentiated	17	0

so that the skin on the convex surface of the pinna can be pulled over the underlying cartilage and sutured to the skin of the concave surface.

Basal-cell carcinoma

The characteristic cell of these tumours is not the basal cell of the epidermis but the more primitive epithelial germ cell lacking desmosomes. The neoplastic cells are small and have little cytoplasm and prominent oval hyperchromic nuclei. The cell is a primitive pluropotential cell and can thus give rise to several cell lines. One such line, derived from the follicular sheath, will produce the trichoepithelioma; a second, derived from the hair papilla, will produce the pilomatricoma.

Characteristically, the cell margins are indistinct. There may be abundant melanin pigment present indicating active melanocytes; this type is particularly common in cats and may mimic melanoma. Spaniels have a breed predisposition to this tumour (Neilsen & Cole, 1960).

Basal-cell tumours are most often observed on the head and forelimbs. They are firm, encapsulated, not fixed and occasionally ulcerate (Figs 6.19, 20 and 21). Regional lymph nodes are usually not involved and metastasis does not occur. A good prognosis can therefore be given, following excision, in dogs and cats.

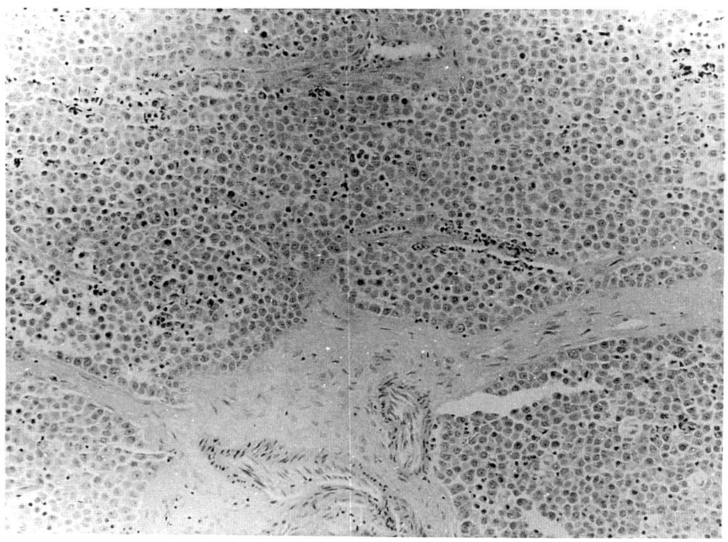

Fig. 6.19. Basal-cell tumour of 4-year-old boxer.

Trichoepithelioma

These primitive basal-cell hair-follicle tumours occur in dogs and cats as usually benign, solitary, slow-growing, often hairless, firm masses, 1–10 cm in diameter. They are grey on the cut surface, with small, white foci. In dogs, trichoepitheliomata may occur most commonly on the dorsal trunk. They are usually non-invasive and metastasis has not been recorded. They are relatively common in dogs and rare in cats.

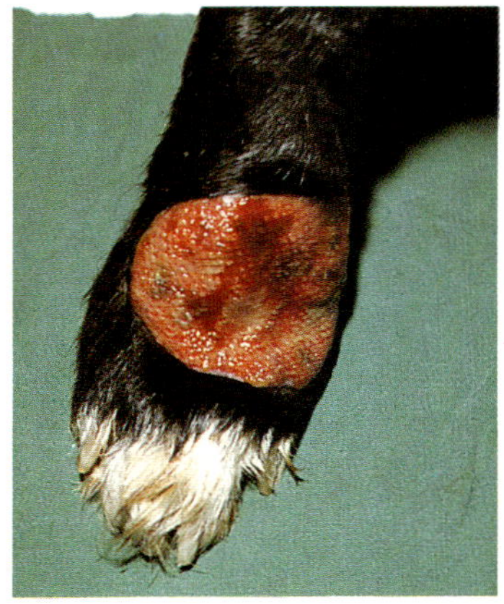

Fig. 6.20. Basal-cell tumour.

Pilomatricoma (Fig. 6.22)

These like the trichoepitheliomata, may be considered variants of the basal-cell carcinoma. They are also benign but are rare in dogs. Poodles and Kerry blue terriers are apparently predisposed (Stannard & Pulley, 1978).

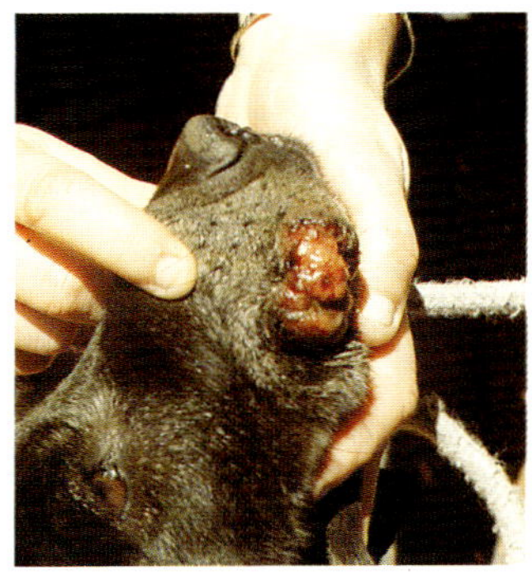

Fig. 6.21. Basal-cell tumour.

Canine viral papillomata

These are common tumours of young immature dogs, not reported in cats, caused by a DNA papovavirus. Transmission is by direct contact, with an incubation period of 30 to 32 days. They are usually multiple and located around the mouth (Fig. 6.23); however, they may be found within the buccal cavity, on the eyelids, limbs and perineal regions. They are smooth, white-grey in colour, about 5 mm in diameter and may be grouped together to form cauliflower-like plaques. These tumours are usually first noticed at the age of 3–4 months. Viral papillomata are host specific, but spread to other young susceptible animals may be rapid. Animals in breeding kennels are therefore at risk.

Histologically, two types are recognized: squamous papillomata with exuberant proliferation of squamous epidermal cells (the more common type) and fibropapillomata with a more extensive collagenous stroma and a less hyperplastic epidermis.

Regression occurs rapidly with disappearance before puberty; however, viral papillomata may persist in immune incompetent dogs.

If they are extensive and interfere with feeding these tumours should be removed: care will be necessary to control bleeding from the broad base of these multiple tumours.

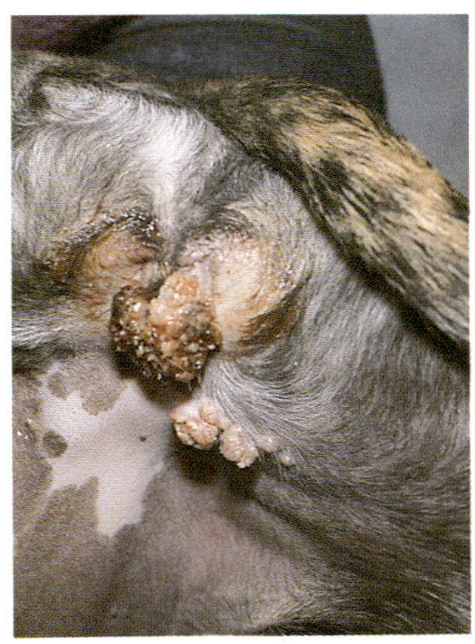

Fig. 6.22. Pilomatrixoma, dog.

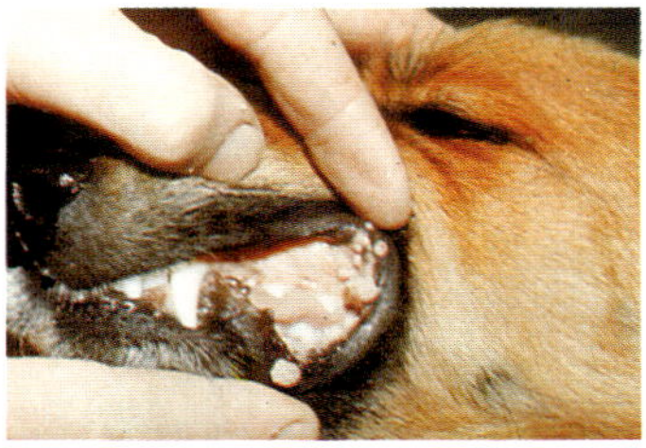

Fig. 6.23. Viral papillomata of a 6-month-old mongrel.

Intracutaneous cornifying epithelioma (keratoacanthoma)

Whilst the latter term is used for humans, the former is preferable for this relatively common benign tumour of the dog: there are similarities but they are not considered identical tumours (Stannard & Pulley, 1978).

The lesions, which may be single or multiple, are most common in mature dogs of 5 years of age or less; they are more prevalent in males than females, and in pure-bred dogs than mongrels (Stannard & Pulley, 1978). These authors found that Keeshonds and Norwegian elkhounds were over-reported.

The tumours are usually located on the trunk and neck. They are firm and often umbilicate with a hard central plug of keratin which is usually irregular with many projections (Fig. 6.24). The central opening has a diameter with a size range of 0.5–4.0 cm; most have an average diameter of 2 cm. Occasionally, there may be no central opening; then the tumour appears to be in the dermis and be cyst-like.

The histopathology is characteristic. The main mass of the tumour consists of the keratin plug, which may be produced in columns and have a feathered appearance (Fig. 6.25). It is produced by a straightforward squamous epithelium, which

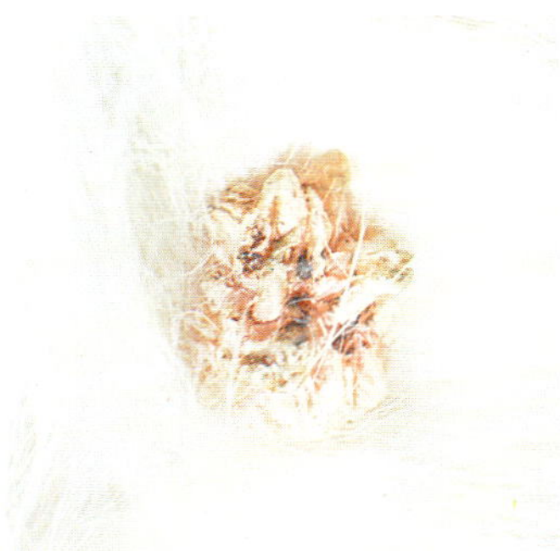

Fig. 6.24. Keratoacanthoma, dog.

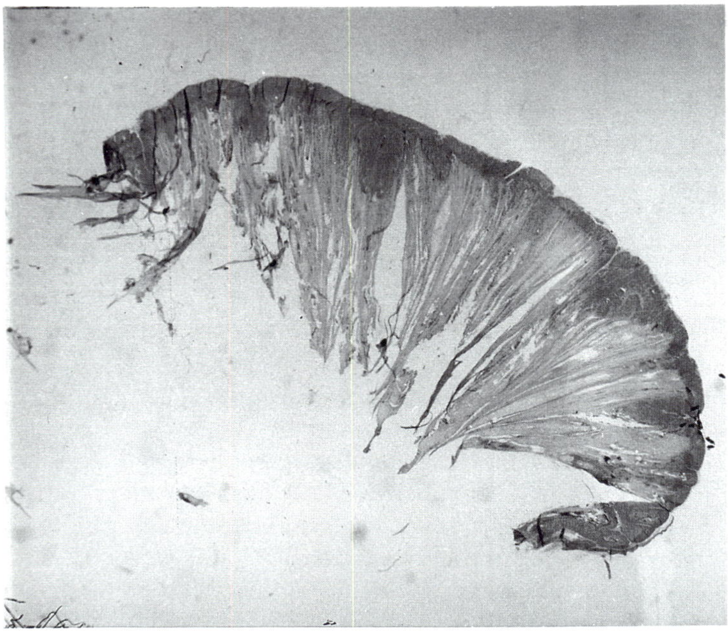

Fig. 6.25. Keratoacanthoma, dog. Low-power section of entire tumour.

is well differentiated with little anaplasia. There is some pseudocancerous insinuation into the dermis but it is limited to the mass of the base of the tumour and does not infiltrate the surrounding normal tissue, as in the squamous-cell carcinoma with which superficially it may be confused.

These are benign tumours so a good prognosis may be given. They should be removed surgically. However, the owner should be informed that there may be recurrence at another site.

In humans, chemical carcinogens are considered important in the aetiology (Ghadially *et al.*, 1963). It is possible that the predisposition of the elkhound type is a result of the effect on the normal epidermis of prolonged contact — with accumulated debris of excessively exfoliated keratinocytes and lipids which plug the hair follicles and become carcinogenic.

Haemangioma (Figs 6.26 and 6.27)

These are benign tumours, usually single, originating in the endothelial cells of blood vessels, most commonly on the extremities. German shepherd dogs, Bernese mountain dogs and boxers are most commonly affected. They are relatively common, usually small (less than 3 cm) and solitary, but are occasionally large. The cut surface is dark brown–red or red in colour. The tumour is composed of many sinuses lined by single layers of spindle-shaped cells with dark nuclei and separated by a fibrous stroma, bluish to reddish black in colour. There may be evidence of thrombi in various stages of organization.

Haemangiomata should be surgically removed with suitable ligation to control bleeding.

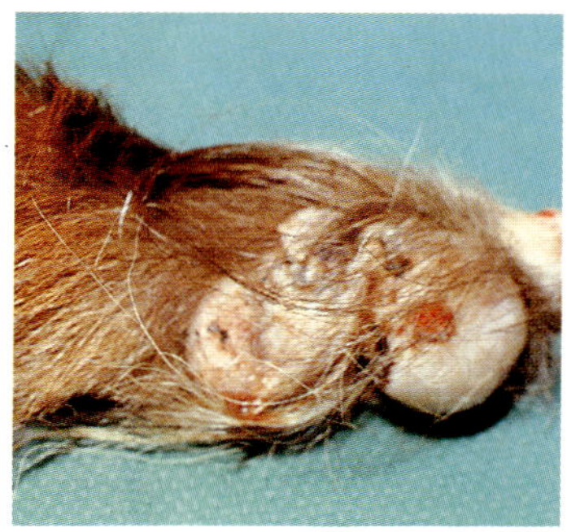

Fig. 6.26. Haemangioma of a dog — tail neoplasia.

Haemangiopericytoma

These tumours are benign, well-demarcated and firm with a diameter of 2–25 cm and most often sited on the limbs. They grow slowly and metastasis is not common. The pericyte has not been definitely established as the origin of the tumour. Canine haemangiopericytomata are considered by Weiss and Frese (1974) to be a subcategory of fibrosarcomata, but the tumours have only a few common characteristics. The extremities are most commonly affected.

Histopathologically distinguishing features are the concentric rings of cells around the blood vessels.

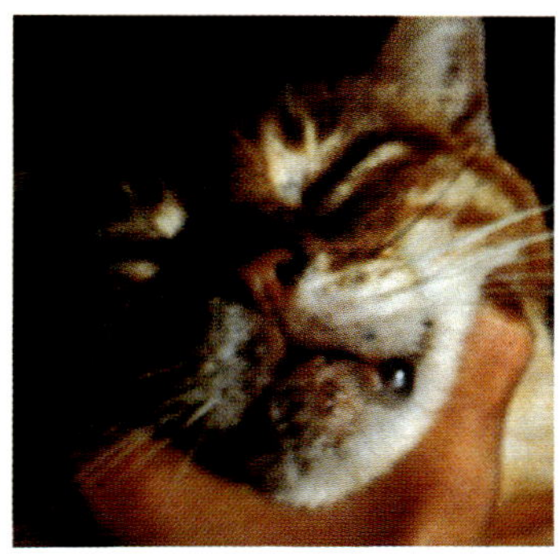

Fig. 6.27. Haemangioma of a cat — mouth neoplasia.

Haemangiosarcoma

These are malignant tumours, usually solitary, often soft and friable. They grow rapidly with ill-defined borders and are composed of polymorphic endothelial cells; erythrocytes will be found in spaces between cells. Characteristically, they ulcerate and bleed easily. Mitotic figures are numerous. They are invasive and metastasis to other organs occurs.

Fibroma and fibrosarcoma

These are relatively common tumours. Fibromata are usually single, encapsulated, circumscribed, but mobile, usually without hair covering. Ulceration is not common. They may be soft to firm, and white to yellow when cut. The cell of origin is the fibroblast. They are not invasive and do not metastasize. Often there is calcification. Simple excision is desirable and a good prognosis may be given.

Fibrosarcomata grow rapidly, attain a large size, invade other tissues, and often ulcerate. They have a fibrous cut surface, and there are often friable areas with focal haemorrhage and necrosis (Fig. 6.28). The tissue is of disorganized interwoven bundles of immature fibroblasts which are fusiform or stellate with dense nuclei, with less collagen than in the fibroma. Giant cells may be present and mitotic figures are numerous (Fig. 6.29).

A grading system for fibrosarcomata has not yet been established. Many mitotic figures indicate potentially high malignancy. Unfortunately, tumours apparently containing few mitotic figures, and therefore apparently benign, may recur and metastasize after apparent excision. However, Bostock and Dye (1980) consider that the mitotic index should be determined for the prognosis (Table 6.8)

THERAPY

Wide surgical excision is indicated because of the infiltrative nature of the tumour. The associated lymph nodes should be removed if enlarged. For tumours in the limbs amputation may be necessary, as tumour regrowth is common. Chemotherapy or radiotherapy are of little benefit.

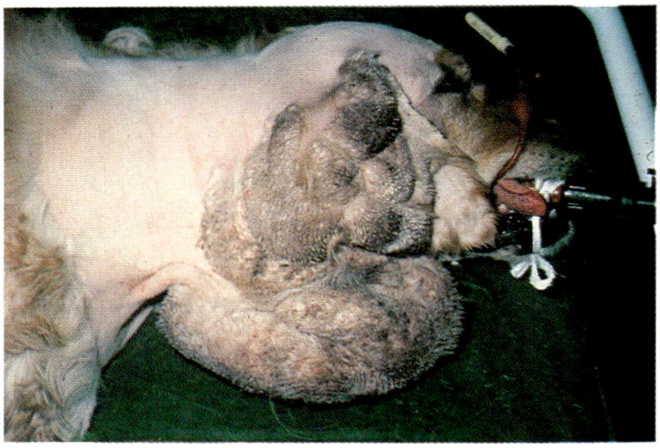

Fig. 6.28. Giant fibrosarcoma of a retriever.

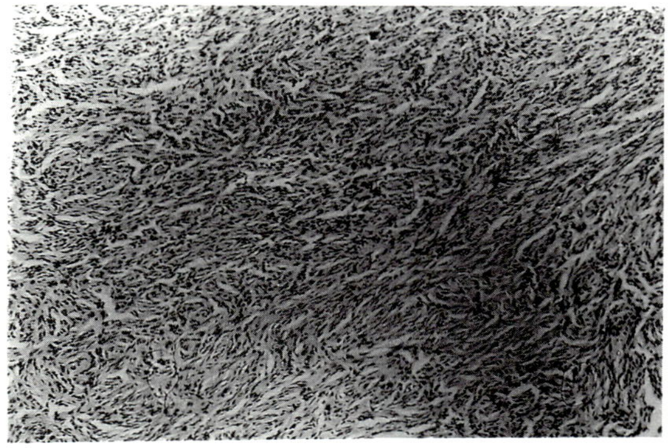

Fig. 6.29. Canine fibrosarcoma.

Table 6.8. Determination of prognosis from mitotic index. (From Bostock & Dye, 1980)

Mitotic index	Median survival time (weeks)	% recurrence within 3 years	% with secondaries
0–8	118	25	1–6
9 or more	49	63	15

Fibroepithelial polyp, skin tag, acrochordon, soft fibroma

The second term is perhaps the most descriptive of these tumours, which are pedunculated, smooth or very wrinkled. They are relatively common in older dogs and cats, particularly in the large breeds of dogs. Skin tags may be single or multiple and may attain a length of 1 cm; they are most frequently seen on the ventral thorax and abdomen. Histopathologically, they have the appearance of papillomata; there may be marked acanthosis and hyperkeratosis. Although unsightly, they are benign. Surgical excision is desirable but advice should be given that recurrence at the other sites is possible.

Transmissible venereal tumours (reticulum-cell tumours)

Transmissible venereal tumours occur only in dogs and have a worldwide distribution. In some countries they are very common (the Bahamas), whilst they are unknown in Sweden. They have a tendency to be most common in intensive breeding units, like hound kennels (Grimes *et al.*, 1964). The cell of origin is not known.

Transmission is usually by coitus and the tumour is nearly

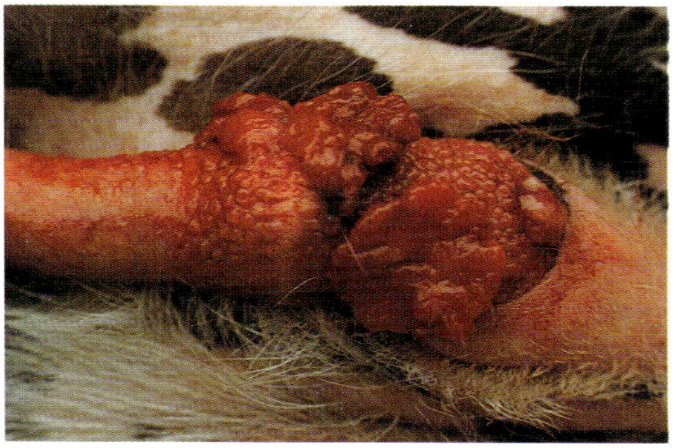

Fig. 6.30. Transmissible venereal tumour around the base of the glans penis of a harrier dog.

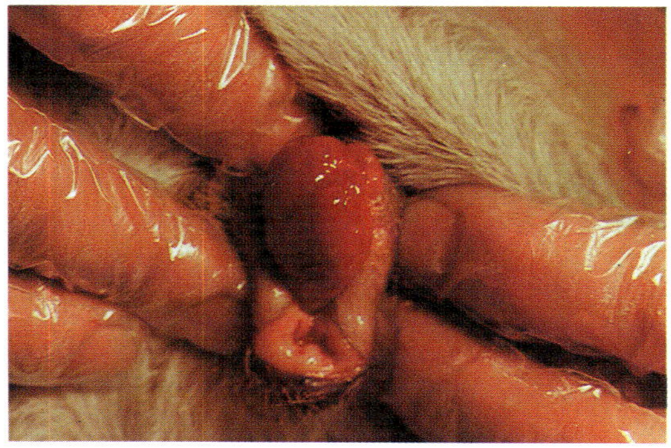

Fig. 6.31. Transmissible venereal tumour protruding through the vulval lips of a harrier bitch.

always located on the external genitalia; however, there are reports of transmission to other sites in the skin, e.g. they may protrude through the preputial orifice and be transmitted by licking, biting or scratching.

They are single or multiple (0.5–10 cm in diameter) and very often cauliflower-like, firm and somewhat friable. In males they are found more commonly at the base of the penis at the crura to the bulbus glandis or glans (Fig. 6.30). In females the most common site is the junction of the vestibule and vagina, where they may protrude through the vulval lips (Fig. 6.31). Uncommonly the tumours may be found on the face and limbs.

The cells are round or ovoid, and the nucleus is prominent with a distinct nucleolus with many mitotic figures.

Metastasis is uncommon. Although some tumours regress naturally, surgical excision is indicated for all cases when first seen. Vincristine, cyclophosphamide or methotrexate therapy give good results.

Schwannoma

Schwannomata are rare tumours of dogs and cats, arising in nerve sheath cells — Schwann cells. They are usually single and found on the limbs. As with most skin tumours, surgical excision is advisable; chemotherapy does not give good results.

Mammary tumours (Fig. 6.32)

These make up 52% of all neoplasms in female dogs, and less than 3% in male dogs. They are extremely rare in male cats but comprise 22% of the total number in female cats (Bostock, 1977). Until 6 years of age, mammary tumours are very uncommon. They are characterized by their marked pleomorphism. There is regional distribution in bitches: neoplasm of the posterior glands is up to four times more common than neoplasia of the anterior glands.

Malignant mammary tumours may sometimes metastasize to the skin lymphatics leading to a rapidly spreading ulcerative condition of the skin with marked irregular thickening of the skin; this development has a hopeless prognosis.

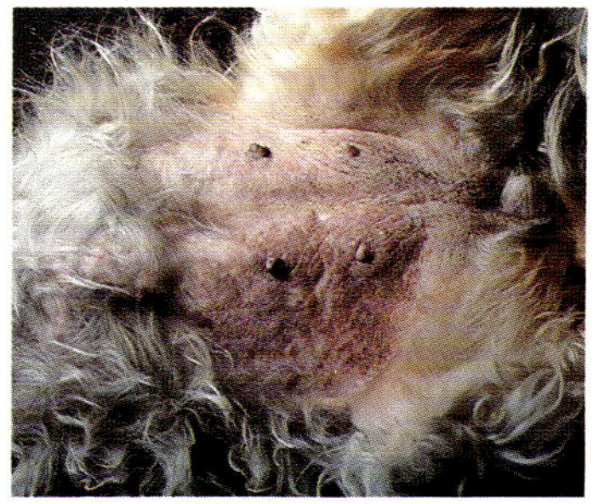

Fig. 6.32. Mammary tumour with dermal involvement.

Myxoma and myxosarcoma

Both tumours are infiltrative and poorly defined; however, they are uncommon in cats and dogs. In character they are benign and metastasis is rare. They result from disorganized fibroblasts which produce mucin. Commonly they recur after surgery because of their infiltrative growth.

Sweat-gland tumours

Tumours of apocrine glands are uncommonly reported in dogs and cats. To date eccrine gland tumours have only been reported in dogs. Apocrine gland tumours may briefly be classified as follows:

Apocrine cystic hyperplasia. In apocrine cystic hyperplasia multiple circumscribed soft masses about 1 cm in diameter are seen, most usually on the head and neck of dogs. By contrast syringoadenomata are single, larger (<4 cm) and firm (Fig. 6.33). Apocrine adenocarcinomata are diffuse, often ulcerated and may simulate pyoderma. All require surgical excision.

Tumours of the ceruminous glands (mixed apocrine and sebaceous glands) are far more common in cats than dogs. They constitute 1–2% of the population of feline tumours. These tumours are mostly malignant (Cotchin, 1961; Schmidt & Langham, 1967). A further danger is that they may simulate the signs of chronic otitis and be mistreated if the clinical examination is not thorough. Examination of the ear canal under general anaesthesia may be necessary to reveal the infiltrating tumour. Examination of the local lymph nodes should be made for potential metastasis, and radiography is indicated for thoracic metastasis.

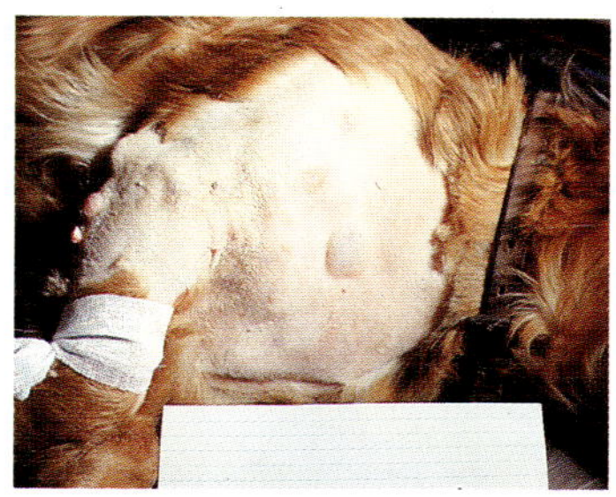

Fig. 6.33. Syringoadenoma on the forelimb of a dog. There is an epidermoid cyst on the chest wall.

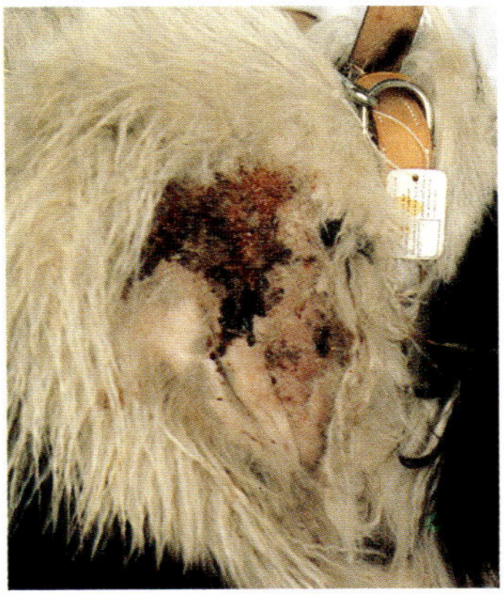

Fig. 6.34. Multiple lymphosarcoma.

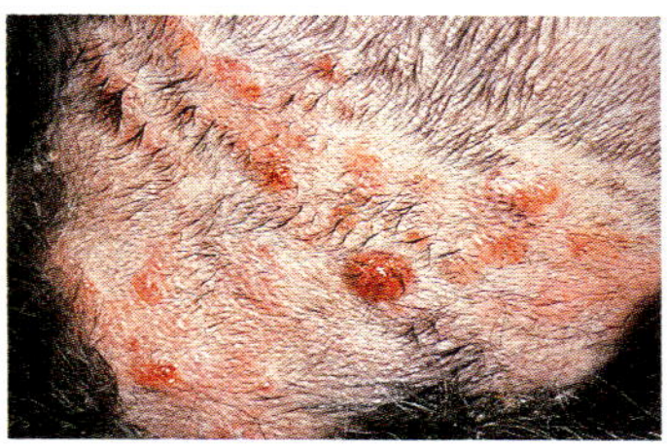

Fig. 6.35. Multiple lymphosarcoma.

Surgical removal is advisable: the lumen of the auditory meatus is exposed by the removal of its lateral wall to permit thorough investigation. Recurrence is common and a guarded prognosis is advisable.

Lymphosarcoma (Fig. 6.34)

Lymphosarcomata involving the skin are rare in dogs and cats. They may be single or multiple. Kelly *et al*. (1972) indicated that the relation of diffuse cutaneous lymphosarcoma to human mycosis fungoides required investigation. The aetiology of lymphosarcoma in dogs has not been determined; in cats the cause is the feline leukaemia virus. The prognosis of cutaneous lymphosarcoma is very grave. For example, of 22 dogs examined and diagnosed as having lymphosarcoma (Brown *et al*., 1980), 17 were destroyed because of rapid progression of the disease; the mean survival time was 398 days and the mean age was 9.5 years.

Lymphosarcoma is usually generalized with small nodules (<1 cm diameter) (Fig. 6.35), pustules and plaques over most of the body. There may be associated ulceration, generalized pyoderma, exfoliative dermatitis and associated pruritus.

Mycosis fungoides is a rare cutaneous disease of humans with a poor prognosis, and Brown *et al*. (1980) classified two dogs in their series as having mycosis lesions on histological examination. The disease may present initially as a pruritic exfoliative dermatitis and may subsequently resemble pemphigus vulgaris and bullous pemphigoid. Basically it is a T-cell lymphosarcoma; histologically it is characterized by small intra-epithelial groups of tumour cells — micro-abscesses. The prognosis for mycosis fungoides is hopeless.

A second rare form of cutaneous lymphosarcoma which may be a type of mycosis fungoides is pagetoid reticulosis described in humans and recently reported in a Scottish terrier (Johnson & Patterson, 1981). This had a chronic inflammatory disease of 1 year duration with the formation of irregular smooth papules of the foot-pad and oral epithelia and were more vesicular in appearance than the lesions observed in canine mycosis fungoides. Fluorescent antibody tests were negative. The authors considered it to resemble pagetoid reticulosis on the basis of a monomorphous neoplastic cell population, the cells multiplying largely within the epithelium.

Both mycosis fungoides and pagetoid reticulosis are considered to be examples of cutaneous T-cell lymphosarcoma.

Leiomyoma

These are benign tumours derived from smooth muscle. They are uncommon, usually single, firm, localized masses in the dermis with a whorled cut surface. When examined by microscope they are seen to be made up of interlacing bundles of typical smooth muscle cells.

Leiomyomata should be surgically excised and a good prognosis may be given.

Plasmacytoma

Prior to the report of Lucke (1987) there has been apparently no report of primary cutaneous plasmacytomata in the cat or dog: the author, however, describes this tumour in 11 dogs and one cat in England. The sites in dogs were the feet, face, lip and ear canal; in the cat the site was just below the eye. All were solitary except in a boxer in which all the feet and the face were affected.

The tumours were firm and raised with partially ulcerated skin and grew rapidly.

Lucke (1987) considers that plasmacytomata should be included in the differential diagnoses of round-cell tumours of canine and feline skin, the prognosis being good. Serum proteins were investigated in one case only (a boxer dog) and found to be normal. The author concluded that this finding, with the benign nature of the tumour, suggests that these are primary skin tumours not related to the malignant disease of myelomatosis.

Cysts

These are benign non-neoplastic growths which probably arise as a result of epidermal faults during embryonic development, or as a result of trauma. They are common in dogs and rare in cats. The contents of cysts may be white to creamy yellow and are usually soft.

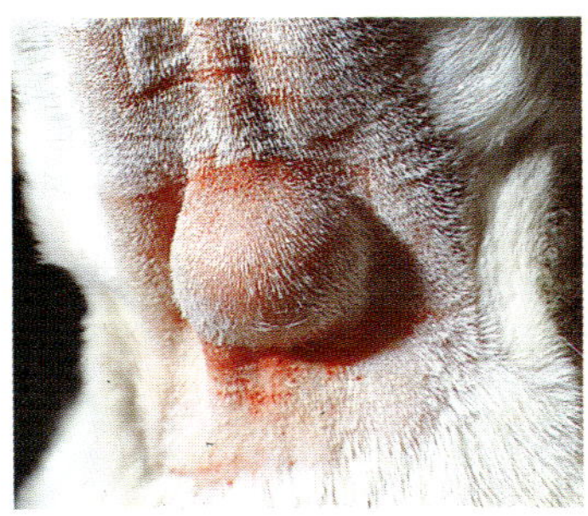

Fig. 6.36. Dermoid cyst on the ventral neck of a 2-year-old Labrador bitch.

Dermoid cyst (Fig. 6.36)

These probably develop during embryonic development. In the Rhodesian ridgeback they are hereditary (see p. 70). They may be single or multiple. The Kerry blue terrier is also predisposed. The dermoid cyst is small (usually about 1 cm in diameter) and firm with a stratified epidermis associated with which are dermal glands and small hair follicles. Dermoid cysts should be surgically excised.

Epidermal cyst

This cyst most probably develops as a result of a puncture wound depositing pieces of epidermis within the dermis where viability and growth continue. They may become secondarily infected. There is no breed predisposition and size is variable (1–4 cm). They may have a central pore and discharge creamy material to the surface. Their lining is a stratified squamous epithelium without adnexae. Therapy is by surgical excision.

Milium

Milia are small, white, firm structures less than 5 mm in diameter. They are usually multiple. They may be congenital or acquired and arise when the pilary orifice of a hair follicle is occluded, either as a developmental anomaly or following trauma or infection. They may be seen in hypothyroidism. Histopathologically they resemble small epidermal cysts.

Cutaneous horns

Cutaneous horns are relatively uncommon and occur in dogs and cats. There is apparently no breed or sex predisposition, but in the opinion of one of the authors they are more common in the Norwegian elkhound. They usually arise spontaneously but may develop at sites of unusual excessive epidermal proliferation, e.g. basal squamous-cell carcinomata, papillomata and lesions of actinic keratosis. Size is variable, usually less than 2 cm. They are thorn-like and project above the surface (Fig. 6.37), and may be smooth or rough. The horn is composed of a mass of compact keratin produced by an acanthotic epidermis with pseudocancerous hyperplasia extending a short distance into the dermis.

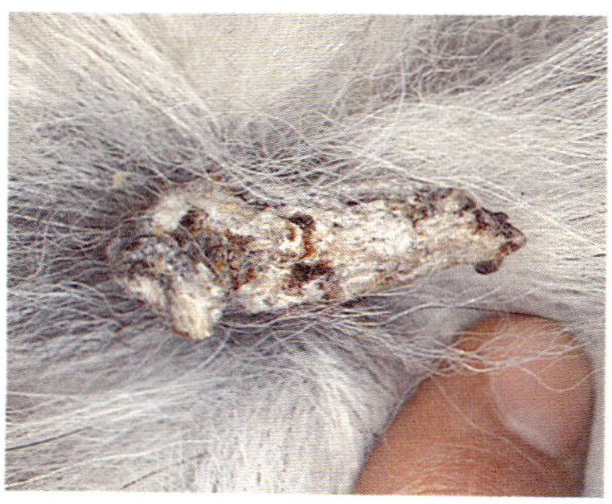

Fig. 6.37. Cutaneous horn on an elkhound.

Cutaneous horns should be surgically excised and submitted for histopathological examination to determine if there is any neoplastic association.

Hyperkeratinization defects

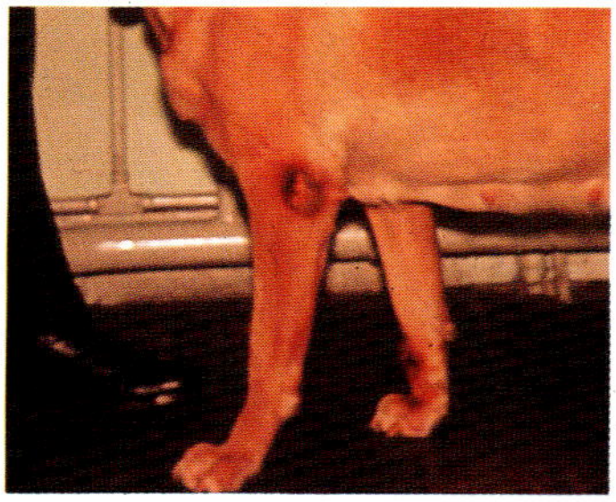

Fig. 6.38. Callus elbow of a Labrador bitch.

Callus (Fig. 6.38)

A callus is a thickened plaque of skin which is a protective response of parts of the body subjected to repeated pressure and friction. They commonly develop over pressure points, particularly in large dogs and obese dogs. However, they commonly occur in small dogs with short hair, like the smooth dachshund, over the sternum and ventral thoracic area, in which cases they may be regarded as normal. They should be distinguished from lesions produced by dermatophytes and arthropod parasites. The colour is greyish brown, the surface is rough and relatively hairless and the shape is round to oval, increasing in size with age. Dogs sleeping on hard surfaces are predisposed to callus formation; however, mature Labrador retrievers, for example, commonly develop them even though bedded on soft material.

Calluses may be ignored after explaining to the owner their nature. Sometimes, they may become secondarily infected, and the dog should be bedded on soft material and the lesion(s) bathed with benzoyl peroxide or 20 volume hydrogen peroxide daily and Siopel ointment applied.

Sporting dogs, particularly the short-haired pointers, may be at risk: often nutrition is poor and the combination of prominent pressure points with hard bedding leads to extensive callus formation over all the pressure points by middle age. The aetiology of the condition must be explained to the owner in order to improve nutrition and husbandry.

The histopathology of uncomplicated callus is of extensive hyperkeratinization with acanthosis; the dermis contains hyperkeratinized follicles which are usually filled with whorls of keratin — milia.

Keloid (Fig. 6.39)

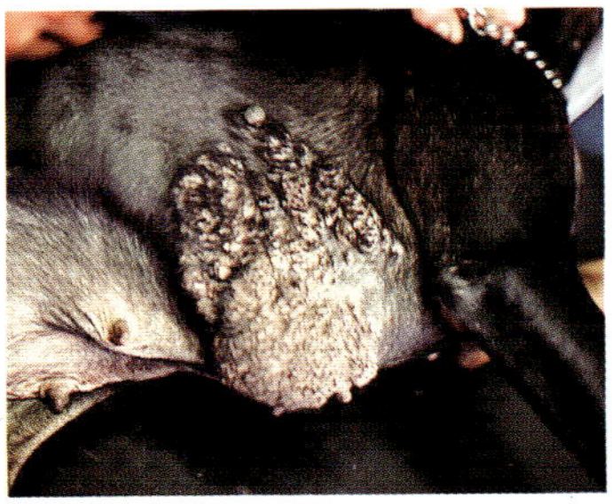

Fig. 6.39. Keloid in a Doberman bitch.

Areas of extensive callus formation at unusual sites have been seen by one of the authors in two dogs, and these bear some resemblance to human keloid.

A 5-year-old great Dane was presented with an extensive lesion 20×12 cm, extending below the left tuber coxa: the area was steel-grey in colour and verrucose without associated pain. There was no history of previous injury and the bitch was not bedded on hard surfaces. Histopathologically the lesion resembled a callus. The mass had grown rapidly in size over the previous 6 months. Following surgical removal there was no regrowth.

The second case was a 5-year-old male smooth-coated pointer. The scrotum was grossly enlarged and pendulous, its lower edge being on a level with the hocks; the testicles were normal. The mass was not painful. There was no history of associated injury during the previous 6 months when the lesion had developed. Castration and removal of the greatly enlarged scrotum was undertaken, and the lesion did not recur.

Calcinosis cutis

This is a term used to describe the deposition of calcium in the skin. It may be localized or generalized and be due to a variety of causes; it is uncommon.

Calcinosis circumscripta is a localized form observed mostly in large breeds of either sex of less than 2 years of age. There is deposition of granular material in the dermis near or over pressure points, which provokes a granulomatous reaction. The skin is raised over the area, which may have a diameter of 10 cm; ulceration may follow with the discharge of a chalk-white gritty substance. The lesion should be excised.

Multiple deposits of calcium are commonly seen in hyper-adrenocorticism and resolution of the primary condition will result in regression of the lesions. They also occur in some cases of chronic renal disease in dogs.

References

Bevier D.F. & Goldschmidt M.H. (1984) Skin tumour in the dog. Part 1. Epithelial tumours and tumour-like lesions. *Compendium of Continuing Education for the Practising Veterinarian*, 3rd edn., p. 389.

Bostock D.E. (1972) The prognosis in cats bearing squamous cell carcinoma. *Journal of Small Animal Practice* **13**, 119–125.

Bostock D.E. (1973) The prognosis following surgical removal of mastocytomas in dogs. *Journal of Small Animal Practice* **14**, 27–41.

Bostock D.E. (1977) Neoplasia of the skin and mammary glands in dogs and cats. In *Current Veterinary Therapy VI* (Ed. Kirk R.W.) pp. 493–505. W.B. Saunders, Philadelphia.

Bostock D.E. (1986) Neoplasms of the skin and subcutaneous tissues in dogs and cats. *British Veterinary Journal* **142**, 1–19.

Bostock D.E. & Dye M.T. (1980) Canine fibrous connective tissue sarcomas. *Veterinary Pathology* **17**, 581–588.

Bostock D.E. & Owen L.N. (1975) *A Colour Atlas of Neoplasia in the Cat, Dog and Horse*. Year Book Medical Publishers, Chicago.

Brodey R.S. (1970) Canine and feline neoplasia. *Advances in Veterinary Science and Comparative Medicine*, **14**, 309.

Brown N.O., Nesbitt G.H., Putnaik A.K. & McEwan E.G. (1980) Cutaneous lymphosarcoma in the dog: A disease with variable clinical and histologic manifestations. *Journal of the American Animal Hospital Association* **16**, 565–572.

Cotchin E. (1954) Further observations of neoplasms in dogs with particular reference to site of origin and malignancy. *British Veterinary Journal* **110**, 218–230.

Cotchin E. (1955) Melanotic tumours of dogs. *Journal of Comparative Pathology* **65**, 115–129.

Cotchin E. (1959) Some tumours of dogs and cats of comparative veterinary and human interest. *Veterinary Record* **71**, 1040–1050.

Cotchin E. (1961) Skin tumour of cats. *Research in Veterinary Science* **2**, 353–361.

Dorn C.R., Taylor D.O.N., Schneider R., Hibbard H.H. & Klanber M.R. (1968) Survey of animal neoplasia in Alameda and Contra Costa Counties California II. Cancer morbidity in dogs and cats from Alameda County. *Journal of the National Cancer Institute* **40**, 307–318.

Engle G.C. & Brodey R.S. (1965) A retrospective study of 395 feline neoplasms. *Journal of the American Animal Hospital Association* **5**, 21–31.

Frese K., Eskers U. & Frank H. (1982) Hauttumoren des Hundes. Pathologie, Klinische und Differential Diagnostische Aspekte. *Deutsch Veterinärmedizinische Gesellschaft*, 188–208.

Ghadially F.N., Barton B.W., & Kerridge D.F. (1963) Etiology of keratoacanthoma cancer. *Cancer* **16**, 603–611.

Gillette E.L. (1976) Radiation therapy of canine and feline tumour. *Journal of the American Animal Hospital Association* **12**, 359–362.

Glick A.D., Holscher M. & Campbell G.R. (1976) Canine cutaneous histiocytoma, ultrastructural and cytochemical observations. *Veterinary Pathology* **13**, 374–380.

Griffiths G.L., Lumsden J.H. & Valli V.E.O. (1985) Fine needle aspiration cytology and histological correlation in canine tumours. *Veterinary Clinical Pathology* **13**, 13–17.

Grimes T.D., Baker K.P. & Winstanley E.W. (1964) Transmissible venereal tumour of dogs. *Veterinary Record* **84**, 124.

Hause W.R., Stevenson S., Menten D.J. & Caper C.C. (1981) Pseudohyperthyroidism associated with adenocarbonate of anal sac origin in four dogs. *Journal of the American Animal Hospital Association* **17**, 373–379.

Hayes H.M. & Wilson G.P. (1977) Hormone-dependent neoplasms of the canine perianal gland. *Cancer Research* **37**, 2068–2071.

Head K.W. (1965) Some data concerning the distribution of skin tumours in domestic animals. In *Comparative Physiology and Pathology of the Skin* (Eds Rook A. & Walton G.S.) p. 615. Blackwell Scientific Publications, Oxford.

Holzinger E.H. (1973) Feline cutaneous mastocytoma. *Cornell Veterinarian* **63**, 89–93.

Johnson J.A. & Patterson J.M. (1981) Canine epidermotropic lymphoproliferative disease resembling *Pagetoid Reticulosis* in man. *Veterinary Pathology* **18**, 487–493.

Kelly D.F., Halliwell R.E.W. & Schwartzmann R.M. (1972) Generalised canine eruptions in a dog with histology similar to human mycosis fungoides. *British Journal of Dermatology* **86**, 164–171.
Lucke V.M. (1987) Primary cutaneous plasmacytomas in the dog and cat. *Journal of Small Animal Practice* **28**, 49–55.
Macey D.W. & Reynolds H.A. (1981) The incidence, characteristics and clinical management of skin tumours of cats. *Journal of American Animal Hospital Association* **17**, 1062–1034.
Moulton, J.E. (1965) *Tumors in Domestic Animals*, 1st edn. University of California Press, Berkeley.
Moulton J.E. (1978) *Tumors in Domestic Animals*, 2nd edn. University of California Press, Berkeley.
Neilsen S.W. & Cole C.R. (1960) Cutaneous epithelial neoplasms of the dog — a report of 153 cases. *American Journal of Veterinary Research* **21**, 931–948.
Owen L.N. (1980) *T.N.M. Classification of Tumours in Domestic Animals*. World Health Organisation VPH/CMO/80.20, Geneva.
Patnaik A.K., Ehler W.S. & MacEwan E.G. (1984) Canine cutaneous mast cell tumor. Morphology grading and survival time in 83 days. *Veterinary Pathology* **21**, 496–474.
Preister W.A. (1973) Skin tumours in domestic animals: data from 12 US and Canadian colleges of veterinary medicine *Journal National Cancer Institute* **50**, 457.
Scott D.W. (1980) Feline dermatology 1900–1978: A monograph. *Journal of the American Animal Hospital Association* **16**, 331–459.
Schmidt R.E. & Langham R.F. (1967) A survey of feline neoplasms. *Journal of the American Veterinary Association* **151**, 1325–1328.
Schneider R. (1978) In *Tumors in Domestic Animals*, 2nd edn. University of California Press, Berkeley.
Seawright A. & Grono L.R. (1964) Malignant mast cell tumour in a cat with perforating duodenal ulcer. *Journal of Pathology and Bacteriology* **87**, 107–111.
Sober A.A., Mihm M.C., Fitzpatrick T.B. & Clark W.H. (1979) Malignant melanoma of the skin and benign neoplasms and hyperplasias of melanocytes in the skin. In *Dermatology in General Medicine*, 2nd edn. (Eds Fitzpatrick T.B., Eisen A.Z., Wolff K., Freedburg I.M. and Austen K.F.). McGraw-Hill, New York.
Stannard A.A. & Pulley L.T. (1978) Tumors of the skin and soft tissues. In *Tumors of Domestic Animals*, 2nd edn. (Ed. Moulton J.E.). University of California Press, Berkely.
Strafuss A.C. & Bozarth A.J. (1973) Liposarcoma in dogs. *Journal of the American Animal Hospital Association* **9**, 183.
Taylor D.O.N., Dorn C.R. & Luis O.H. (1969) Morphologic and biologic characteristics of the canine hystiocytoma. *Cancer Research* **29**, 83–92.
Van den Ingh T.S.G.A.M. (1973) Hindtumoren bij de hund. *Tidjschrift Diergeneesk* **98**, 538.
Weiss E. & Frese K. (1974) Tumours of the skin. *VII Bulletin of the World Health Organisation* **50**, 79–100.
Whitehead J.E. (1967) Neoplasia in the cat. *Veterinary Medicine/Small Animal Clinician* **62**, 357–358.
Wilcock B.P., Jager J.A. & Zink M.C. (1986) The morphology and behaviour of feline cutaneous mastocytomas. *Veterinary Pathology* **23**, 320–324.

7 / Neurological and Behavioural Disorders

Psychosomatic dermatoses (psychogenic dermatoses, neurodermatitis, dermatitis artefacta)

These are conditions in which the damage is self-inflicted in the absence of pathogenic stimuli, probably as a result of stress, discomfort or boredom. Any breed of cat or dog can be affected, although some forms are often seen in particular breeds. Dogs and cats are normally active, inquisitive, free-ranging creatures who dislike being restrained. Modern living conditions often deny this so that energetic creatures may be confined for long periods in small flats without company or stimulation. Sporting dogs may be subject to short periods of intense interesting activity then consigned to small kennels without company. Frustration and boredom may be sublimated to some extent by conditional behaviour, such as compulsive licking or biting, which over a comparatively short period may lead to extensive skin lesions. Sublimated activity may also result from changed circumstances, e.g. the death of an owner, or of another animal which has been a constant companion, or the acquisition of another pet or the birth of a baby on which attention is lavished with the consequent comparative neglect of the subject.

In the clinical examination of such cases it is obviously essential to eliminate other possible causes, e.g. ectoparasitism, local or referred pain and systemic disease. Whilst individual animals may be particularly hyperaesthetic or nervous most cases result from bad management.

All cases of apparent psychosomatic dermatosis require careful counselling to determine the history of the case, after which a thorough clinical examination is essential.

Anal licking

Persistent licking of the anus or perineum occurs particularly in small breeds of dogs. It is not recorded in cats. From initial erythema there is a sequence of acanthosis with hyperpigmentation, hyperkeratosis and subsequent lichenification. Causes other than psychological disturbances must be eliminated; of these, anal sac impaction is the most important. Repeated emptying of the sacs in this condition does not result in cessation of anal licking, whilst anal sac ablation has no effect.

Possible psychological reasons should be investigated and alleviated if this is possible. An Elizabethan collar and the daily administration of 2 mg/kg megestrol acetate may be helpful. However, this drug must not be given for long periods.

Acral lick dermatitis (lick granuloma, Labrador granuloma)

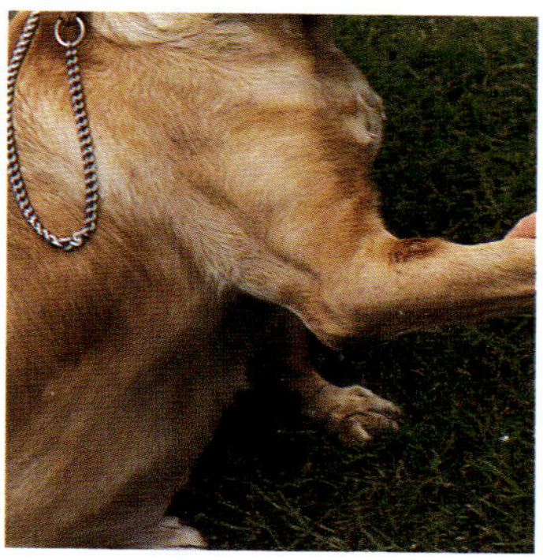

Fig. 7.1. Acral lick dermatitis.

None of these terms is particularly apposite. The word 'acral' refers to the extremities, yet the most common location of this granuloma is on the anterior aspect of a fore- or hindlimb near the carpus or tarsus. Very occasionally, parts of the trunk and tail accessible to licking may be the site. Usually only one limb or site is affected. All breeds of dog may be affected, with a predilection for the larger breeds, particularly gun dogs. Affected animal are commonly 5 years old and more usually male.

When presented, the lesion is of variable size — 2 to 10 cm — and the surrounding hair is stained brown. The lesion is a raised, thickened plaque with variable ulceration (Fig. 7.1). It does not appear to be painful. Acral lick dermatitis has some clinical and histopathological similarities to the human lichen simplex chronicus, a disease of unknown aetiology (Soter & Fitzpatrick, 1987).

Acral lick dermatitis is to be distinguished from the acral mutilation syndrome, a rare hereditary condition reported in puppies of the English pointer and short-haired German pointer. In these, loss of sensory perception of the extremities in puppies aged 3–5 months results in persistent licking and chewing of the feet with severe mutilation.

In the lesions of acral lick dermatitis sinuses may form with secondary infection. The differential diagnoses should be foreign body granuloma, carbuncle, fungal infection, neoplasia and callus. Histopathology shows a chronic granulomatous reaction without specific features.

THERAPY

The underlying cause, whether psychotic or boredom, must first be eliminated otherwise licking will recommence after therapy, whether medical or surgical. If small enough, the lesion may be surgically removed, whilst cryosurgery may be used for quite large lesions. Obviously the patient should be restrained from removing sutures by fitting an Elizabethan collar. Following surgery 2 mg/kg megestrol acetate is administered, diminishing the dose over several weeks. Prolonged progestogen therapy is not satisfactory for bitches. Tranquillizers may be used but are less satisfactory. Tranquillizing therapy may also be used in combination with intralesional corticosteroids (methyl prednisolone) or topical corticosteroid. The latter (1% hydrocortisone) has been used in combination with 90% DMSO to aid penetration; however, DMSO is a carcinogen and rubber gloves must always be used when applying the preparation. The prognosis is guarded; there will be recurrence at the same site or another site unless the predisposing factors are eliminated. Veith (1986) considered that each case should be approached and investigated as a separate clinical entity.

Flank sucking

In flank sucking, the left, right or both flank folds are persistently licked and/or sucked with resulting thickening, hyperpigmentation and finally extensive lichenification involving the ventral abdomen and inguinal region (Fig. 7.2). Some animals may hold the folds in their mouth for long periods. It is most commonly seen in mature Doberman pinschers of either sex, but also occurs in other large breeds. There is no evidence to suggest referred pain from intestinal infestation (e.g. trichuriasis) or from lesions in the spinal column.

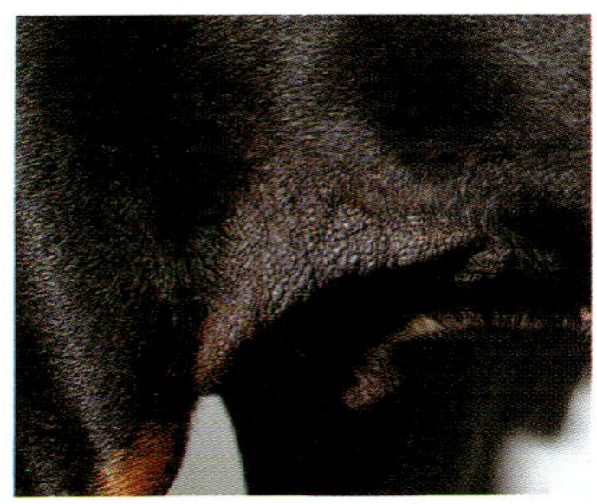

Fig. 7.2. Flank sucking.

As with other psychosomatic disorders, possible predisposing factors are to be eliminated. Tranquillizers are unsatisfactory but in two separate cases involving Doberman pinschers (one bitch) satisfactory remission was achieved with a megestrol acetate dose rate of 1.5 mg/kg for 1 month when treatment ceased.

The owners were also advised to provide more exercise and activity for their dogs. Nine months after treatment had ceased there had been no recurrence.

Feline neurodermatitis

This is a chronic dermatitis with alopecia resulting from persistent licking of an area of the skin in an animal psychologically stressed. It is more common in Siamese and Burmese cats.

The areas of skin most commonly affected are those that can be licked easily — the mid-dorsum of the back, axillary and inguinal areas of the inner aspect of the hindleg (Fig. 7.3).

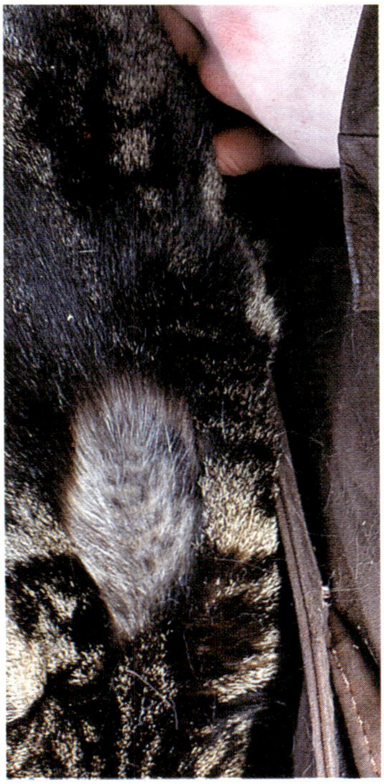

Fig. 7.3. Feline neurodermatitis.

The area is initially moist; subsequently the hair is broken and exfoliates, the skin is inflamed and thickened and feels rough. The remaining hair becomes darker. Persistent licking over a long period may lead to eosinophilic granulomata.

DIAGNOSIS

An examination of the clinical history may reveal a reason for psychological stress, e.g. a house move, birth of a new baby, an aggressive dog within the district or household, the addition of a dominant cat to the family or loss of dominance in the environment.

It is necessary to eliminate ectoparasitic causes and dermatophytosis. Feline endocrine alopecia is usually symmetrical, the hairs are inactive so that they are easily plucked out, and they have clubbed roots with normal tips. In contrast, hair from an affected area in neurodermatitis is less easily pulled out; some or all roots will show activity and will have bulbous roots, whilst the hairs will be broken with ragged ends (Fig. 7.4).

THERAPY

Neurodermatitis will be aggravated by ectoparasitism, therefore therapy must be prescribed to eliminate parasites and prevent reinfestation. The psychological stimulus should be investigated and the problem discussed with the owner.

Elizabethan collars exacerbate the psychological stress and are not really satisfactory.

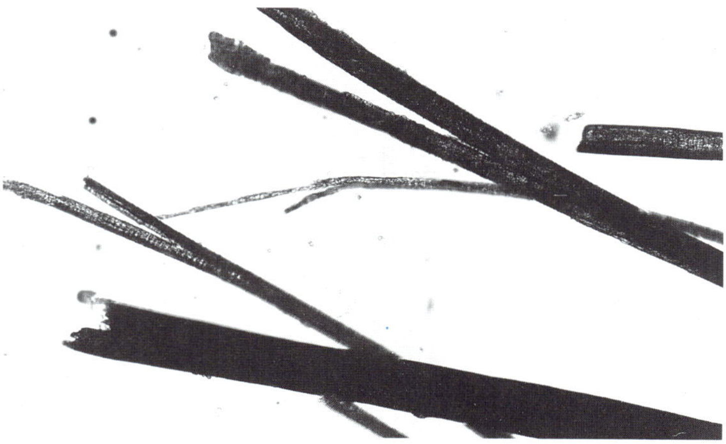

Fig. 7.4. Broken hair tips from the pelage of a psychotic cat.

Megestrol acetate is satisfactory and is to be preferred to sedatives such as phenobarbitone and tranquillizers such as diazepam. The dose rate is 5 mg daily, given by mouth for 1 week, then the dose is halved week by week until licking is controlled. The danger of prescribing megestrol acetate for a long period must be appreciated: its prolonged use is contra-indicated in cats because of the danger of iatrogenic diabetes mellitus. The application of anti-inflammatory, bitter-tasting ointments to the lesion or lesions is not good practice, for these will be immediately licked off.

Tail biting

Tail biting is particularly common in young dogs with long, feathered tails and in older large dogs which are closely confined. In the former, the habit will usually stop after puberty. In older dogs the usual reason is boredom and the vice will be broken if the husbandry is corrected. For both, the possibility of ectoparasitism, particularly otodectic mange, should be investigated.

Sucking of the tip of the tail is seen in cats as a result of boredom, the fur and skin becoming wet but without excoriation. It occurs in closely confined cats — allowing more freedom and combating boredom will break this vice.

References

Soter N.A. & Fitzpatrick T.B. (1987) In *Dermatology in General Practice*, 3rd edn. (Eds Fitzpatrick T.B., Eisen A.Z., Wolff K., Freedburg L.M. & Austen K.F.) p. 1370. McGraw-Hill, New York.

Veith L. (1986) Acral lick dermatitis in the dog. *Canine Practice* **13**, 15–22.

8 / Allergic and Autoimmune Diseases

Urticaria and angioedema

Urticaria (literally 'nettle rash') results from capillary and small arteriolar dilatation with transudation into the dermis and the formation of itchy papules (hives) or wheals. If the reaction is hypodermal, large, itchy swellings result and angioedema may occur with urticaria. Numerous stimuli may cause these reactions: they may be internal or external, immunological or non-immunological.

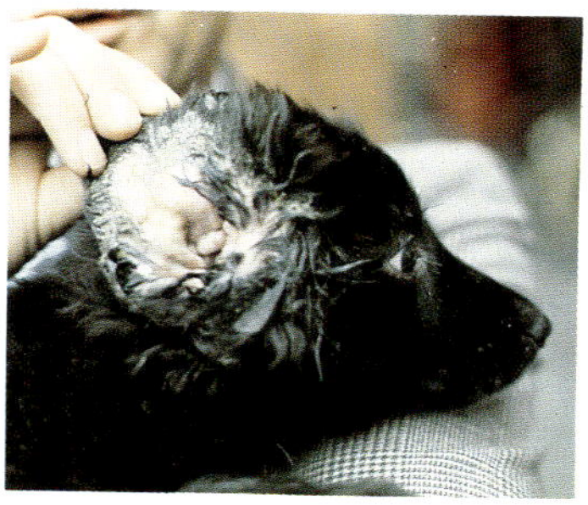

Fig. 8.1. Oedema of ear with transudation — juvenile pyoderma.

EXTERNAL CAUSES

These include nettle stings, insect bites and stings, jellyfish stings, *Sarcoptes* mites, heat, cold, pressure (dermographism), and light.

INTERNAL CAUSES

Examples are food, drugs, infection (e.g. juvenile pyoderma) (Fig. 8.1), antisera, vaccines, blood transfusions, atopy, oestrus, allergen injections, intestinal parasites, and genetic (hereditary angioedema).

CLINICAL SIGNS

Urticaria and angioedema are seen less commonly in cats than dogs. The onset is usually acute. In angioedema the swelling may be extensive and dramatic with marked swelling of the head, neck and forelimbs; serum leakage from the distended tissues may occur after a few days. In urticaria the swelling is superficial, less dramatic and often accompanied by pruritus; the hair may appear tufted.

DIFFERENTIAL DIAGNOSES

These include cellulitis, lymphoedema associated with generalized demodicosis, lymphoreticular neoplasia, oedema may result from manipulation of some mast-cell tumours.

DIAGNOSIS

This may be difficult and the history and a thorough clinical examination will be helpful, bearing in mind the possible aetiological factors. Examination of hives may reveal central puncta, skin scrapes may reveal *Sarcoptes* or *Demodex*. However, in many cases it will not be possible to determine the cause.

The histopathology is not specific; there is dilatation of the vascular network and associated oedema with moderate infiltration of inflammatory cells.

TREATMENT

Where life is threatened as a result of oedema of the upper respiratory tract, an adrenaline injection (1 : 1000 <0.5 ml) given intramuscularly or subcutaneously is advisable. Antihistamines are not of value for the treatment of angioedema and urticaria. Prednisolone (2 mg/kg) may be given orally or by intramuscular injection. In all cases thorough investigation is desirable to identify and remove the stimulus where possible.

Allergic diseases

Allergy is the result of an immunologically mediated reaction to an environmental allergen manifested by clinical reactions on exposure to the allergen. It is to be contrasted to immunological defence against pathogens, toxins and neoplasms, in which there is recognition of the foreign nature of the antigens with the activation of humoral and cellular mediators of inflammation. The immunologically mediated response of inflammation is common to both; in the former, however, the environmental allergen is not usually harmful.

The types of the immunological reactions in allergy have been classified by Gel *et al.* (1975). Types II and III are immediate allergic reactions, Type IV is a delayed hypersensitive reaction.

TYPE I

IgE antibodies attached to mast cells and basophils react with allergens resulting in the release of vasoactive substances and subsequent tissue damage. Examples are atopy, anaphylaxis, angioedema, urticaria and flea allergy.

TYPE II

IgG or IgM antibodies react with allergens on target cells activating complement with resulting cell lysis. Examples are pemphigus and pemphigoid, drugs.

TYPE III

IgG or IgM form complexes with complement and allergen. These are attractive to neutrophils, which release enzymes and cause tissue damage, e.g. serum sickness, drug eruption, lupus erythematosus.

TYPE IV

In Type IV reactions a hapten (an incomplete allergen) in combination with a tissue protein (e.g. collagen) forms a complete allergen which, after processing by Langerhans' cells, monocytes or macrophages, sensitizes T lymphocytes. Upon subsequent challenge by the identical allergen, the sensitized T lymphocytes release lymphokines with resulting tissue damage.

Examples are contact-allergic dermatitis, flea allergy, and drug eruption.

Atopy

Atopic allergy is a Type I hypersensitive reaction to environmental allergens in genetically susceptible animals with the production of IgE antibodies and the release of mediators; the action of these mediators in tissue is responsible for the clinical signs of atopy. The atopic patient may be susceptible to one or more allergens; the house-dust mite, *Dermatophagoides pteronyssinus,* is the most important. Human and animal dander, pollen and fungal spores are also involved. Atopy is commonly caused by drug allergy. There is some evidence that canine atopy is hereditary (Scott, 1981).

Willemse (1984) reported that only five of 46 atopic dogs had a positive response to the Prausnitz–Kustner (PK) test, whilst only three of these were dogs with a positive nasal response to pollen.

CLINICAL SIGNS

Most cases first show chronic signs as young adults of 1–3 years. The major sign of atopy is marked pruritus, which may be intense, often with severe self-excoriation. The pruritus is usually non-seasonal in northern Europe; in warmer countries it is often seasonal indicating the presence of potent pollen allergens, e.g. the pollen of ragweed (which is not found in Europe). If the pruritus is seasonal an association with pollen should be considered. The pruritus is usually generalized with marked signs on the head; there is muzzle rubbing and pawing, conjunctivitis with spectacle alopecia, and otitis externa (Fig. 8.2). The skin folds and flexures, axillary and inguinal areas are particularly affected (Fig. 8.3). There is erythema and there may be papules, pyoderma and secondary alopecia. In chronic cases hyperpigmentation and lichenification may be marked, particularly along the ventral trunk as a result of persistent excoriation with the hindfeet, which may induce enlargement of the nipples. The skin and coat feel hot and dry; there may be moderate alopecia.

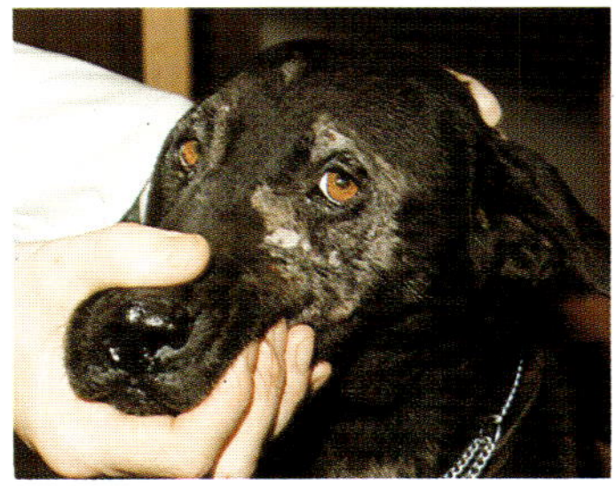

Fig. 8.2. Acanthosis, alopecia and hyperpigmentation — chronic atopy.

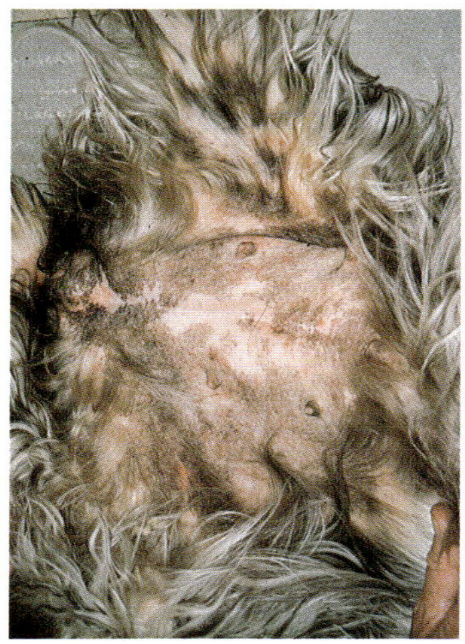

Fig. 8.3. Inguinal lesions, English setter — atopy.

DIAGNOSIS

The differential diagnosis includes all dermatoses associated with marked pruritus: flea hypersensitivity, food allergy, sarcoptic mange, hookworm dermatitis, contact sensitivity, seborrhoeic dermatitis, generalized pyoderma and subcorneal, pustular dermatosis. With contact dermatitis the clinical signs are localized to the areas of the body in contact with the sensitizer, usually the ventral trunk. The histopathology and laboratory findings are not specific. Willemse (1984) found no evidence of increased circulating eosinophils or tissue eosinophils in nasal smears of atopic dogs.

The diagnosis is made on the clinical history, signs and positive intradermal reactions to environmental allergens; however, it must be remembered that the skin of some normal animals will also give positive reactions to challenge.

Intradermal tests

The skin of the allergic animal is hypersensitive, therefore minimal preparation of the test area is essential. A difficulty with the severe case will be the availability of an area of skin not scarred by self-excoriation and papular erythema; for that reason it may only be possible to undertake a small number of tests at any one time.

When tested, the patient should not have been treated with corticosteroids within the past week; the widespread and unavoidable use of depot corticosteroids should be borne in mind. To determine the sensitivity of the skin it may be challenged, after preparation, with 0.05 ml of 0.0001 histamine phosphate injected intradermally. This will produce a wheal up to 2 cm in diameter in sensitive skin within 30 minutes. If no reaction is seen, the tests should be postponed.

With the dog in lateral recumbency an area of uninvolved skin of the desired size is clipped with 2 mm electric clippers. The hair is lightly brushed off; no cleaning should be undertaken. If the patient is uncooperative, control is achieved using xylazine hydrochloride, at the recommended dosage and with the usual safeguards.

Sites for injection are identified 2 cm apart in rows separated by 2 cm.

Allergens and controls are prepared in disposable 1 ml syringes each fitted with a 25 standard wire gauge (s.w.g.) × 15 mm needle, 0.05 ml being injected intradermally to produce a palpable blob at each site, and marked on a grid record.

Allergens. Commercial allergens are available; examples are those produced by Veterinhal and Miles Laboratories (DHS). Some allergens have quite a short shelf life and for that reason some specialists produce their own allergens. Two controls are used: one containing the vehicle for the allergens alone, the other being histamine phosphate (0.01%). It is important to use allergens produced for veterinarians. For example, Willemse (1984) reported that the skin threshold concentration in 45 normal dogs for house dust, house-dust mite and human dandruff extracts were the same as those for humans, while those for animal dandruff, pollen and fungi were 10 times higher in the dog.

Reactions are read and recorded 20 minutes, 1 hour and 4 hours after injection and are considered positive if the wheal diameter is at least half that of the positive control.

THERAPY

The avoidance of allergens is not possible, but the exposure to them should be minimized; for example, atopy may be exacerbated by ectoparasitic infestation, particularly flea infestation, and therefore should be prevented. The most common allergen is house dust and the environment indoors must be kept as dust free as possible; access to bedrooms should be prevented at all times. Other common household allergens are cat dander, feathers (pillows, cage birds) and newsprint. When first presented the atopic case may have a grossly thickened skin which is dry and pruritic. This will benefit from bathing with a mild non-allergenic soap, rinsing in tepid water containing a little baby oil, and patting dry with a cotton towel or blowing dry with a hair dryer. Prednisolone orally is effective for the control of atopy: the dose rate is 2 mg/kg each morning for 1 week with a change to alternate morning therapy.

Hyposensitization

A series of injections containing various dilutions of the allergens to which the patient is allergic is undertaken using alum precipitated allergen solutions (Veterinhal, HAL Allergen Laboratories). The course begins with a dilution of the allergen which does not provoke a reaction when injected intradermally. Injections are then once or twice weekly at increasing strengths until the highest dosage the patient can tolerate without reaction is reached. The maintenance dose is thereafter injected at monthly intervals depending upon the clinical response. Injections are given in the interscapular region using a tuberculin syringe or 1 ml syringe fitted with a 25 s.w.g. needle. The patient is observed for 20 minutes after each injection for signs of adverse reaction. There may be some swelling at the sites of injection for up to 24 hours. If the swelling is unusually large, the next dose should be reduced. Anaphylactic reactions during the course of hyposensitization are rare. Adrenaline 1:10 000 is given intravenously, repeating at 30–60 minute intervals if necessary.

Willemse (1984) reported a significant improvement in 16 of 27 (59.3%) atopic animals subjected to hyposensitization therapy; other authors have published results indicating better therapeutic benefit (Nesbitt, 1978; Scott, 1981).

Food allergy

Hypersensitive reaction (Type I) to food is uncommon in dogs and cats. It is a much overdiagnosed condition. There may be urticaria, anaphylaxis and pruritic dermatitis. There is no correlation of age, sex or breed with incidence. However, severe urticarial reactions are more common in dogs less than 6 months old. The clinical signs are variable and non-seasonal. Usually there is evidence of alimentary involvement with vomiting and/or diarrhoea. There may be depression. There is generalized non-seasonal pruritus usually with erythema and papules; self-excoriation may result in pyoderma or localized pyotraumatic dermatitis (Figs 8.4–7). Chronic cases may have an exfoliative dermatitis or seborrhoeic dermatitis. In juvenile cases there is extensive oedema of the pinna, muzzle, neck and limbs.

DIAGNOSIS

The differential diagnosis is any condition with generalized pruritus, ectoparasitism, atopy, and miliary dermatitis of cats.

The histopathology is not helpful. Intradermal tests are of no value in the diagnosis of food allergy other than for juvenile urticarial reactions to food allergens. There are no specific changes in the haematology. Food allergy can only be determined when pruritus subsides after the elimination of the

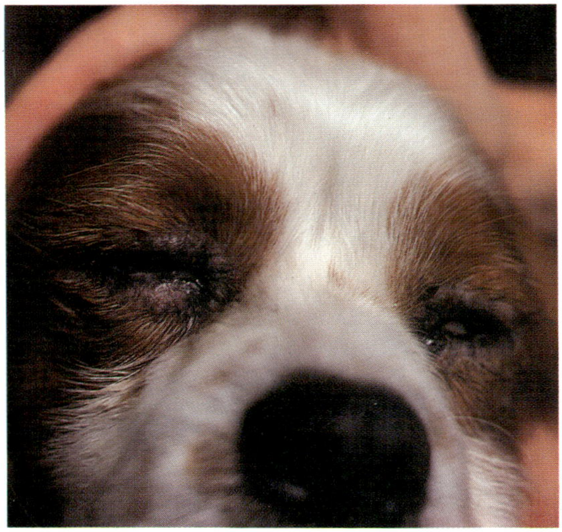

Fig. 8.4. King Charles spaniel, periorbital alopecia with oedema of eyelids — food allergy.

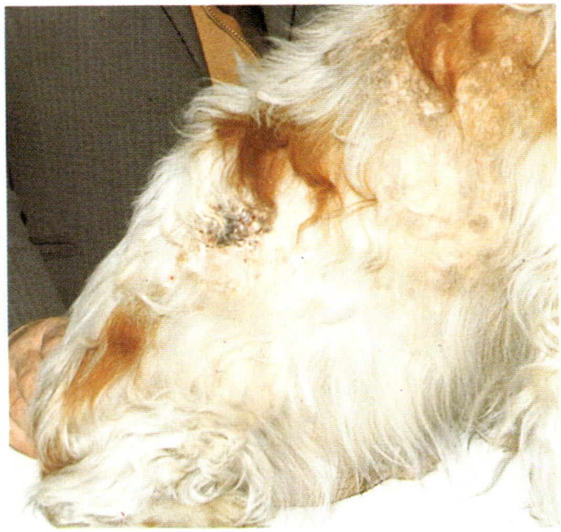

Fig. 8.5. King Charles spaniel, generalized pruritus and self-excoriation — food allergy.

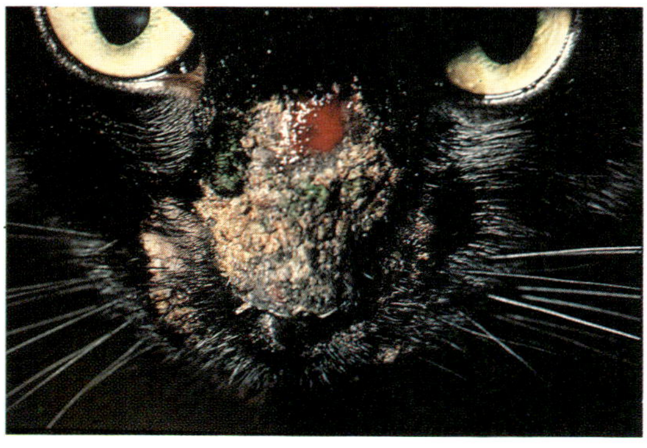

Fig. 8.6. Exfoliative dermatitis and ulceration — milk allergy.

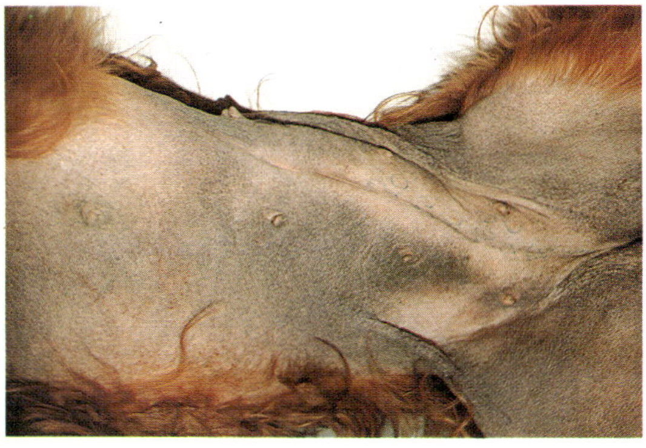

Fig. 8.7. Hyperpigmentation and alopecia — secondary to food allergy.

allergen from the diet. This entails the rigid adherence to a commercial hypo-allergenic diet for at least 3 weeks. The procedure requires careful cooperation with the owner and there are obvious difficulties in controlling the dietary intake of the patient in a household with other animals. For that reason hospitalization may be advisable. In food allergy there is diminution of pruritus within 2 weeks of removal of the allergens from the diet.

THERAPY

Strict adherence to a hypo-allergenic diet will ensure a good prognosis. Additional items of food may be added singly, with a period of 2 weeks elapsing before the next item is added. Such items should contain one food only and not be mixtures, e.g., white fish, chicken and rabbit, but not biscuits or tinned food. Dieting to control food allergy is, however, difficult and oral prednisolone may be necessary at minimal levels to control pruritus and its associated clinical signs. Failure to control the clinical signs with corticosteroid therapy should lead the clinician to review the diagnosis. There are numerous causes of pruritus — food allergy is one of the least important.

Bacterial hypersensitivity

A presumed hypersensitive reaction to staphylococcal antigen has been reported (Baker, 1974; Scott *et al.*, 1978). There may be pruritus with pyoderma, and target lesions may be seen — these are, however, non-specific, being circular, irregular or annular, of variable size initially with central erythema; subsequently there is hyperpigmentation with flaking collarettes. Lesions may heal spontaneously leaving permanent pigmented spots. The differential diagnosis is bacterial pyoderma, subcorneal pustular dermatosis, seborrhoeic dermatitis, flea hypersensitivity and pustular demodicosis. The histopathology is not diagnostic. It is reported that the diagnosis may be confirmed by the demonstration of a delayed response (Arthus response) to specific staphylococcal toxoid after 24 and 72 hours. Normal dogs will usually produce a 'positive' dermal reaction within 18 hours when challenged with toxoid but will not develop an Arthus reaction. Muller *et al.* (1983) further report a satisfactory response to biological therapy with Staphoid AD in 67% of dogs.

Alternatively, therapy with the antibiotic indicated by sensitivity tests should be implemented for at least 3 weeks, in conjunction with shampooing using 2.5% benzoyl peroxide at 3-day intervals. A guarded prognosis should be given.

Hypersensitivity to internal parasites

A number of different intestinal parasites have been presumed to be related to skin diseases exhibiting pruritus (protozoa, ascarids, tapeworms) in humans and animals; however, such cases are not well documented in the latter. Clinical signs reported have been generalized pruritic papular dermatitis, generalized seborrhoea with pruritus, urticaria with pruritus, or pruritus with self-excoriation. Differential diagnoses are ectoparasitism, seborrhoeic dermatitis and atopic dermatitis.

A circumstantial diagnosis can be made based on the history, clinical signs, faecal evidence of intestinal parasites and the absence of signs on elimination of the parasites (Chamberlain, 1974).

Contact-allergic dermatitis

This is an uncommon pruritic papular dermatitis, usually of the relatively hairless, thin-skinned parts of the body of dogs. It is rare in cats. Persistent self-excoriation results in lichenification and hyperpigmentation of the affected area. It is to be distinguished from the more common primary irritant contact dermatitis.

Whilst in humans there is extensive documented evidence proving the association of numerous contact allergens with contact-allergic dermatitis, there is little documentary evidence in the veterinary literature, many reports are of an empirical nature unsubstantiated by patch tests. Information, however, has been gained by the experimental application to guinea pig skin of dinitrochlorobenzene (DNCB), which reacts with skin components to form haptens. The antigen consists of hapten combined with a protein carrier, the hapten entering the skin and combining with the carrier in the cell wall of a macrophage or Langerhans' cell. Following induction and elicitation a Type IV delayed reaction develops on subsequent exposure to the hapten. There is necessarily a latent period of days, months or years before reaction occurs following induction. Gaafar and Krawiec (1974) experimentally induced hypersensitivity to DNCB in dogs by intradermal injections with subsequent contact challenge.

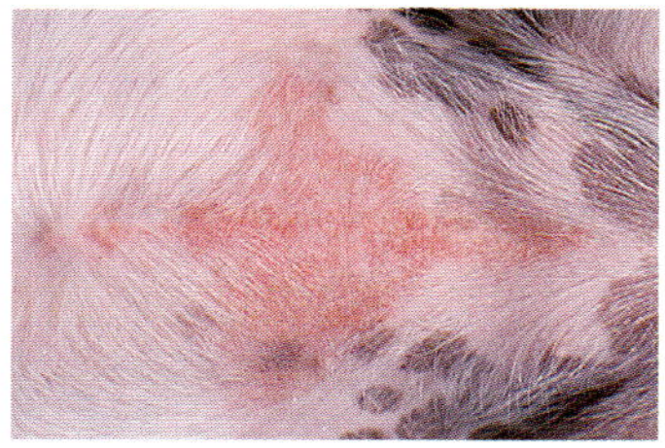

Fig. 8.8. Contact-allergic dermatitis, ventral abdomen, reaction to carpet cleaner.

CLINICAL SIGNS

Where the contact allergen is in the environment the lesions are first seen on the thin-skinned relatively hairless parts of the body (the foot pads and the nipples are usually spared) (Fig. 8.8). If the allergen is contained in a spray, lotion, ointment, bath or powder the whole body may be affected. In some cases the lesions may be confined to the neck because of a collar, or to the thorax through contact with a harness; examples of allergens include the insecticides used in flea collars, the chromium salts used to tan leather, or the chromium plated or nickel connections or medallions on collars or harnesses. Lesions confined to the lips indicate a reaction to chew toys or feeding bowls.

Initially, there is erythema, with pruritus, licking and/or excoriation of the affected area following. Papules and vesicles are quickly obliterated, the skin becomes hot and thickened with rugae in chronic cases thus causing lichenification and hyperpigmentation. The nipples may be enlarged as a result of persistent excoriation with the hindfeet.

DIAGNOSIS

Patch testing is used in the diagnosis of human contact-allergic dermatites but no practical method is available for the veterinarian. In the open patch test method reported and recommended by Walton (1977) suspect allergens are paired onto an area of normal skin and examined daily for 5 days. In the author's experience the test is unsatisfactory.

DIFFERENTIAL DIAGNOSIS

Atopy, focal hypersensitivity, sarcoptic mange, hookworm dermatitis, contact dermatitis and pelodera dermatitis may resemble contact-allergic dermatitis and must be excluded. In the first three there is generalized pruritus with associated clinical signs, whereas in most cases of contact sensitivity it is the ventral parts of the body or other relatively hairless areas that are affected. Peloderma dermatitis and hookworm dermatitis are also most often seen on the ventral surfaces and the contact surfaces but examination of the clinical history, signs and histopathology will help to distinguish these. In contact dermatitis the reaction progresses far more rapidly and is severe with extension into the hairy part of the skin.

Unfortunately histopathology of contact-allergic dermatitis is not specific.

THERAPY

The owner should be questioned about exposure to potential contact allergens. The patient's environment itself ideally should be examined by the veterinarian. A diary should be kept to determine if there is any waxing or waning of the lesions indicating intermittent exposure — for example, contact with soft furnishing cleaned by a carpet cleaner in a particular room, or contact with leather upholstery in a car, occasional visits to work premises.

The rational therapy is avoidance of the allergen(s), when identified, that may be responsible. Absorption of allergen is aided by moisture, therefore the coat should be kept dry — a cotton coat may be tolerated. Prednisolone 2 mg/kg daily for 1 week may be necessary, reducing the alternate-day dosage as necessary. Topical betamethasone cream may be used with care — excessive use may lead to iatrogenic Cushing's disease. Hyposensitization is not successful.

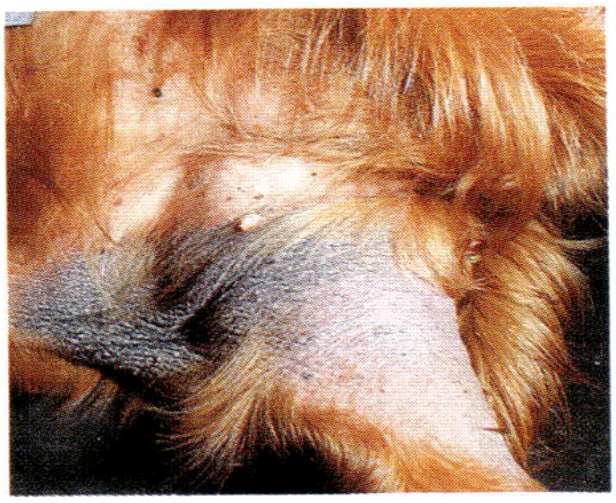

Fig. 8.9. Flea-allergy dermatitis in a red setter; acanthosis with hyperpigmentation.

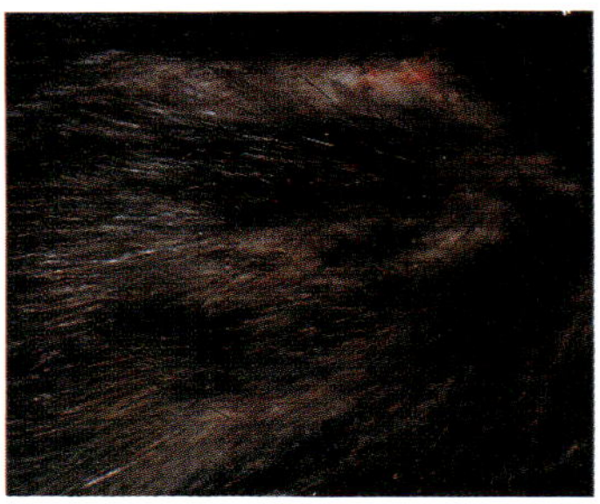

Fig. 8.10. Miliary dermatitis in a cat.

Flea-allergy dermatitis (FAD) (flea hypersensitivity, papular urticaria)

In the UK the dermatitis resulting from hypersensitive reactions to flea bites is the most common cause of skin disease. The clinical signs may continue throughout the year as a temperate climate permits fleas to survive and breed all year round.

CLINICAL SIGNS

There is an intensely pruritic papular dermatitis with a characteristic distribution of lesions, in both cats and dogs. These are most marked along the dorsum from the interscapular region to the tail base and ventrally in the axilla, belly, inguinal and perineal regions. In some cases the entire trunk is affected.

In the early case the first sign may be a bilateral area of excoriated hair on the shoulders and subsequently papules may be observed. Persistent licking, biting and scratching produces extensive erythema, alopecia, and acanthosis. A papular crustaceous, nodular, hyperpigmented dermatitis is seen in the dog (Fig. 8.9). Seborrhoea is common. Pyotraumatic dermatitis ('hot spots', 'wet eczema') is common in the dog.

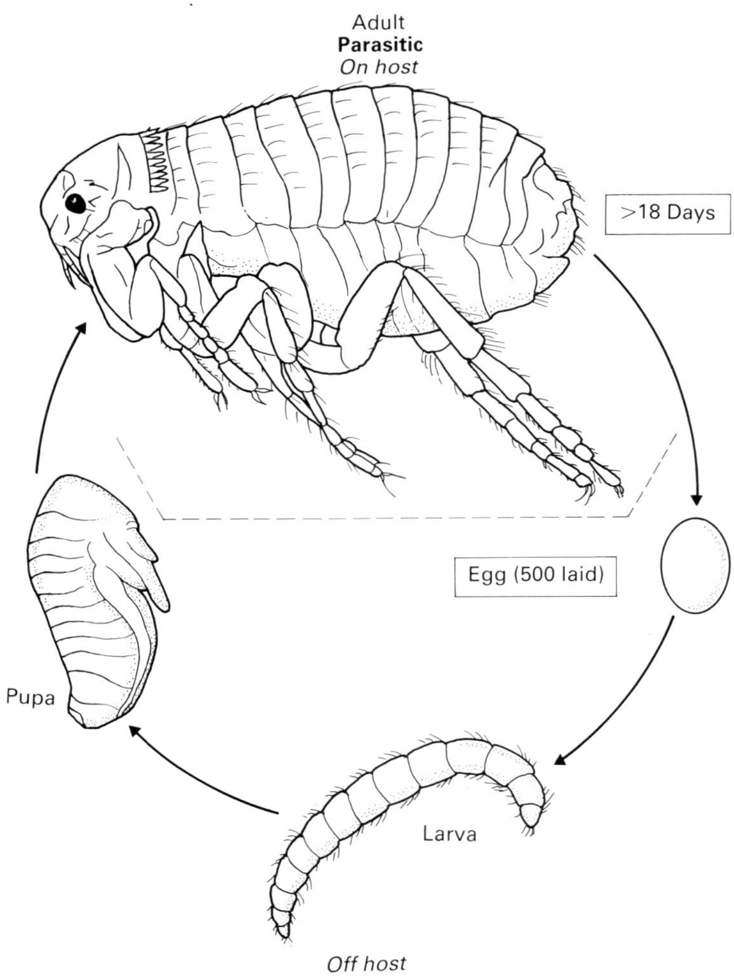

Fig. 8.11. The life cycle of the dog and cat flea. A single adult flea may produce up to 500 fleas in a life time. The time from hatching of a flea to egg production may be as short as 18 days or it may be many months.

Whilst the distribution of the lesions is similar in cats and dogs, in cats the individual lesions are smaller and arranged in groups of papules about 3 mm in diameter. These quickly rupture to release serous fluid and sometimes blood with rapid encrustation. The coat feels hot and sticky from prolonged licking and hair is broken at these sites (feline miliary dermatitis) (Fig. 8.10).

In both dogs and cats clinical signs appear after the first year but cases may occur in young animals. Without adequate therapy the clinical signs persist throughout life with increasing intensity in the warmer months.

DIFFERENTIAL DIAGNOSIS

Other allergic diseases produce extensive papular pruritic dermatitis, but flea-allergy dermatitis has a characteristic distribution. Lice and *Cheyletiella* also cause marked pruritus but close inspection will reveal these parasites.

The absence of fleas on the body does not remove flea allergy as a cause: the allergic subject will react for a long period to saliva deposition in the skin in the absence of the parasite. The response to challenge with fresh flea extract intradermally is an immediate type reaction and is of considerable diagnostic value (Setrié, 1965, Baker, 1971). Commercial whole flea extracts are available (Veterinhal); these have a comparatively short life. Whole flea extracts and flea 'saliva' extracts may be prepared in the practice laboratory with the minimum of equipment (Baker & Mulcahy, 1986). At present intradermal tests for the identification of flea allergy in cats are unsatisfactory. The histopathology is non-specific although increased numbers of eosinophils are seen.

CONTROL AND THERAPY

Whilst anti-inflammatory agents may be used to control the severe pruritus and associated clinical signs of FAD the basis for successful therapy must be the prevention of access to the patient of fleas. Herein there is considerable difficulty: fleas are ubiquitous in the urban and rural environment. It is known that several different species feed on dogs and cats and carry in their saliva the hapten responsible for the development of the allergic response.

A number of techniques are available for the control of fleas. Their effectiveness depends on the susceptibility of the fleas to the various parasiticides, the efficiency of their application, their residual action, and treatment of all animal contacts. This may not be possible when infected animals, wild or stray, visit the environs of the patient. The occasional finding of human fleas on dogs and cats may of course indicate a human source of infestation, although *Pulex irritans* can successfully breed on dogs.

Control measures should be commenced before peak breeding activity during the warmer months of the year.

The entire household should be vacuum-cleaned weekly with a parasiticide placed in the vacuum box. The household should be sprayed with an effective parasiticide; synthetic pyrethroid may give a residual effect for 60 days. Particular attention should be given to bedding areas and favoured resting sites.

A particular problem may arise when infested domestic or feral dogs or cats have access to the patient's home environment, for single bites may precipitate the itch–scratch cycle.

Flea collars will not prevent biting and should not be considered in isolation.

The effectiveness of insecticides is variable; whilst most are effective, few have residual effects. However, Coopers' 'Head to Tail Shampoo' will give 100% control for up to 2 weeks and will prevent biting during that time (Baker & El Harrem, in press).

If infestation continues the services of a professional exterminator should be sought.

Several reports of hyposensitization for the treatment of FAD have been published, claiming good results, but none of these prior to that of Halliwell (1981) was a clinically controlled study. Halliwell considered that his results did not justify the hyposensitization vaccines he used for the therapy of FAD. Hyposensitive vaccines available are as follows: Greer (Greer Laboratory, Lennoir, North Carolina, USA); Hauer Lockhart (Kansas City, Missouri USA); Hollister-Pleur (Spokane, Washington, USA).

The juvenile hormone methoprene (Acclaim) is now marketed. It delays metamorphosis of insect larvae and death results. The residual effect is 90 days. Since it has no action on adult fleas it should be and is used in combination with effective parasiticides. Methoprene is available as a dual-purpose spray (Ceva Ltd) with synthetic pyrethroids. The contents of one can should be sufficient for the average-sized house; however, all rooms should be sprayed. Pyrethroids are very toxic to fish and should not be used near ponds or aquaria.

Consideration should be given to the prevention of pollution of the environment by injudicious use of parasitides. Some texts advocate extreme use without thought being given to the harmful effects this will have on non-parasite life forms sharing the environment. Adult fleas remain on their hosts to feed (Osbrink & Rust, 1984; Baker & El Harrem, in press). The flea problem can be controlled by the treatment of all the possible hosts with a residual insecticide, with the identification of breeding fleas and their elimination, together with regular vacuum cleaning of soft furnishings.

Toxic epidermal necrolysis

This is a rare, severe ulcerative disease of the skin and mucosa of dogs and cats. The aetiology is not determined but it may be associated with drug therapy, and malignancy. In humans sulphonamides, penicillin, barbiturates, diphenylhydantoin and allopurinol are among the many drugs reported to cause this condition.

CLINICAL SIGNS

The initial signs may be lethargy, fever and stiffness, shortly followed by severe painful vesicles and bulla formation, localized or generalized. The buccal mucosa and mucocutaneous sites are nearly always affected. Sloughing is rapid to reveal a fiery red dermis. There may be generalized pain: the affected animal moves reluctantly and handling may be resented. Nikolsky's sign is present.

DIAGNOSIS

The sudden onset of a severe, painful ulcerative condition is characteristic. The differential diagnosis should, however, include pemphigus vulgaris and bullous pemphigoid. Haematology is not helpful; eosinophilia does not occur.

The diagnosis is made on the basis of the history, recent medication, clinical signs and the histopathology; a biopsy should be taken from an active early lesion if possible. While there may be little remarkable in the dermis, there is upper dermal oedema with subepidermal vesicles and marked hydropic degeneration of the epidermis.

As the condition may be secondary to systemic disease, a thorough clinical examination should be made. Attempts to reproduce the signs by remedication with a suspect drug are most undesirable.

THERAPY

The prognosis is guarded, although in cases associated with drug reactions it is good. Betamethasone (0.25 mg/10 kg) is given on the first day intramuscularly, with fluid therapy if required and with antibiotics. Subsequently prednisolone 2 mg/kg b.i.d. is given. Good nursing care is essential. The condition is painful, therefore the animal should be placed on a soft bed and fed soft food. Emollient creams should be applied to the ulcerated areas and chloramphenicol eye ointment applied to the eyes.

In uncomplicated cases, recovery may extend over 3 weeks.

Autoimmune diseases

DIAGNOSIS OF AUTOIMMUNE SKIN DISEASE (AISD)

The diagnosis of AISD presents difficulties: cases may be submitted for examination at various stages of the disease, whilst lesions may be complicated by the effects of self-excoriation and chronic inflammatory reactions. The characteristic lesions of AISD may therefore not be observed. A thorough search of the entire body is essential to detect early non-excoriated lesions. Animals may be kennelled to permit subsequent examination.

Immunoglobulin in the patient with AISD may be demonstrated using direct immunofluorescence staining of frozen skin biopsy sections, using a cryostat (Lever & Schaumberg-Lever, 1983). However, the method has several disadvantages: cryostat sections may deteriorate during processing, and sections cannot be counterstained so that biopsy specimens must be divided for routine histological processing, whilst immunofluorescence staining is transient.

These difficulties have been a stimulus for the development of other techniques. The peroxidone antiperoxidase (PAP) technique developed by Steinberger has greatly improved the capability and sensitivity of immunostaining. Peroxidase labelling is visible using light microscopy, whilst the sections may be counterstained with routine stains like haematoxylin.

The PAP procedure has been evaluated by Suter *et al.* (1984) who compared immunofluorescence and the immunoperoxidase method in canine pemphigus. In the PAP study of Moore *et al.* (1987), 15 of 16 cases of AISD demonstrated immunoreactions for IgG or C3; IgG was the most commonly localized immunoglobulin (14 of 15 cases). This is of interest when compared to the study of Werner *et al.* (1983) who reported 52% positive results in AISD examined by the direct immunofluorescence method. However, the PAP technique requires considerable practice, it also shows reactivity in many cases of canine skin diseases. It must be included with the history, clinical signs, and general histopathological interpretation. The technique is most useful for the diagnosis of AISD where inflammatory changes are minimal.

A method more sensitive than PAP staining is the avidin–biotin peroxidase technique. For example, Haines *et al.* (1986), using this procedure, revealed intercellular and basement-membrane immunoglobulin deposits in 27 of 28 dogs considered to have AISD by clinical and histopathological evaluation. Immunostaining was not present in five biopsies of normal skin or in biopsies from four dogs with non-inflammatory dermatoses.

Pemphigus

This is a group of uncommon autoimmune diseases involving superficial or deep lesions of the skin. The mucous membranes, including the buccal cavity, may also be affected. There may or may not be accompanying pruritus. Lesions are considered to be the result of serum autoantibodies (IgA) reacting with antigen or antigens in the intercellular spaces between epidermal cells of the skin or mucosa. Wolff and Schreiner (1971) demonstrated ultrastructural localization of pemphigus autoantibodies within the surface of keratinocytes in human patients.

Hashimoto *et al.* (1983) reported the mechanism of the process of separation of epidermal cells (acantholysis): pemphigus antibody when incubated with epidermal cells releases plasminogen activator. There are no statistics available for bullous disease in dogs and cats but Muller *et al.* (1983) reported that pemphigus accounts for 0.28% of all canine skin disorders seen at the New York State College of Veterinary Medicine. The term bullous disease is not descriptive for pemphigus in dogs and cats as blisters quickly rupture due to the thinness of the hirsute epidermis, healing with a crust, a scaly collarette or leaving an ulcer. Moore *et al.* (1987) reported that all of 44 dogs with autoimmune skin disease (AISD) showed varying amounts of epidermal spongiosis. In Ireland pemphigus is more common in Collie breeds and German shepherds. In humans pemphigus has been described in all races but the disease is more common in people of Mediterranean origin (Lever *et al.*, 1983).

HISTOPATHOLOGY

There is characteristic cleft formation in the immediate suprabasal epidermal region with some basal cells still attached to the basement membrane. There may be a variable dermal infiltrate of lymphocytes, plasma cells and neutrophils unless the disease is diagnosed in its early stages. The epidermis is generally acanthotic in affected areas. Scrapes from the floor of fresh blisters or recent erosions may reveal Tzanck cells (free, rounded epidermal cells) when stained with Giemsa's stain. Although not specific for pemphigus, the finding of large numbers of Tzanck cells, with the characteristic history and clinical signs, is most suggestive of pemphigus.

THERAPY

Corticosteroid therapy is effective in most cases of pemphigus, and it is probable that some reported poor results are due to too low an initial dose. This initial dose must be high, up to 4 mg/kg daily. The owner must be instructed with regard to the nature of the disease, the prognosis and side effects of corticosteroid therapy. During high-dose therapy the possibility of opportunist infections in an immunocompromised patient must be considered. High-dose therapy may be gradually reduced according to response to alternate-day therapy. Severe pemphigus is a life-endangering problem, and without adequate treatment death will follow.

In the author's experience there is no alternative to the initial use of high-dose glucocorticoids in severe pemphigus. However, consideration may be given to supplementation with immunosuppressive drugs like methotrexate and cyclophosphamide so that in some cases corticosteroid therapy may be withdrawn after a suitable period. Azathioprine (Imuran, Wellcome) may also be used once the signs are controlled by corticosteroid therapy at a daily rate of 2 mg/kg; if the response is good, corticosteroid therapy may be substantially reduced. The antileprosy drug dapsone (Avlosulfon, ICI) should also be considered: the human literature reports its value in pemphigus therapy although there are no published reports in the veterinary literature. The dose is 1 mg/kg daily. This drug is hepatotoxic in prolonged high doses.

Gold therapy may be considered valuable as an alternative to glucocorticoids or immunosuppressant drugs like azathioprine. Its mode of action is not understood. Sodium aurothiomalate is first given with a test injection intramuscularly: 1–2 mg for cats and for dogs less than 11 kg, and 5–10 mg for dogs weighing more than 11 kg. Weekly injections of 0.5 mg/kg are given until there is clinical response, usually at 6–10 weeks, when injections may be given at 2-weekly intervals for 4 weeks followed by monthly injections for 6 months, when therapy may be discontinued. During the early stages of therapy, corticosteroids may also be necessary. The authors have not observed drug reactions to gold therapy for pemphigus although these have been observed in human patients.

In the acute stages of the disease, topical wet dressings are beneficial and when buccal lesions are severe soft foods should be given.

Exposure to bright sunlight should be avoided, sun tan lotions may be beneficial but will require regular renewal. Clioquinol hyrdocortisone cream (Vioform, Ciba) alone with sun avoidance may be sufficient therapy for some cases of pemphigus erythematosa.

PEMPHIGUS VULGARIS

This is the most commonly occurring type of pemphigus. It occurs in dogs and cats. There is no reported breed, age or sex predilection; however, in Ireland (pemphigus vulgaris) as in other types of pemphigus, is more commonly seen in the collie breeds and German shepherd dog.

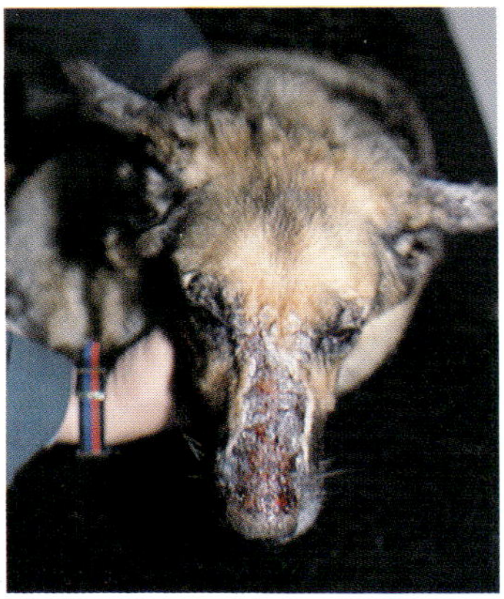

Fig. 8.12. Pemphigus vulgaris, buccal ulceration.

It is the most severe form of pemphigus, characterized by extensive weeping lesions. In nearly all cases there is severe ulceration of the buccal cavity and lips (where secondary infection may cause halitosis) and sites of mucocutaneous junctions, planum nasale, entrance to the nostrils, vulva, anus, prepuce and eyelids (Fig. 8.12). Pruritus may be present. There is usually severe involvement of the axillary and inguinal regions, hence the earlier descriptive term of this disease, hidradenitis suppurativa. Affected animals are depressed and may show diminished appetite.

Routine laboratory examination does not show any characteristic abnormalities. The Nikolsky sign is usually present.

PEMPHIGUS VEGETANS

This is a rare variant of pemphigus vulgaris with only occasional reports in the literature in the dog (Scott, 1977). In its early stages the lesions and histopathology are identical to pemphigus vulgaris; subsequently exuberant warty granulations are produced at the site of erosions.

PEMPHIGUS FOLIACEUS

The lesions in pemphigus foliaceus are more superficial and less severe than in pemphigus vulgaris. It occurs in cats and dogs. Whilst shallow erosions may be seen early in the course of the disease, more usually there is diffuse extensive crusting and scaling, hence foliaceus — the scales appearing leaf-like. The mucocutaneous areas are not usually involved. The first signs may appear on the head, particularly inner aspects of the pinna, and feet, with subsequent involvement of other parts of the body. Later the pads may become hardened with verrucose hyperkeratotic areas around their periphery (Fig. 8.13).

Pruritus may occur, and there may be depression.

The immune response is located higher in the epidermis than in pemphigus vulgaris, cell separation occurring in the epidermis with cleft formation just below the stratum corneum. There may be a dermal infiltrate of neutrophils and eosinophils.

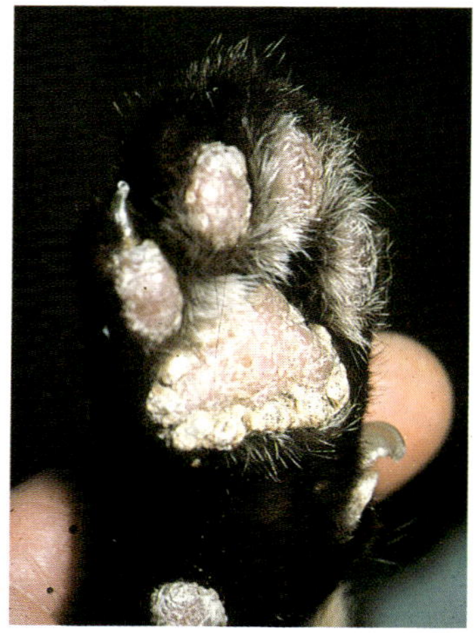

Fig. 8.13. Pemphigus foliaceus, pedal lesions in a cat.

PEMPHIGUS ERYTHEMATOSUS

This is a more localized form of pemphigus foliaceus, with epidermal erosion and accompanying erythema and alopecia of the face and ears, often with secondary pyoderma. There may be pruritus, the buccal cavity is not involved and affected animals are not depressed. The planum nasale and adjacent area are usually affected with depigmentation. The planum nasale may be severly ulcerated and eroded (Fig. 8.14). As with other forms of pemphigus the lesions of unprotected areas, like the face, are worse in bright sunny weather. As collies show a breed predilection the term 'collie nose' has been given; another synonym is nasal solar dermatitis. As with other forms of superficial autoimmune disease collarette lesions may be seen.

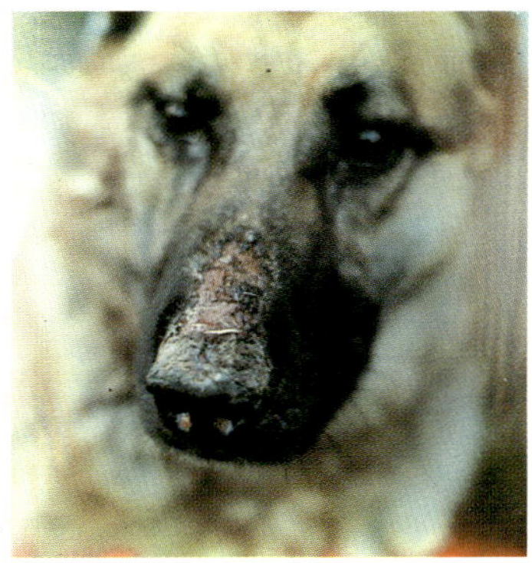

Fig. 8.14. Pemphigus erythematosus.

In humans there are clinical and immunological similarities to the more severe disease lupus erythematosus. Histopathologically there is no difference between pemphigus erythematosus and pemphigus foliaceus.

The differential diagnoses for pemphigus foliaceus and pemphigus erythematosus are bacterial pyoderma, dermatomycosis, seborrhoeic dermatitis and demodicosis.

The diagnosis of pemphigoid is made on the basis of clinical history, signs examination of Tzanck preparations serial

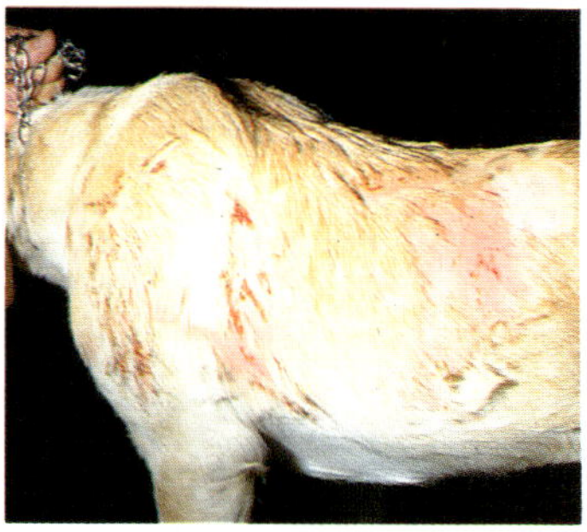

Fig. 8.15. Bullous pemphigoid in a Labrador dog.

sections prepared for light microscopy and immunofluorescence studies with FITC antidog IgG, most cases show intercellular deposits of IgG in the epidermis.

BULLOUS PEMPHIGOID

This is a rare ulcerative disease of the cat and dog thought to result from reactions between autoantibody and antigen or antigens in the lamina lucida of the basement membrane involving complement activation, neutrophil and eosinophil attraction, release of proteolytic enzymes and cleavage at the dermoepidermal junction. In Ireland, bullous pemphigoid is most commonly seen in dogs of the collie breed. As in other autoimmune diseases of the dog and cat, blisters are uncommonly seen: cases are usually presented with severe extensive erosions of the skin, usually in axillary and inguinal regions and often with lateral extension (Fig. 8.15). The buccal cavity also usually shows severe ulceration, and the other mucocutaneous areas may be affected.

Affected animals are depressed and in pain. Often there is pruritus in association with secondary pyoderma and halitosis.

Histopathology of early lesions shows vacuolation immediately below the basement membrane with subsequent cleft formation without acantholysis. There is associated dermal infiltration with lymphocytes, monocytes, eosinophils and neutrophils. Direct immunofluorescence staining reveals IgG at the basement membrane zone.

The diagnosis of bullous pemphigoid rests upon the history and clinical signs.

The therapy for bullous pemphigoid is as for other forms of pemphigus; dapsone may be effective in some cases. In the author's cases there has been good response to prednisolone given orally, initially at a daily rate of 2 mg/kg. Scott *et al.* (1982), however, report that most cases in their experience require more aggressive therapy, e.g. nine dogs were treated with 3 mg/kg prednisolone twice daily, but two were destroyed because of unacceptable side effects, and another two died with acute pancreatitis after 7–10 days of therapy.

Scott *et al.* (1982) reported more favourable results with cyclophosphamide, azathioprine or chlorambucil.

As with other bullous diseases, careful documentation of established cases will reveal in future much useful information with regard to the clinical course, response to therapy and prognosis.

Dermatitis herpetiformis

This is a rare, very pruritic, papular vesicular disease in which the lesions tend to be symmetrically distributed on the extensor surfaces of the body. In humans it is usually accompanied by gluten sensitivity, often asymptomatic. However, a strict glutenfree diet results in improvement of skin lesions. In humans IgA antibodies may be demonstrated immediately below the basement membrane. The term 'herpetiformis' indicates the herpes-like grouping of the lesions.

Halliwell *et al.* (1977) reported a very pruritic papulocrustous dermatitis in a mongrel dog with a 'subepidermal' vesicular dermatitis with numerous eosinophils. The histopathology resembled that in human dermatitis, with response to oral dapsone therapy as in humans. Although the response to dapsone is circumstantial evidence for a diagnosis of dermatitis herpetiformis, this drug is not solely specific for the condition. The aetiology remains to be determined.

Subcorneal pustular dermatosis

This is a rare chronic and recurrent pustular disease of dogs of unknown aetiology with sterile pustules in the stratum corneum containing numerous neutrophils. Affected dogs respond to therapy with dapsone.

There have been too few cases reported to indicate age or sex predisposition. Although apparently healthy, patients have recurrent crops of small vesicles, or pustules, predominantly on the trunk. These may enlarge but are, however, of short duration and rupture to leave circular, dry, scaly crusts. Peripheral spreading results in macules with collarettes. Pruritus may be present. Established cases may have an extensive seborrhoeic dermatitis (McKeefer & Dahl, 1977; Baker, 1980).

The histopathology is subcorneal pustules containing predominantly neutrophils without bacteria or evidence of acantholysis. The underlying epidermis is little affected although diapedesis is seen, and a perifollicular neutrophilic infiltrate is present. Tests for immunoglobulins in the epidermis are negative.

The differential diagnosis is seborrhoeic dermatitis, demodectic mange, pemphigus foliaceus and bacterial pyoderma. Examination of the pustules fails to reveal numerous bacteria, whilst absence of immunofluorescence in the epidermis distinguishes it from pemphigus.

THERAPY

Dapsone by mouth is considered to be specific therapy for this disease. The dose rate is 2 mg/kg daily. The response may be slow and resolution may not be effected for 4 weeks; thereafter the dose rate may be according to progress. In some cases it may be withdrawn (Schwartzman *et al.* 1977).

Dapsone is potentially hepatotoxic and the clinician must examine the case regularly during dapsone therapy for signs of drug-related disease. A guarded prognosis should be given for relapses may occur.

Systemic lupus erythematosus (SLE)

SLE is a rare disease of unknown aetiology (probably multifactorial), which affects both dogs and cats. There is autoantiody production which may affect many systems of the body, including the skin, producing a complex of clinical signs. It is a chronic progressive inflammatory disease. In 1971 the American Rheumatism Association published criteria for the classification of human patients with SLE, and stated that a person shall be said to have SLE if any four or more of the listed 14 manifestations are present. Shetland collies and collies are reported to be more commonly affected than other breeds.

CLINICAL SIGNS

A feature of SLE is the variability of the clinical signs, which may be episodic. Initially there is usually a febrile reaction with one or more painful, swollen joints, there may or may not be cutaneous signs, and polyarthritis, proteinuria, anaemia and lymphadenopathy may also be present. The skin lesions are also variable and are seen in about one-third of cases; pruritus is not constant. There may be bullous ulceration of the skin, foot pads and mucocutaneous areas with discoid lupus erythematosus. Generalized seborrhoeic dermatitis may be seen, and hyperpigmentation and hyperkeratosis may occur.

DIAGNOSIS

The clinical signs are variable and diagnosis requires an examination of the history, clinical signs and laboratory data. Systemic lupus erythematosus may imitate many skin diseases.

There is hydropic degeneration of the dermo-epidermal

junction with the demonstration by direct immunofluorescence of immunoglobulins around the epidermal basement membrane. If there is glomerulonephritis, the urine will contain large amounts of globulin. The presence of the LE cell in peripheral blood or skin sections was originally considered the most important diagnostic test but can be demonstrated in only about 60% of cases. It is a neutrophil containing a homogeneous mass of cytoplasmic basophilic material. There may be anaemia and Coomb's test may be positive. Of more value is the antinuclear antibody (ANA) test with peripheral nuclear fluorescence.

DIFFERENTIAL DIAGNOSIS

This is a disease that may mimic many others. The multisystem involvement demands thorough clinical examination of every animal presented for dermatological examination. An animal presented with a fever and a plethora of clinical signs may be misdiagnosed as suffering from infection.

TREATMENT

The clinical signs may be exacerbated by sunlight; therefore exposure should be minimized.

Prednisolone is administered at a dose rate of 2 mg/kg daily initially to control the clinical signs, with reduction to alternate-day therapy at this dose rate if possible.

Cytotoxic drugs (cyclophosphamide, azothioprine) may be prescribed. The side effects of these drugs should be explained to the owner before prescription. Chloroquine and dapsone therapy are prescribed for humans but no published records of animal treatment are available.

Affected animals require thorough clinical examination because of the potentially high risk of infections.

Discoid lupus erythematosus (Fig. 8.16)

This is a rare skin disease of dogs which is characterized by raised erythematous lesions on the face without the systemic signs of SLE, of which it is considered a benign variant. As with other bullous diseases it is most often seen in the collie breeds and German shepherd dogs. The cause is not known but it is, however, exacerbated by sunlight. There is deposition of immunoglobulin and complement in the dermo-epidermal

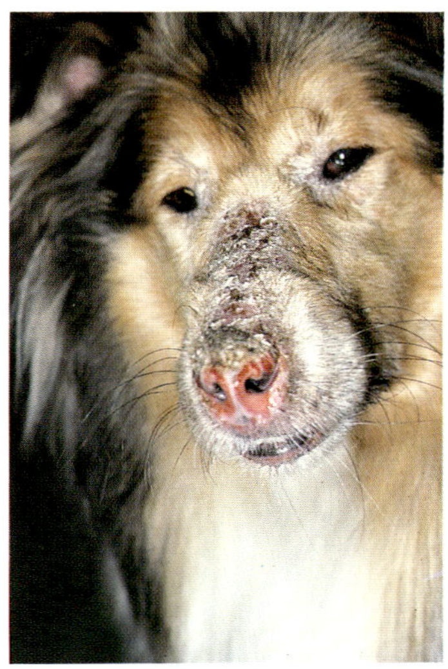

Fig. 8.16. Discoid lupus erythematosus.

junction of lesions as revealed by direct immunofluorescence.

CLINICAL SIGNS

The first lesions are seen on the planum nasale where there is loss of pigment and subsequently scale formation. The epidermis is lost over a variable area to expose the reddened dermis and there is spreading along the bridge of the muzzle. Occasionally there is ulceration of the pinna and lips. Chronic lesions may be predisposed to squamous-cell carcinoma formation.

HISTOPATHOLOGY

The basal cell of the epidermis is apparently the target in discoid lupus erythematosus, with hydropic degeneration, vacuole formation and focal necrosis. The normal transfer of melanin to keratinocyte is disturbed, the pigment being taken up by histiocytes in the dermis. The basement membrane may appear thickened. Numerous mononuclear cells infiltrate the upper dermis and surround the appendages with a small number of plasma cells. Polymorphonuclear leucocytes are absent. When subjected to direct immunofluorescence, immunoglobulin and/or complement in the region of the basement membrane are revealed.

DIFFERENTIAL DIAGNOSIS

This includes pemphigus erythematosus, SLE and toxic epidermal necrolysis. Diagnosis is based upon the histopathology.

THERAPY

Avoid exposure to direct sunlight. Prednisolone 2 mg/kg daily is administered, diminishing as control is achieved. A good prognosis may be given. It is important to continue avoidance of sunlight even when clinical signs are not apparent; the benefit of sunscreen applications may be then considered.

References

Ackerman L. (1986) Pemphigus and pemphigoid in dogs and cats. Part 2: A clinical survey. *Modern Veterinary Practice* **67**, 358–360.

Baker E. (1974) Staphylococcal disease. *Veterinary Clinics of North America* **4**, 107.

Baker K.P. (1971) Intra-dermal tests as an aid to the diagnosis of skin diseases in dogs. *Journal of Small Animal Practice* **12**, 445–452.

Baker K.P. (1980) Sub-corneal pustular dermatosis seen in dogs. *Veterinary Record*.

Chamberlain K. (1974) Allergy. *Veterinary Clinics of North America* **4**, No. 1, 29–39.

Cluff L.E. (1965) The inflammatory response of skin to bacterial invasion. In *Skin Bacteria and their Role in Infection* (Eds Masbach H.I. & Hildick-Smith G.). McGraw-Hill, New York.

Gaafar S.M & Krawiec D.R. (1974) Chemical sensitisers and contact dermatitis. *Journal of the North American Animal Hospital Association* **10**, 133–138.

Gel P.G.H., Coombs R.R.A. & Lachman P.J. (1975) *Clinical Aspects of Immunology*. Blackwell Scientific Publications, Oxford.

Haines D.M., Cooke E.M. & Clarke E.G. (1986) Avidin–biotin–peroxidase complex immunohistochemistry to detect immunoglobulin in formalin fixed skin biopsies in canine autoimmune skin disease. *Canadian Journal of Veterinary Research* **51**, 104–109.

Halliwell R.E.W. (1981) Hyposensitisations in the treatment of flea bite hypersensitivity: Results of a double-blind study. *Journal of the American Animal Hospital Association* **17**, 249–253.

Halliwell R.E.W., Schwartzman R.N., Ihrke P.J., Goldschmidt M.H. & Wood M.G. (1981) Dapsone treatment of pruritic dermatitis (dermatitis herpetiformis and subcorneal pustular dermatosis) in dogs. *Journal of the American Veterinary Medical Association* **170**, 697–703.

Hashimoto K., Shafran K.M., Webber P.A., Lazarus G.S. & Singers K.H. (1983) Anti cell surface pemphigus auto-antibody stimulates plasminogen activator activity of human epidermal cells. *Journal of Experimental Medicine* **157**, 259–272.

Lever W.F. & Shaumberg-Lever G. (1983) Non-infectious vesicular and bullous dermatitis. *Histopathology of the Skin*, pp. 92–135. J.B. Lippincott, Philadelphia.

McKeever P.J. & Dahl (1977) A disease of dogs resembling human subcorneal pustular dermatosis. *Journal of the American Veterinary Medical Association* **170**, 704–708.

Moore F.M., White S.D., Carpenter J.L. & Torchon E. (1987) Localisation of immunoglobulin by the peroxidase method in autoimmune and non-autoimmune canine dermatopathies. *Veterinary Immunology and Immunopathology* **14**, 1–9.

Muller G.R., Kirk R.W. & Scott D.W. (1983) *Small Animal Dermatology*. W.B. Saunders, London.

Nesbitt G.H. (1978) Canine allergic inhalant dermatitis, a review of 230 cases. *Journal of the American Veterinary Association* **172**, 55–60.

Schwartzman R.M., Halliwell R.E.W., Irke D.J., Goldschmidt M.H. & Wood M.G. (1977) Dapsone treatment of pruritic dermatitis (dermatitis herpetiformis and sub-corneal pustular dermatitis) in dogs. *Journal of the American Veterinary Association* **170**, 697–703.

Scott D.W. (1977) Pemphigus vegetans in a dog. *Cornell Veterinarian* **67**, 374–384.

Scott D.W. (1981) Observations on canine atopy. *Journal of the American Animal Hospital Association* **17**, 91–100.

Scott D.W., McDonald J.M. & Schultz R.D. (1978) Staphylococcal hypersensitivity in the dog. *Journal of the American Animal Hospital Association* **14**, 767–779.

Scott D.W., Manning T.O., Smith C.A. & Lewis R.M. (1982) Observations on the immunopathology and therapy of canine pemphigus and pemphigoid. *Journal of the American Veterinary Medical Association* **180**, 48–52.

Setric V. (1965) Clinical and experimental investigations in allergic diseases of domestic animals. 1. Chronic allergic dermatitis of dogs. *Veterinarski archiv Zagreb* **35**, 278.

Suter M.M., Palmer D.C., Zindel S. & Schenk S. (1984) Pemphigus in the dog: comparison of immunofluorescence and immunoperoxidase method to demonstrate intercellular immunoglobulins in the epidermis. *American Journal of Veterinary Research* **45**, 367–369.

Walton G.S. (1977) Allergic contact dermatitis. In *Current Veterinary Therapy VI*. (Ed. Kirk R.W.) p. 571. W.B. Saunders, London.

Werner L.L. (1983) Diagnosis of autoimmune skin disease in the dog. Correlations between histopathologic, direct immunoflourescent and clinical findings. *Veterinary Immunology and Immunopathology* **5**, 47.

Willemse A. (1984) *Investigations on Canine Atopic Dermatitis*. Drukkerig Elinkwirk, Utrecht.

Wolff K. & Schreiner E. (1971) Pemphigus autoantibodies: ultra structural localisation within the epidermis. *Nature* **229**, 59–61.

9 / Diseases of the Endocrine System

Disorders associated with endocrine system malfunction are characterized by changes in the hair coat, giving rise to abnormal character, growth rate, distribution and colour as well as other, often subtle, changes in the skin and adnexa.

In addition to those changes affecting the hair and skin, clinical signs involving other systems may suggest disease of endocrine origin.

Hormones secreted by the endocrine glands act as regulating factors controlling physiological processes which maintain the biological normality of the organism.

This situation of endocrine physiological equilibrium has been likened to an orchestra whose players are, as far as the skin is concerned, the thyroid, adrenal, ovary and testis with the pituitary/hypothalamus the conductor. Once there is disharmony amongst the players (endocrine malfunction) or the conductor (pituitary/hypothalamic disease) then the resulting discord is reflected in abnormalities of the skin and other body systems.

The production of the hormonal secretions of the testis, ovary, adrenal and thyroid glands is dependent upon the secretion of the relevant trophic hormones by the pituitary gland and of the appropriate hypothalamic releasing factors. Mechanisms of production and control of the releasing factors are as yet not clearly understood.

From the complex interdependence of gland, pituitary and hypothalamus, the initiation of endocrine skin disease can be described as:

1 Primary — due to a lesion or dysfunction of the target organ, thyroid, adrenal, testis or ovary.

2 Secondary — due to disordered production of the relevant stimulating factor from the pituitary.

3 Due to hypothalamic malfunction by abnormal production of releasing factors.

In relation to the skin and adnexa the adenohypophyseal secretions of importance are:

TSH	thyroid-stimulating hormone
ACTH	adrenocorticotrophic hormone
GH	growth hormone — somatotropin
FSH	follicle-stimulating hormone
LH	luteinizing hormone
MSH	melanocyte-stimulating hormone
Prolactin	

Clinical aspects of endocrine disease

It can be seen from the complexity of the aetiology of skin disorders of endocrine origin that a wide variation of clinical signs may be produced. A detailed medical history relevant to all systems, not the skin alone, is therefore essential as an aid to definitive diagnosis.

A number of clinical features are, however, common to the hormonal skin disorders: bilaterally symmetrical alopecia, hyperpigmentation of the area of hair loss and the absence of primary pruritus (pruritus may arise from secondary infection).

Canine hypothyroidism

This is a common condition of the dog which has not yet been confirmed in the cat.

Nesbitt (1983) quotes the bulldog, golden retriever, Irish setter, Basenji, great Dane, Doberman, poodle, dachshund, Schnauzer and boxer breeds as being predisposed to the disease. The onset may be at any age but usually is in middle to old age (6–10 years), earlier in the giant breeds.

AETIOLOGY

The more commonly encountered causes are: primary — thyroid atrophy, lymphocytic thyroiditis (90%); secondary/tertiary — congenital/acquired hypopituitarism (10%).

HISTORY

The onset is usually insidious, with clinical signs varied in both intensity and variety. Changes in the coat, absence of pruritus and behavioural abnormalities are common.

CLINICAL SIGNS

General

There are varying degrees of depression or lethargy, ranging from virtually no obvious temperamental or behavioural change to severe changes resulting in dullness, poor response to stimuli and disinclination to move. There is obesity with marked increase in the thickness of the skin folds of the neck. The skin is cold and there may be reduced body temperature. The heart rate is slowed and there is a slow, weak pulse and low-voltage ECG. Exercise tolerance is progressively reduced, and the patient gives the impression that every step taken is an effort — it does not pick its feet up when walking, and when taken for exercise will frequently lay down to rest.

Examination of the feet shows that the dorsal surfaces of the nails particularly those of the forefeet, are worn due to poor gait.

Myopathy

There is reduced reproductive action, loss of libido and irregular oestrus or anoestrus. The alimentary tract signs may include constipation, diarrhoea, and vomiting.

A feature of canine hypothyroidism is hypercholesterolaemia, which is shown physically as corneal lipidosis — white 'snowflake', often circular, corneal opacities.

Skin signs

The coat is dry, lustreless, and coarse with readily epilated hair. Alopecia is bilaterally symmetrical, particularly at sites of wear (Fig. 9.1). Areas may be multifocal or total and in some patients complicated by secondary pyoderma.

Where alopecia is marked, inactive hair follicles are plugged with keratinous debris to form comedones, and the skin surface is dry, scaly, seborrhoeic and has a 'sandpaper-like' feel (Fig. 9.2). The skin is thickened and myxoedematous, with lichenification and hyperpigmentation particularly on the dorsal surface of the body. Accentuation of skin folds of the face may give rise to a tragic/pitiful expression — 'tragic facies'.

DIFFERENTIAL DIAGNOSIS

Because of the great variation in clinical signs shown in hypothyroidism in the absence of skin signs the elimination of debilitating disease is essential.

Where coat and skin signs are established, differentiation from other endocrine disorders has to be made by clinical observation and haematological and blood biochemical investigation to eliminate adrenal, ovarian, testicular and pituitary disease.

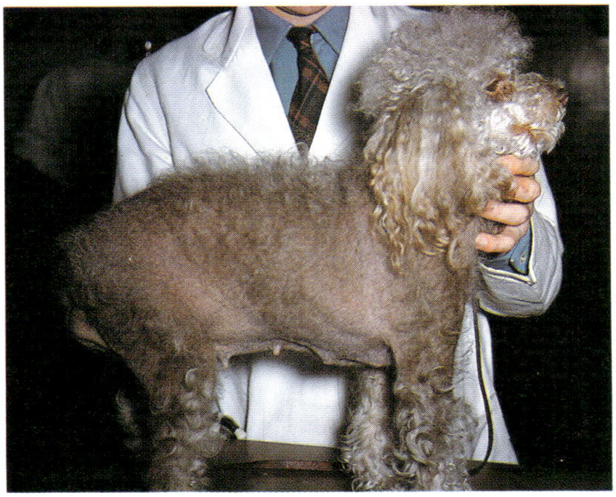

Fig. 9.1. Bilateral alopecia of body — hypothyroidism.

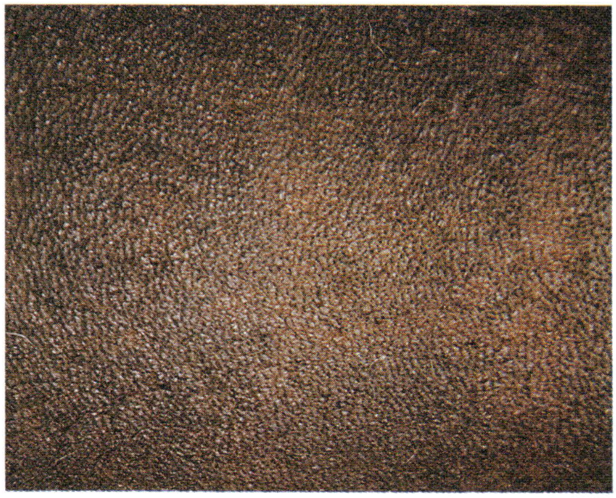

Fig. 9.2. Total alopecia with hyperpigmentation — hypothyroidism.

DIAGNOSIS

This is based on clinical signs with full haematological or blood biochemical work up and specific thyroid function test. Skin biopsy may assist diagnosis.

Haematology

There may be a normochromic normocytic anaemia and lowered haemoglobin concentration.

Blood biochemistry

Serum cholesterol. Although raised in other endocrine disorders a value of >15.6 nmol/l following starvation, presampling for 24 hours, is highly suggestive of hypothyroidism.

Serum T3 and T4 estimations. These may be unreliable.

TSH stimulation test. This is the most reliable test presently available.

1 A resting serum or plasma sample is taken for baseline values.

2 5 i.u. TSH is administered intravenously.

3 After an interval of 4 hours a further serum or plasma sample is taken.

Minimal response indicates hypothyroidism: normally the thyroxine level would increase two to three times.

Thyroid biopsy. This requires the services of a histologist experienced in the interpretation of thyroid histopathology.

Skin histopathology. This reveals orthokeratotic hyperkeratosis and melanosis in the skin; telogen arrest, follicular atrophy, dilatation and keratosis of the hair follicles (Fig. 9.3); and a thickened dermis with increased dermal mucin (care must be taken in interpretation of biopsies from the Shar Pei breed where increased mucin may be demonstrated in normal biopsies) and sebaceous gland atrophy.

THERAPY — REPLACEMENT

Recommendations are for stable, standardized preparations of triiodothyronine (T3) or thyroxine (T4) rather than natural dessicated thyroid extract.

Thyroxine (Eltroxin, Glaxo)

This is given orally at a dose rate of 10–20 μg/kg twice daily for 3 weeks after which time the patient is reassessed. Signs of overdosage, although uncommon, may be restlessness, panting, tachycardia, cardiac murmur, polyphagia, polyuria, diarrhoea, and vomiting.

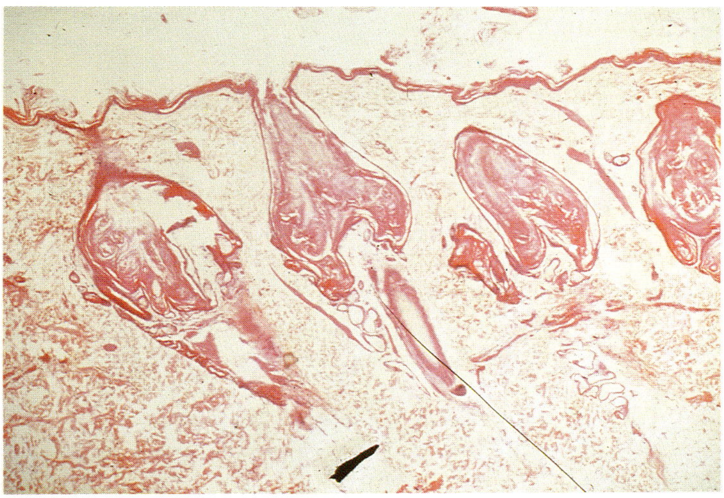

Fig. 9.3. Hyperkeratosis, dilated plugged hair follicles — hypothyroidism. Dog skin stained by haematoxylin and eosin.

Treatment, provided the dosage is tolerated, is continued and further monitoring at 2 and 3 months after initial treatment is advised. Assessment after 3 months determines the need to increase the dose or review the diagnosis. Whilst the systemic signs respond quickly, the response of the skin may be delayed and there may be little improvement or hair growth for several months. Replacement hormone therapy will be required for life.

Triiodothyronine (Tertroxin, Glaxo)

This entails a similar regimen to T4 but the dose of this preparation is 6 μg/kg t.i.d. Observation of the patient for overdosage is as for thyroxine.

Dessicated thyroid extract

This preparation is of low and variable potency and therefore of unpredictable biological activity and shelf life; it is better avoided.

Hyperadrenocorticism (canine Cushing's syndrome)

This is a usually chronic disorder characterized by the presence of excess circulating glucocorticoids. It is relatively common in the dog but rare in cats.

In symptomatology it may be mild to severe, and chronic or rapid in onset depending upon its aetiology.

AETIOLOGY

Pituitary dependent

There is excess production of ACTH due to neoplasia or hyperplasia of the pituitary gland. Hypersecretion causes bilateral hyperplasia of the adrenal cortex.

Peterson (1984) states that this accounts for 85–90% of cases of hyperadrenocorticism.

Adrenocortical tumour

This is a benign or malignant, spontaneous, mostly unilateral adenocarcinoma. Peterson (1984) considered that 10–15% of cases were within this category.

Iatrogenic — Cushing's syndrome, focal cushingoid skin atrophy

The most usual cause is the excessive use of glucocorticosteroids to control pruritus for other therapeutic purposes.

Ectopic ACTH syndrome

This is very rare.

PREDISPOSITION

In the USA Muller *et al*. (1983) stated that hyperadrenocorticism is more common in the boxer, Boston terrier, poodle and dachshund. Workers in Europe are not agreed on any particular breed incidence.

No predisposition by sex has been reported; the disease is, however, more frequently encountered in the middle to old age group. Pituitary-dependent hyperadrenocorticism has been seen in dogs as young as 1 year of age.

HISTORY AND CLINICAL SIGNS

A detailed history may well determine the premonitory signs before more obvious, well-established signs are noted by the owner.

Peterson (1984) considered the predominant clinical signs to be polyuria, lethargy and hair loss. In order of importance all the signs of hyperadrenocorticism are:

1 Polyuria/polydipsia.
2 Pendulous abdomen.
3 Hepatomegaly.
4 Hair loss.
5 Lethargy.
6 Polyphagia.
7 Muscle weakness.
8 Anoestrus.
9 Obesity.
10 Muscle atrophy.
11 Comedones.
12 Panting.
13 Testicular atrophy.
14 Hyperpigmentation of the skin.
15 Calcinosis cutis.
16 Facial nerve palsy.

Polyuria, polydipsia and polyphagia may be noticed up to a year prior to the occurrence of more obvious signs. Abnormal behaviour relative to these can be:

1 Progressive increase in fluid requirement, seeking water or other fluids, drinking from bath, toilet, ponds and puddles.
2 Increased frequency of urination, need to empty during the night with spontaneous urination soiling kennel, bedding, house. In severe cases this also occurs during daytime.
3 Worrying for food, thieving in the home, raiding garbage bins.

SYSTEMIC EFFECTS

Musculoskeletal system

The glucocorticoid excess causes catabolism, muscle wasting and inhibition of fibroblast activity with collagen atrophy, e.g. poor wound healing and scar breakdown.

Associated clinical signs are lethargy, poor exercise tolerance, lordosis, pendulous abdomen and abdominal enlargement (Fig. 9.4). Palpation of the abdomen may reveal hepatomegaly.

Wasting of the musculature of the head, shoulders, hindquarters and thighs is more marked at these sites than elsewhere.

Reproductive system

Females produce excess androgen from the adrenal producing clitoral enlargement. The female remains in anoestrus.

Hyperadrenocorticism causes testicular atrophy in males.

Immune system

Hyperadrenocorticism causes immunosuppression with increased susceptibility to infection, particularly of the respiratory and urinary systems and skin.

Skin and appendages

Although all affected animals do not show alopecia, progressive thinning of the hair on the body, with sparing of the head, ears and distal limbs, even the tip of the tail, is common, with a true bilateral symmetry (Fig. 9.5).

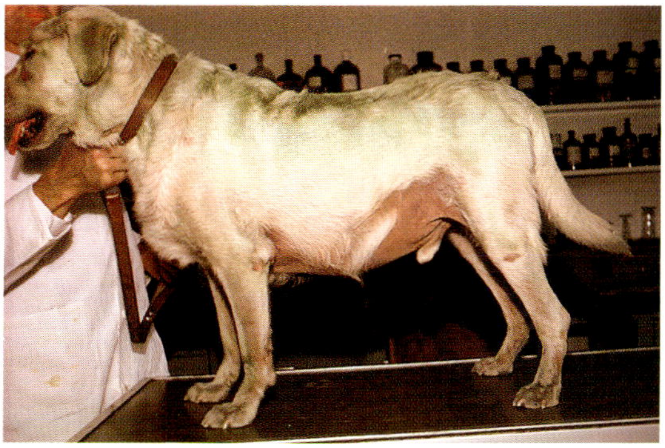

Fig. 9.4. Hyperadrenocorticism of a dog. Lordosis, pendulous abdomen and prepuce, patchy alopecia.

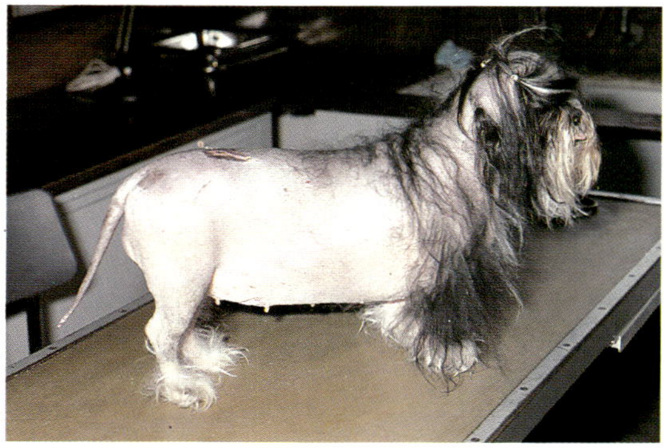

Fig. 9.5. Alopecia of body with extremities and head spared — hyperadrenocorticism.

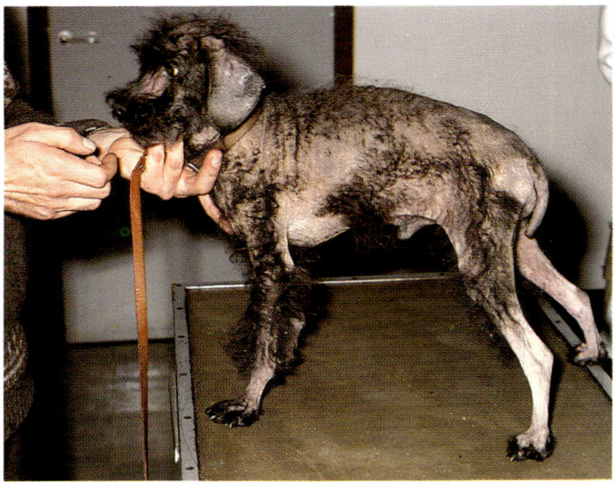

Fig. 9.6. Generalized partial alopecia — hyperadrenocorticism.

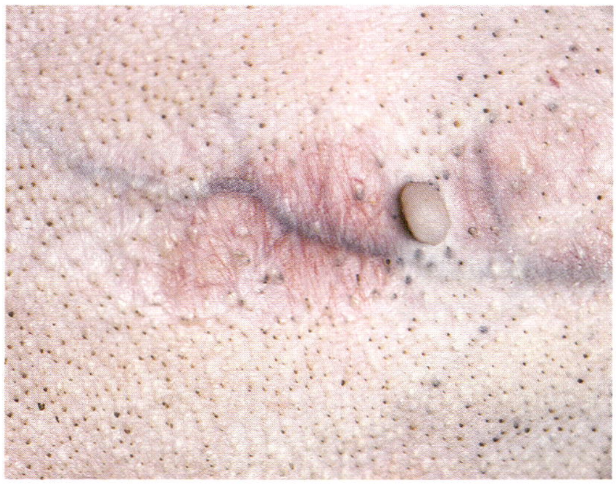

Fig. 9.7. Comedones, thinned skin with prominent subcutaneous blood vessels, collagen atrophy — hyperadrenocorticism.

Short-haired dogs may show a less specific pattern of hair loss, having a generalized 'mothy' appearance with shortening of the hair rather than bilaterally symmetrical alopecia (Fig. 9.6).

The hair coat is lustreless, dry and brittle and in some cases also takes on an abnormal colour, e.g. the yellow Labrador retriever coat takes on a ginger colour and in some cases also a tendency to curl.

Varying degrees of hyperpigmentation and macule formation occur in the skin; the texture is dry, scaly and inelastic.

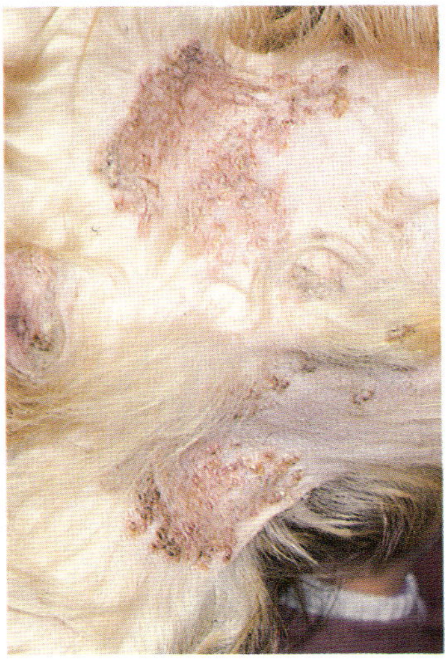

Fig. 9.8. Diffuse calcinosis cutis of abdominal skin — hyperadrenocorticism.

In some long-standing cases the skin is extremely thin. Comedones are common and often a prominent feature, particularly on the skin of the abdomen (Fig. 9.7).

The skin bruises readily, damage heals slowly and old abdominal scars may be seen to be breaking down.

Secondary pyoderma and other concurrent infective diseases may cause pruritus and self-trauma. Hyperadrenocorticism is not a pruritic disease.

Protracted cases may progress to a stage of mineralization of soft tissues — i.e. bronchi, kidney, skin — the presence and extent of which may be determined radiologically although the results of investigation may be somewhat variable.

Calcinosis cutis. This form of mineralization varies considerably and skin deposits are seen as areas of fine, white, amorphous granules in the dermis (Fig. 9.8). This is often seen where there is marked skin thinning and loss of hair coat (abdomen, thorax). Tensing the skin shows this to be linear or as striae.

More discrete granular or plaque-like accumulations may be over the withers, neck and other areas of the dorsum. Although these are predilection sites, calcinosis can also occur at other sites, e.g. skin of the abdomen, thorax, groin.

Where dense deposits are laid down, a foreign-body reaction with rejection and ulceration takes place, leaving white/yellow granular material exposed or dried on the surface of the lesion (Fig. 9.9). Creamy white exudate from areas of early ulceration may suggest deep pyoderma, and culture of this material is often repeatedly sterile.

The mineralized character of the exposed material may be suggested by scraping the surface with the tip of a scalpel blade or hypodermic needle to produce a grating sound.

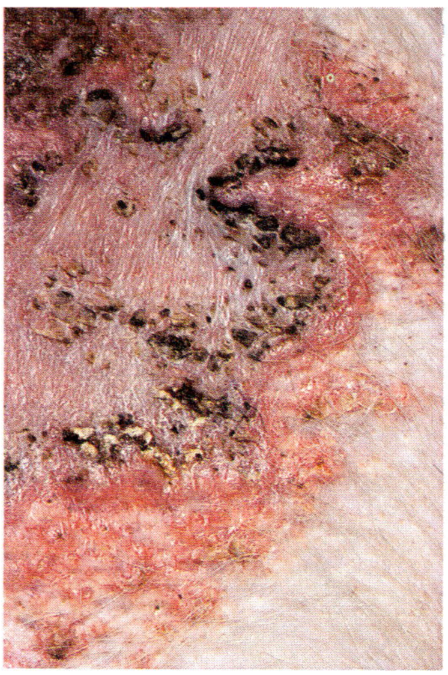

Fig. 9.9. Calcinosis cutis erythema, scarring, granular calcified masses on skin surface — hyperadrenocorticism.

DIFFERENTIAL DIAGNOSIS

1 Other causes of polydipsia/polyuria/polyphagia, e.g. kidney disease, diabetes mellitus.

2 Other causes of abdominal distension — normal or abnormal — e.g. pregnancy, cardiac disease.

3 Other causes of alopecia — endocrine disease, e.g. Sertoli-cell tumour, hypothyroidism.

4 Calcinosis circumscripta — mainly giant breeds, e.g. foot and oral lesions.

DIAGNOSIS

The variability of clinical signs often makes definitive diagnosis difficult.

Haematology. There is mild leucocytosis and neutrophilia with lymphopenia and eosinophilia.

Blood biochemistry. Serum alkaline-P (SAP) is significantly increased. There is also a rise in alanine amino transferase (ALT).

There may be mild hyperglycaemia and perhaps even diabetes mellitus. Resting T3 and T4 levels are low, TSH test is normal and there is raised serum cholesterol.

Urine. The specific gravity of the urine is low — less than 1.007.

Cortisol. This is raised to 0.8–3.0 μg/dl.

ACTH-response test. This determines the abnormality but not the cause. A pre-injection sample of 5 ml whole blood is taken into a heparinized tube. For dogs up to 9 kg bodyweight 10 i.u. of ACTH gel is administered intramuscularly or 0.1 mg tetracosactrin. A repeat blood sample is taken into a heparinized tube 4 hours after injection of ACTH or 1.5 hours after tetracosactrin.

For dogs over 9 kg bodyweight the above method is used but with 20 i.u. of ACTH gel or 0.2 mg of tetracosactrin.

The test is unsatisfactory because a large number of hyperadrenocorticoid cases due to adrenal cortical neoplasia will show the same response as normal dogs. Dogs with normal adrenocorticoid activity will show increased cortoid levels following the test, many cases with adrenal neoplasia and all cases with pituitary dependant hyperadrenocorticism will show a much greater increase in cortisol levels. Cortisol values increased to more than 20/100 ml will nearly always be diagnostic whilst values above 35/100 ml will always be diagnostic.

Dexamethasone suppression test (DST). Two methods are available — low dose and high dose. The former determines whether the patient has hyperadrenocorticism, the latter determines the specific cause.

For *low-dose* DST, a resting pre-injection blood sample is

taken for cortisol estimation then 0.01 mg/kg dexamethasone is administered intravenously or intramuscularly. After 8 hours a further sample for plasma is taken. Suppression is normal, no suppression indicates hyperadrenocorticism.

For *high-dose* DST, a resting pre-injection sample is again taken for plasma. After the administration of 0.1 mg/kg dexamethasone intravenously or intramuscularly, a postinjection sample is taken 4 hours later. A lack of significant suppression of the cortisol level at 4 hours indicates adrenal neoplasia; suppression at 4 hours indicates pituitary-dependent adrenal hyperplasia.

A number of methods are available and vary in the dosage of dexamethasone and timing of blood sampling. The basic principle of highand low-dose tests is the same and the reader is referred to the reference list at the end of the chapter.

Skin biopsy. This is an aid to diagnosis but is not diagnostic as such.

The epidermis is thin and there is follicular keratosis and plugging with telogen arrest. Hair-follicle and sebaceousgland atrophy are seen and there is also collagen atrophy and calcinosis.

TREATMENT

Adrenalectomy is only of value in adrenal neoplasia. In bilateral adrenal hyperplasia, adrenalectomy entertains major hazards. There is a high mortality rate with this treatment. Adrenal supplementation is essential.

Hypophysectomy is surgically difficult except for the well-experienced surgeon. Glucocorticoid supplementation and medication with o.p. DDD (mitotane) are required. DDD should be administered at the rate of 50 mg/kg daily for 10 days, then weekly for 2 weeks, and at fortnightly intervals thereafter. Regrettably this product has now been withdrawn from the UK market where it has no product licence. Mitotane is now available from Idis Ltd (Gruffydd-Jones, 1989). Mitotane is cytotoxic and should be handled only when wearing gloves. Of the alternative drugs, ketoconazole is promising but requires clinical assessment (Gruffydd-Jones, 1989). One report (Fieldman & Nelson, 1987) gave a dose rate of 30 mg/kg daily with clinical improvement in 15 cushinoid dogs.

It is advisable to wean the animal from a high cortisol state to a low cortisol state by giving cortisol, otherwise known as hydrocortisone (e.g. in the form of 'Hydrocortone tablets'), at a dose rate of 1.5 mg/kg per day, starting on the third day of mitotane treatment and finishing on the 17th day.

Although unlikely, if the animal should collapse soon after starting treatment give an injection of corticosteroid immediately, preferably as a soluble preparation (e.g. 'Betsolan soluble').

Prognosis in all cases is guarded as not all calcinosis cutis resolves and sudden death may occur.

Iatrogenic hyperadrenocorticism

Long-term glucocorticoid therapy for pruritic skin disease will give rise to all the clinical signs of naturally occurring hyperadrenocorticism.

Withdrawal of medication and treatment with 0.2–0.5 mg/kg once daily on a reducing scale over 6–12 weeks is required.

Focal cushingoid skin atrophy (focal hyperadrenocortical skin atrophy)

The subcutaneous injection of long-acting corticosteroid preparations, particularly those recommended for deep intramuscular use, may in some patients give rise to local lesions of skin atrophy. These become totally hairless patches, circular in outline and over 5 cm in diameter. The skin is markedly thinned and subcutaneous blood vessels are visible. They are seen particularly over the withers and hindquarters since these are common injection sites.

Attempts to cure the condition by surgical removal of the affected skin and central subcutaneous tissue have proved ineffective.

Hypopituitarism, pituitary dwarfism

This is a congenital disease of dogs caused by lack of growth hormone, often accompanied by thyroid, adrenocortical and gonadal disorders. There is a particular predisposition for the German shepherd breed, in which it has been shown to be a simple autosomal recessive trait (Zanesco *et al.*, 1984).

CLINICAL SIGNS

There are no clinical signs until approximately 2 months of

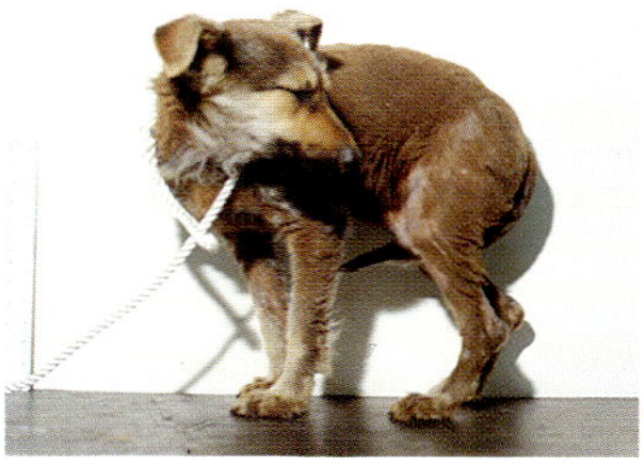

Fig. 9.10. Pituitary dwarf. German shepherd.

age. There is poor skeletal development at 1 year of age and affected dogs may be half the height and weight of their littermates (Fig. 9.10). The epiphyses of long bones fail to close until 3 years of age, there is failure of calcification of the os penis and delayed eruption of permanent dentition. Genital development is poor and the prepuce is pendulous. Pituitary dwarfs are usually timid and may be aggressive.

Skin and appendages

There is poor coat development, with the puppy coat (down hair) retained and few guard hairs at 2–4 months of age. Progressive bilateral trunk alopecia occurs, with hyperpigmentation at 9–12 months particularly involving the friction areas. Seborrhoea is present and the epidermis peels off, therefore secondary bacterial infection is common.

DIAGNOSIS

The differential diagnosis is congenital hypothyroidism.

Assays for T3 and T4 may be subnormal, the TSH-response test shows an increase in T4 and the ACTH-response test shows normal plasma cortisol, but increasing the intravenous injection of insulin stimulates a prolonged hyperglycaemia. The administration of 10–30 μg/kg clonidine and 100–300 μg/kg xylazine in the growth hormone response test produces no rise in plasma growth hormone levels.

SKIN HISTOLOGY

The epidermis is thinned and hyperkeratotic and hyperpigmented; the follicles are dilated with keratosis and there is telogen arrest. The sebaceous and apocrine glands atrophy and there is a reduction in the size of dermal elastic fibres (Scott, 1982; Zanesco *et al.*, 1984).

THERAPY

There is a variable response to therapy. Most affected animals do not improve. The therapy is a course of injections of either porcine or bovine growth hormone. Bovine GH 10 i.u. subcutaneously or porcine GH 2 i.u. subcutaneously on alternate days has been used experimentally. The main disadvantages of the therapy are that growth hormone is very expensive and that repeated injections of foreign protein may cause hypersensitivity reactions or diabetes mellitus (Eigenmann, 1986a). There will, of course, be no increase in stature if therapy is commenced subsequent to closure of the growth plates.

Where other endocrines are involved adrenocortical and thyroid supplementation may also be required.

The prognosis is poor.

Growth-hormone deficiency of mature dogs

This disorder has a predisposition for spitz breeds, e.g. keeshond, chow, and also the Pomeranian, poodle and Lhasa Apso. It occurs mostly in male dogs of 1–2 years of age. The cause of the condition in unknown (Eigenmann, 1986a, b).

CLINICAL SIGNS

The general physical condition is good. Clinical signs are confined to the skin and coat, where there is non-pruritic, progressive bilaterally symmetrical alopecia of the trunk, tail, posterior thigh, neck and pinnae (Fig. 9.11). The hair that is retained is dry, lustreless and brittle in texture. The skin is hyperpigmented at areas of hair loss and in some dogs there is seborrhoea.

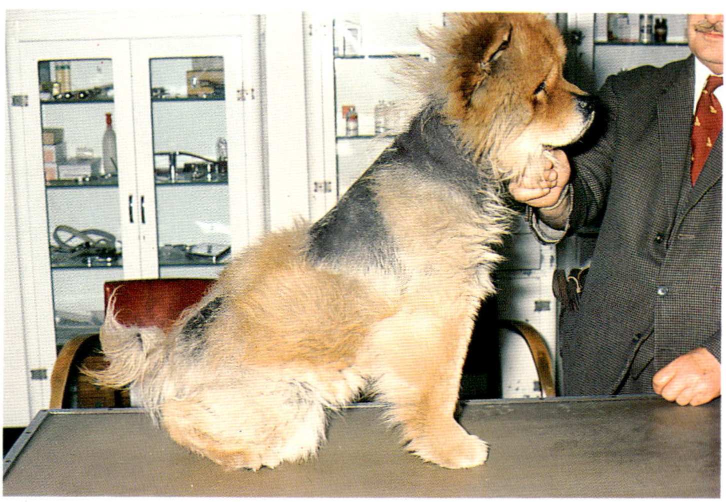

Fig. 9.11. Adult growth hormone insufficiency in a chow. There is bilaterally symmetrical alopecia with hyperpigmentation.

DIFFERENTIAL DIAGNOSIS

The condition must be distinguished from hypothyroidism, hyperadrenocorticism, and male and female gonadal disorders associated with bilaterally symmetrical alopecia.

DIAGNOSIS

The clonidine and xylazine tests reveal that most affected animals have a complete growth hormone deficiency and others have only a partial deficiency.

Adrenal and thyroid function tests are normal.

SKIN HISTOLOGY

The histopathology reveals epidermal thinning with hyperkeratosis, atrophic catagen-type hair follicles, 'flame follicles' with tricholemmal keratin penetrating the follicle wall, follicular plugging and melanosis. Two-thirds of cases have been shown to have reduced dermal elastin.

THERAPY

Bovine or porcine growth hormone has been used, but such treatment is very expensive and can result in foreign protein hypersensitivity and/or diabetes mellitus. 2.5–5.0 i.u. of bovine or porcine growth hormone is administered subcutaneously on alternate days for 10 injections, or 0.1 i.u./kg is administered three times a week for 5 weeks (Eigenmann, 1986b). Response should be seen after an interval of 3 months.

Hypersomatotrophism (acromegaly)

This disorder is more common in the female dog. It is caused by hypersecretion of growth hormone in the adult due to pituitary hyperplasia and also by progestogen therapy in the bitch. The disorder is associated with the reproductive cycle and the condition develops in oestrus.

CLINICAL SIGNS

The thickness of skin increases due to hypertrophy of soft tissue. This leads to the formation of exaggerated skin folds of head, neck, trunk and abdomen. There is also an increase in oral and pharyngeal soft tissue resulting in inspiratory stridor. The interdental spaces increase in size, while other features are polydipsia, polyuria, and general fatigue.

DIAGNOSIS

This disorder may be revealed by hyperglycaemia, raised serum alkaline phosphatase, lowered packed-cell volume and radiography. The growth hormone value may remain raised during glucose tolerance test where 1 g of glucose per kg bodyweight is administered intravenously.

There is epidermal hyperplasia, hyperplasia of the epidermal appendages and increases in dermal collagen and mucin.

THERAPY

Ovariohysterectomy, or cessation of progestogen therapy is necessary.

Sertoli-cell tumour

Oestrogen production due to neoplasia of Sertoli cells of the testis of the ageing dog is more frequent in those animals having abdominally or inguinally retained testis or testes (Fig. 9.12), most being over 7 years of age.

Dogs with scrotal testes are, however, not precluded from being affected by this disease. A small proportion of cases (3.5%) show metastasis from malignant lesions.

Although any breed may be affected there is a predisposition for the boxer, sheltie, poodle and miniature schnauzer.

A proportion of affected dogs will show evidence of feminization, e.g. attractiveness to male dogs, gynecomastia. A similar clinical picture may be seen in dogs medicated with oestrogen orally or by injection.

CLINICAL SIGNS

There is an essentially non-pruritic alopecia of the male dog, insidious in onset with a progressive course.

At initial examination, the first sign may be a pendulous prepuce with or without gynecomastia (Fig. 9.13); the coat may lack lustre and show evidence of thinning.

Progressive bilaterally symmetrical alopecia with hyperpigmentation of the hairless areas (Fig. 9.14) involves the perineum, posterolateral thighs and abdomen, eventually extending to the lateral thorax and neck. The degree of hair loss is variable at these sites, some patients only showing general poor coat quality and alopecia with skin hyperpigmentation confined to the area of collar rub around the neck.

Palpation of the testes for the presence of a lesion may be unrewarding or not confirm any abnormality until the disease has been present for some time. It is possible for a highly active lesion to be so small that it may remain entirely undetectable by palpation.

Careful palpation of the scrotum, abdomen and inguinal region for the retained testis or testes, and of the scrotal testes for abnormalities may be sufficient to suggest the diagnosis; the unaffected testicle becomes atrophic. Some dogs may show concurrent prostatitis or prostatic hyperplasia.

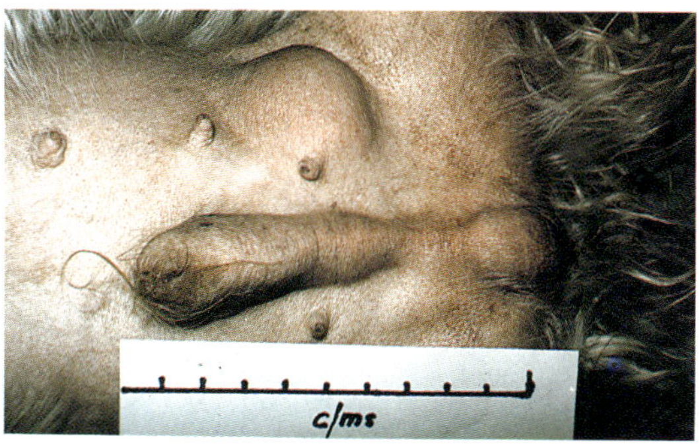

Fig. 9.12. Inguinal testis — Sertoli-cell tumour.

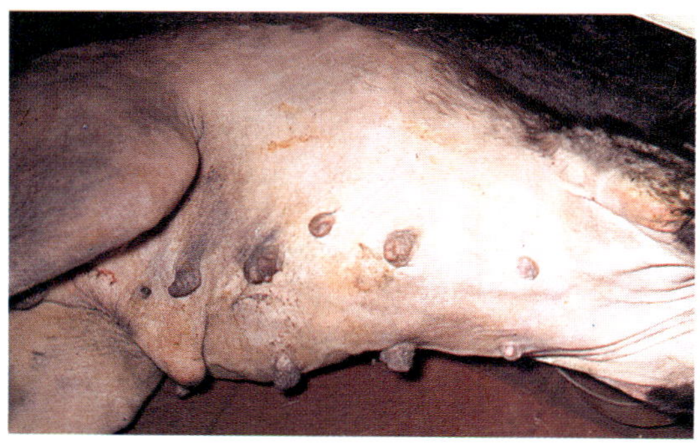

Fig. 9.13. Gynecomastia — Sertoli-cell tumour.

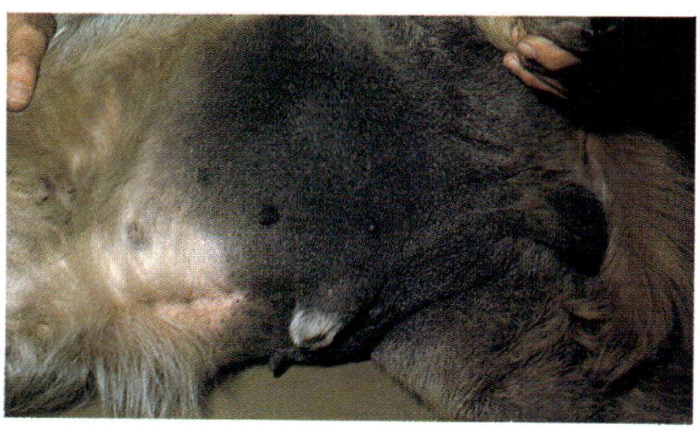

Fig. 9.14. Ventral hyperpigmentation and alopecia — Sertoli-cell tumour.

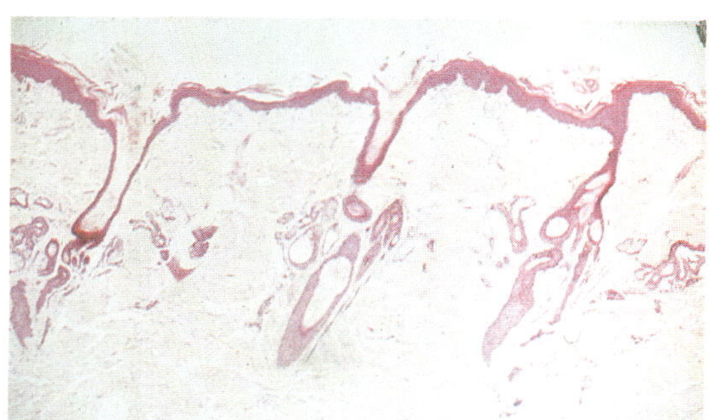

Fig. 9.15. Sertoli-cell neoplasia. Haematoxylin and eosin.

HISTOPATHOLOGY

The skin shows changes similar to other endocrine alopecias: there is orthokeratotic hyperkeratosis, dilatation of follicles with keratin plugging, sebaceous-gland atrophy and telogen arrest (Fig. 9.15).

DIFFERENTIAL DIAGNOSIS

A seminoma may occasionally be associated with feminization, male feminizing syndrome and other causes of bilaterally symmetrical alopecia.

THERAPY

Affected dogs should be castrated.

Hair regrowth usually takes place over a period of 3 months.

Male feminizing syndrome

This is a rare disease of unknown aetiology affecting middle-aged to aged male dogs of any breed. Studies have failed to show any endocrine dysfunction as being responsible (Mattheeuws & Comhaire, 1975).

CLINICAL SIGNS

The general physical condition of the dog is normal. Signs involving the skin are bilaterally symmetrical alopecia with hyperpigmentation mainly of the perineal and genital areas, extension to other sites e.g. the flanks, ventral abdomen, thorax and neck, is commonly affected by other endocrinopathies.

There is also an associated seborrhoea and ceruminous otitis, which may be pruritic.

The testes are palpably normal and the dog is not a cryptorchid.

Feminization is indicated by gynecomastia and behavioural changes, e.g. attractiveness to male dogs, lack of libido.

DIFFERENTIAL DIAGNOSIS

This condition must be differentiated from Sertoli-cell tumour, hypothyroidism, other seborrhoeic diseases, other chronic pruritic diseases and allergy.

DIAGNOSIS

The testicular histology does not confirm the presence of the Sertoli-cell tumour or other tumour. Plasma testosterone and oestradiol are normal, spermatogenesis may or may not be normal and thyroid function is normal.

TREATMENT

1 Castration
2 *Medication*. Oral testosterone 1 mg/kg every other day (maximum total dose 30 mg) followed by maintenance doses once or twice a week.
Depot testosterone (Breen & Reedy, 1975) at 2.2 mg/kg as a single dose repeated at 6-monthly intervals.
3 Benzoyl peroxide shampoo or other antiseborrhoeal shampoo.

Testosterone-responsive dermatosis of the mature dog

The aetiology of this condition is unknown, but castrates, cryptorchids and dogs with normal or abnormal testicles may be affected (Grant, 1986).

CLINICAL SIGNS

There is bilaterally symmetrical, usually non-pruritic, alopecia of male dogs of any breed. Hair loss commences in the genital and perineal regions, extending to involve the medial aspects of the thighs, ventral abdomen and flanks without hyperpigmentation. The coat is dry and lustreless. The skin is thin, lacking in elasticity and there is seborrhoea.

Skin histopathology

There is telogenization of follicles, follicle atrophy and dilatation, sebaceous-gland atrophy, orthokeratotic hyperkeratosis and follicular plugging.

DIFFERENTIAL DIAGNOSIS

This disease should be differentiated from other endocrinopathies, e.g. hypothyroidism, Sertoli-cell tumour, hyperadrenocorticism.

DIAGNOSIS

Diagnosis is made on clinical evaluation and elimination of other alopecic disorders of the ageing male dog.

TREATMENT

Medication consists of testosterone 1 mg/kg (up to 30 mg total dose) daily with maintenance doses every other day.

Endocrine alopecia of the female dog ('canine ovarian imbalance')

It has become the practice to refer to the bilaterally symmetrical alopecias, considered to be endocrinopathies, of the mature bitch or of the bitch spayed prior to the first oestrus, as 'ovarian imbalance Type I' and 'Type II' respectively.

These conditions have been attributed to hyperoestrogenism (Type I) and hypoestrogenism (Type II) although as yet there is little biochemical evidence to support this aetiology.

It is known that alopecia has been induced experimentally by the administration of oestrogen (Jabara, 1962) as well as when oestrogen has been administered therapeutically (Barsanti *et al.*, 1983).

The aetiology of either syndrome remains unclear.

Type I

This syndrome affects middle-aged to aged bitches of any breed with a history of irregular oestrus or pseudocyesis.

CLINICAL SIGNS

The alopecia varies in degree, affecting the perineal and genital areas, with lichenification, hyperpigmentation and seborrhoea, ceruminous otitis and greasy skin. There is enlargement of the nipples.

DIFFERENTIAL DIAGNOSIS

This includes thyroid and adrenal disorders characterized by alopecia and seborrhoea.

DIAGNOSIS

The diagnosis can only be made on symptomatology as definitive tests are not available. Skin biopsy shows changes consistent with an endocrinopathy.

TREATMENT

Ovariohysterectomy will produce a noticeable improvement though this will take several months. Meanwhile care of the coat and skin by bathing is necessary using benzoyl peroxide shampoos or other antiseborrhoeals.

Type II

This syndrome mainly affects bitches spayed before the first oestrus. It may occur at any age but is considered to be uncommon.

CLINICAL SIGNS

It is non-pruritic, non-seborrhoeic with partial alopecia progressing to form discrete areas of hair loss on the perineum, medial and posterior thighs and genital area, eventually involving the ventral abdomen, thorax, neck and ears. Although the bitch's coat is generally soft in character and somewhat immature, hair loss does not progress to involve the dorsal surfaces.

Incontinence has been an associated finding in some patients.

DIFFERENTIAL DIAGNOSIS

As for Type I.

TREATMENT

This involves oestrogen therapy — 0.1 to 1.0 mg diethyl stilboestrol once daily by mouth for 3 weeks; discontinue for 1 week and repeat the routine until hair growth occurs. Maintenance doses of stilboestrol may then be given, 0.1–1.0 mg, once or twice a week, reduced if signs of oestrus are noted. Care should be taken to avoid toxicity, e.g. bone-marrow depression. Stilboestrol has now been withdrawn from the UK market.

Bilateral flank alopecia of short-haired female dogs

This is a common condition of some short-haired breeds, particularly the Doberman, Labrador, boxer and dachshund. It mainly affects mature entire bitches and its symptomatology does not conform to that of ovarian imbalance Type I. The aetiology is unclear.

Eigenmann *et al.* (1984) suggested that this is a manifestation of local rather than systemic hyperoestrogenism due to an increase in (oestradiol) E2 receptors at the affected sites. A recent study (Thomsett & Allen, unpublished) carried out on 45 bitches affected with this condition showed no abnormal levels of circulating oestrogen or progesterone to be present.

CLINICAL SIGNS

Patients are physically normal other than a poor coat and poor skin. Some bitches show irregular oestrus. There is nonpruritic alopecia, in some cases remaining as sparseness of hair rather than total hair loss, with hyperpigmentation of the area of the sublumbar fossa. The area of hair loss is often scaly and some animals may show evidence of a mild seborrhoea throughout the coat. Hair loss may progress to involve the lateral thorax and particularly follow a linear pattern along the outline of the ribs (Fig. 9.16).

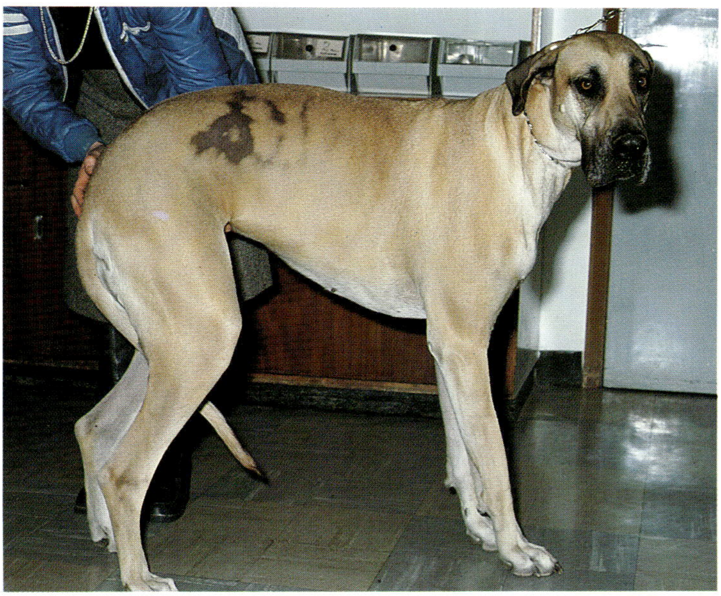

Fig. 9.16. Bilateral flank alopecia of female dog — great Dane showing linear configuration.

DIAGNOSIS AND TREATMENT

Diagnosis is made on the presence of focal hyperoestrogenism. The prognosis is poor as there is no effective treatment. Pregnancy has been suggested.

Canine diabetic dermatosis

In an extensive survey of canine diabetes mellitus in the UK, Foster (1975) reported that 7% of cases had skin lesions. Diabetic dermatosis has recently been described in the dog and shows some similarity to the condition known to occur in humans (Walton *et al.*, 1986).

CLINICAL SIGNS

There is erythema, crusting and alopecia of the perioral and periocular regions and genital area. Erythematous bullae are present and there is ulceration of the skin of the muzzle. Hyperkeratosis of the pads occurs with associated pain and irritation. Secondary bacterial and fungal infection is common.

Severe liver disease may produce marked skin pathology. An early presenting sign may be diffuse hair loss (Baker, 1986).

DIFFERENTIAL DIAGNOSIS

The condition must be distinguished from zinc-responsive dermatosis, systemic lupus erythematosus and pemphigus foliaceus.

DIAGNOSIS

Diagnosis is made mainly on knowledge of the history and signs of the disease consistent with diabetes mellitus; confirmation is sought from laboratory parameters. The histopathology of the skin reveals parakeratotic hyperkeratosis; upper dermal oedema and inter- and intracellular oedema with clefting are characteristic.

Miscellaneous canine alopecias

Tail-gland alopecia (tail-gland hyperplasia)

Nearly all dogs possess a glandular area of skin on the dorsal surface of the proximal one-third of the tail. At this site there are numerous large sebaceous and hepatoid glands which secrete waxy material onto the skin surface. The role of this secretion is unclear but it is thought to be concerned with identification or territorial marking.

The hair follicles also differ from those producing the general body coat inasmuch as they are single, not compound, and produce stouter hairs. A similar but more extensive area is recognized along the dorsal mid-line of the tail of the cat.

CLINICAL SIGNS

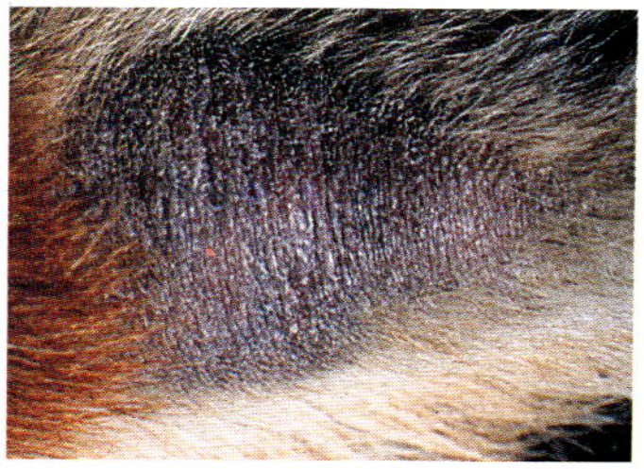

Fig. 9.17. Tail-gland alopecia with hyperpigmentation.

Thinning hair or total hair loss with or without hypertrophy of the glandular area gives rise to an oval alopecic patch, often with hyperpigmentation of the skin, on the dorsum of the tail 3–5 cm from the tail root (Fig. 9.17). The condition is rarely pruritic but may become so when seborrhoea and secondary pyoderma occur.

The patches may mistakenly be regarded as being due to friction when the dog sits.

THERAPY

The therapy is symptomatic using antiseborrhoeals, e.g. selenium sulphide or benzoyl peroxide shampoos. It is claimed by some that progestagen therapy may be beneficial in the cat.

Progesterone-induced alopecia

Some nursing bitches and those in the latter stages of pregnancy may develop a diffuse non-pruritic alopecia of the ventral chest, abdomen and medial thighs not accompanied by hyperpigmentation (Baker, 1986).

DIFFERENTIAL DIAGNOSIS

The condition must be distinguished from other hormonal alopecias of the female dog and iatrogenic alopecia following progestagen therapy.

THERAPY

Once the litter is weaned, hair growth should return to normal. Progestagen therapy should be discontinued.

Feline alopecia

Congenital alopecia, psychogenic alopecia and that associated with ectoparasitism are referred to elsewhere and are only mentioned here for differential diagnosis.

Telogen effluvium

Hair loss due to synchronization of hair follicles in the telogen stage of the hair growth cycle may occur as a result of severe stress or illness.

Regrowth of hair may be delayed for 4–6 months. Once growth commences hair cover should return to normal within 8–12 weeks. Aetiology of the condition is not clearly understood.

TREATMENT

No specific treatment is available. Recourse to hormone therapy should be avoided and the owner persuaded to be patient and await regrowth of hair.

Feline endocrine alopecia

This is a non-pruritic, symmetrical alopecia of cats affecting all ages, sexes and breeds.

AETIOLOGY

While many opinions as to the cause have been put forward, the definitive aetiology has not been determined. Ihrke (unpublished data; Thoday, 1986) has suggested that the aetiology cannot be hormonal because affected animals fitted with an Elizabethan collar to prevent them self-traumatizing their skin and coat have been seen to make a spontaneous recovery.

CLINICAL SIGNS

The cat is normal apart from the coat which has bilaterally symmetrical alopecia. There is diffuse coat thinning of the perineal and genital region and in some cases loss of hair from the tail and caudal thighs extending to the ventral abdomen. Extension to the flanks may occur in severe cases, with hair loss from the area between elbow and carpus on the forelimbs. Concurrent with the extensive hair shedding may be problems associated with hair balls and intestinal disorders.

DIFFERENTIAL DIAGNOSIS

The condition should be differentiated from miliary dermatitis, psychogenic alopecia, telogen effluvium, superficial fungal infections and demodicosis. Ectoparasitic causes of alopecia in the cat are accompanied by self-excoriation. In both thin and psychogenic alopecia the hair is broken and shows lick marks.

DIAGNOSIS

The history is important for diagnosis. T3 and T4 assays are all in the normal range for the cat but the histopathology reveals a reduction in the number of primary follicles with the remainder of the primaries and secondaries all in the telogen phase. Hair plucked from the affected areas show inactive club roots with normal hair tips, when examined microscopically.

THERAPY

A variety of treatment regimens have been used for which success has been claimed. In the absence of a definitive aetiology all are therefore empirical. The following have been used, in some cases to effect.

Megestrol acetate (Ovarid, Pitman Moore) (oral). 5 mg twice a week until evidence of hair growth is seen. Maintenance treatment is then given at 2.5–5 mg once a week.

Progesterone. 100 mg administered by subcutaneous injection as a single dose, repeated in 4 months if necessary (Grant, 1986).

Testosterone phenylpropionate. 5 mg subcutaneously once every 2 weeks.

Liothyronine sodium. Although evidence that affected cats are hypothyroid is lacking it is claimed that 70% of cases will respond to liothyronine therapy for this condition at the following oral dosage: 0.3 mg daily for 3 months then 0.3 mg twice a week or 20 μg b.i.d. increased by 10 μg b.i.d. every third day to a maximum dose of 50 μg b.i.d.

Feline iatrogenic alopecia

The administration of megestrol acetate in high dosage to ovariectomized cats has been shown to cause mammary development and interfere with hair replacement over the ventral abdomen and medial thighs with extension to the sternal thoracic area (Chen & Bellenger, 1987).

References

Baker K.P. (1986) Hormonal alopecia in dogs and cats. *In Practice* **8**, 71.

Barsanti J.A., Medlau L. & Latimer K. (1983) Diethyl stilboestrol induced alopecia in a dog. *Journal of the American Veterinary Medical Association* **182**, 63–64.

Breen P.T. & Reedy L.M. (1975) Endocrine and metabolic dermatoses. *Proceedings of the American Animal Hospital Association* **42**, 131.

Chen J.C. & Bellenger C.R. (1987) Obese appearance, mammary development and retardation of hair growth following megoestrol acetate administration to cats. *Journal of Small Animal Practice* **28**, 1161–1167.

Eigenmann J.E., Poortman J. & Koeman J.P. (1984) Oestrogen induced flank alopecia in the female dog. Evidence of local rather than systemic hyperoestrogenism. *Journal of the American Animal Hospital Association* **20**, 621–624.

Eigenmann J.E. (1986a) Disorders associated with growth hormone oversecretion—diabetes mellitus and acromegaly. In *Current Veterinary Therapy XI. Small Animal Practice* (Ed. Kirk R.W.) pp. 1006–1014. W.B. Saunders, London.

Eigenmann J.E. (1986b) Growth hormone deficient disorders associated with alopecia in the dog. In *Current Veterinary Therapy XI. Small Animal Practice* (Ed. Kirk R.W.) pp. 1015–1018. W.B. Saunders, London.

Feldman E.C. & Nelson R.W. (1987) *Canine and Feline Endocrinology and Reproduction*. W.B. Saunders, Philadelphia.

Foster S.J. (1975) Diabetes mellitus. A study of the disease in the dog and cat in Kent. *Journal of Small Animal Practice* **16**, 295–315.

Grant D.I. (1986) *Skin Diseases in the Dog and Cat*. Blackwell Scientific Publications, Oxford.

Gruffydd-Jones T.J. (1989) Medical management of Cushing's syndrome in dogs. *The Veterinary Record* **124**, 317–319.

Jabara A.G. (1962) Some tissue changes in the dog following stilboestrol administration. *Australian Journal of Experimental Biology and Medical Science* **40**, 293–307.

Mattheeuws D. & Comhaire F. (1975) Oestradiol and testosterone in male dogs with alopecia and feminisation without testicular neoplasia. *British Veterinary Journal* **131**, 65.

Muller G., Kirk R.W. & Scott D. (1983) *Small Animal Dermatology*, 3rd edn. W.B. Saunders, London.

Nesbitt G.H. (1983) Canine and feline dermatology. A systematic approach, Lea and Febiger, Philadelphia.

Peterson M.E. (1984) 'Hyperadrenocorticism' — in *Veterinary Clinics of North America. Small Animal Practice* **14**, no. 4. 731–749.

Scott D.W. (1982) Histopathologic findings in the endocrine skin disorders of the dog. *Journal of the American Animal Hospital Association* **18**, 173–183.

Thoday K.L. (1986) Differential diagnosis of symmetric alopecia in the cat. In *Current Veterinary Therapy XI. Small Animal Practice* (Ed. Kirk R.W.) pp. 545–553. W.B. Saunders, London.

Walton D.K., Center S.A., Scott D.W. & Collins K. (1986) Ulcerative dermatosis associated with diabetes mellitus in the dog. A report of four cases. *Journal of the American Animal Hospital Association* **22**, 79–88.

Zanesco S., Schwalder P., Zapf J., Girard J., von Tscharner C. & Eigenmann J.E. (1984) Pituitary dwarfism in the German Shepherd dog with particular reference to diagnosis. *Kleintierpraxis* **29**, 3–8, 9, 11–14.

10 / Nutritional Diseases with Cutaneous Manifestations

Between 25 and 30% of the daily protein intake is required for the normal nutrition of the skin.

The occurrence of nutritional skin disorders in small domesticated animals is now rare due to the ready availability of prepared balanced proprietary animal feeds.

Except for animals in the less affluent countries and those where quality proprietary foods are not available it is said that dietary deficiencies are so uncommon that they are only seen in animals on diet trial studies.

Skin signs associated with poor diet or the reduction in availability of nutrients due to concurrent disease processes, e.g. malabsorption syndromes, are more likely to be encountered than actual deficiency states.

Protein deficiency

As in protein/calorie deficiency of humans the condition is seen in animals under conditions of malnutrition associated with concurrent disease, e.g. neoplasia or actual starvation.

Clinical signs vary with the degree of protein deficiency and concurrent deficit in energy nutrients, and a combination of a number of the following may be noted — hyperkeratosis, hyperpigmentation of the skin, depigmentation of the hair with a prolonged shedding period. The hair coat is generally poor with brittle hair and patchy alopecia. The differential diagnosis of protein/calorie deficiency is determined by investigating meticulously the management of the patient with special attention to details of dietary components and proportions of protein, carbohydrate and fat.

Any history of concurrent chronic illness which may precipitate starvation will complement the result of a detailed physical examination of the patient leading to a definitive diagnosis. Treatment with special diets and management of disease processes, e.g. malabsorption, should control if not cure the condition.

Fat deficiency

Dietary fat is an essential energy source for both the dog and cat; it provides up to 40% of energy requirements for the latter species. In addition fats provide the essential fatty acids — linoleic, linolenic and arachidonic — which are necessary for the production of cell membranes as well as for the synthesis of prostaglandins.

The cat has a specific enzyme deficiency in respect of N6 desaturase preventing the metabolism of linoleic acid. It thus needs a dietary source of linoleic and linolenic as well as arachidonic acids.

Fat-deficient diets are said not to be uncommon in the USA (Ihrke, 1988), where packaging and storage of petfoods under suboptimal conditions leads to rancidity or leaching of fats and oils through absorbent packaging.

Deficiency of dietary fat may therefore arise not just from absence of a dietary component but also from disease processes interfering with fat digestion, as in pancreatic and hepatic disease and intestinal malabsorption syndromes.

The clinical manifestation of essential fatty acid (EFA) deficiency is variable and may present as a combination of a number of the following signs — dull lustreless coat, alopecia, seborrhoea, impetigo, otitis, lichenification and interdigital exudation.

TREATMENT

Fat deficiency is treated by supplementation with oral EFA in the form of evening primrose oil or a combination of evening primrose oil and fish oil as capsules or liquid or, if such a preparation is not available, then a combination of vegetable oil and animal fat.

Essential fatty acids in atopic disease

There is evidence that dietary supplementation with high doses of EFA in the form of evening primrose oil is beneficial in the treatment of atopic skin disease in the dog, although this is not a fat-deficiency disease. Dosage is three capsules (550 mg/10 kg) daily (Lloyd and Thomsett, unpublished data).

Vitamin deficiencies

Vitamin deficiencies are rare and are only likely to be encountered in situations where vitamin-deficient foods are being fed or in animals with concurrent disease resulting in low vitamin intake or minimal absorption and metabolism.

Where proprietary foods show reduction in vitamin content due to processing, any shortfall is made good by vitamin enhancement of the product before sale.

Vitamin B

B-complex vitamins are essential, for example as constituents of coenzymes in carbohydrate and protein metabolism.

They are important for the maintenance of skin and coat health.

Vitamins A, D, E

All these are important for the maintenance of skin and coat health.

Vitamin A

Hypovitaminosis A is unlikely to occur in the developed countries and is rare even where owners do not have the benefit of readily available quality commercial petfoods.

Vitamin A-responsive dermatosis has been described by Ihrke and Goldschmidt (1983) and characterized by an incidence of 1 in 40–50 cocker spaniels. The lesions involve gross follicular plugging due to a follicular hyperkeratosis and respond to the daily oral administration of 10 000 i.u. vitamin A for up to 8 weeks duration.

Vitamin E

Where animals are fed diets high in fats (e.g. high fish content cat food), particularly polyunsaturates as well as sulphur-containing amino acids, there is an increased requirement for Vitamin E.

Poorly packaged and stored prepared foods with adequate vitamin content at the time of manufacture may become deficient and so induce a hypovitaminosis which presents clinically as a suppression of T-cell immunity with signs similar to severe canine demodicosis.

In cats, hypovitaminosis E may present as a pansteatitis with painful subcutaneous and intra-abdominal fat nodules.

DIAGNOSIS

The diagnosis of pansteatitis is confirmed by histological examination of fat nodules which show a panniculitis and the presence of ceroid in lipocytes, macrophages and giant cells.

TREATMENT

This consists of dietary supplementation with 10 mg/kg vitamine E once daily.

Zinc-deficiency dermatoses

Zinc is a component of over 100 metalloenzymes and plays an important role in the maintenance of skin health. It is essential for the normal production of keratin.

In humans a deficiency state associated with disordered zinc metabolism of genetic origin, acrodermatitis enteropathica, was described by Moynahan (1974) and since that time a wide variety of dermatological and other human ailments have been associated with disordered zinc absorption or utilization.

In the UK zinc-deficiency dermatosis of pigs was well documented shortly after World War II, being attributed to the feeding of high-fibre (phytate)/high-calcium diets with consequent poor zinc availability.

With these conditions well known, it was therefore not long before a zinc-deficiency dermatosis was recognized as occurring spontaneously in dogs.

Zinc-deficiency dermatosis had been induced experimentally well before the paper on the naturally occurring disease was published by Kunkle (1980), who described two conditions.

Syndrome one

The predilection is for Alaskan malamutes, Siberian huskies, Doberman pinschers and great Danes — mainly fast growing puppies although some adults were involved (Degryse *et al.*, 1987). Lesions were seen clinically as alopecia, crusting and scaling with suppuration around the orifices — of great similarity to acrodermatitis enteropathica of humans.

Some dogs showed crusting over the bony prominences of the limbs with hyperkeratosis of the pads (Fig. 10.1).

Greatest similarity with the human condition was seen in the malamute where a specific genetic defect in intestinal absorption of zinc has been demonstrated.

In addition to genetic defects in zinc utilization, high cereal (phytate)/high-calcium diets bind zinc reducing its availability in the dog as in other species, leading to clinical signs

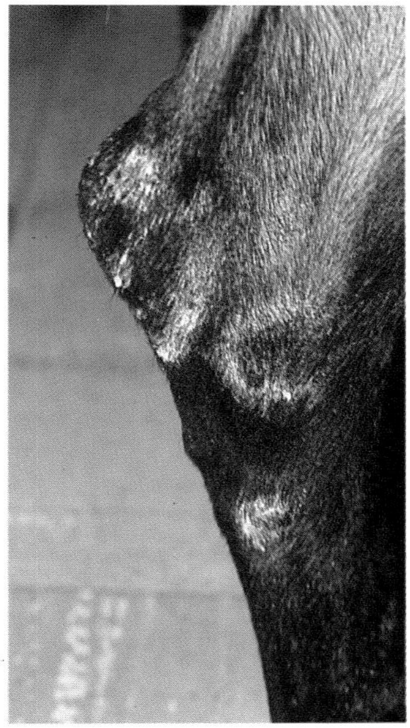

Fig. 10.1. Zinc-deficiency dermatosis — annular crusted lesions on hock.

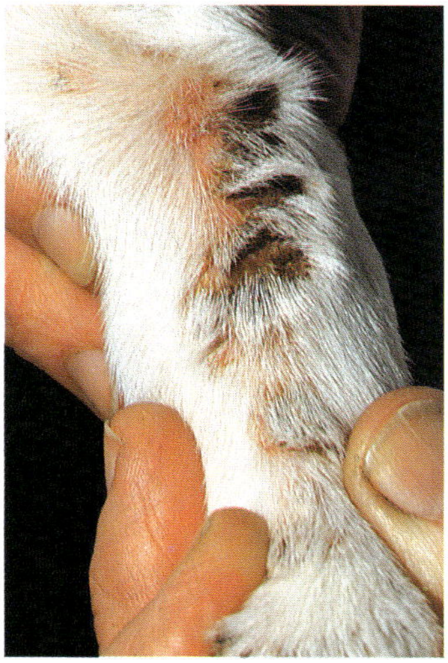

Fig. 10.2. Zinc-deficiency dermatosis of a beagle puppy — crusted erythematous lesion on forelimb.

of deficiency such as unthriftiness. Van den Broek and Thoday (1986) described zinc-deficiency dermatosis in a group of Labrador retrievers where the condition was considered to be a combination of reduced availability due to a high-fibre/high-calcium diet and a demonstrable absorption defect.

In addition to greying of the hair, widespread hyperkeratotic/parakeratotic lesions were seen, particularly on the limbs. The condition was confirmed by serum and hair zinc assays before and after treatment by zinc supplementation of the diet.

Syndrome two

This is seen in rapidly growing puppies of a number of breeds, e.g. great Dane, German shepherd, doberman pinscher, beagle, German short-haired pointer, and standard poodle, particularly on high-fibre diets and diets rich in soyabean meal with calcium supplementation.

The degree of severity has been shown to vary even among littermates and a variety of clinical signs can be seen: poor growth rate, general malaise, loss of appetite, and formation of hyperkeratotic plaques having the appearance of pyoderma crusts on the limbs, periorbital skin, and over bony protuberances, as well as hyperkeratosis of the planum nasale.

One author (Thomsett) has seen this manifestation of zinc dermatosis to particularly affect laboratory beagle colonies maintained on high-fibre diets, notably dry complete foods, under otherwise ideal conditions of husbandry (Fig. 10.2).

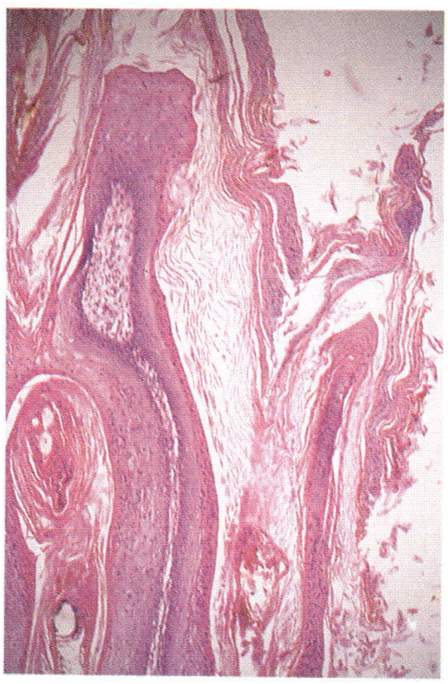

Fig. 10.3. Zinc-deficiency dermatosis of a beagle — parakeratotic hyperkeratosis.

DIAGNOSIS

The diagnosis is made following an investigation of management, clinical examination of the patients, with histological examination of skin biopsies showing parakeratotic hyperkeratosis as a significant feature (Fig. 10.3).

Estimations of serum and hair zinc may be undertaken although great variation in values can be obtained.

Response to treatment with zinc confirms the diagnosis.

TREATMENT

Dietary imbalances are corrected and zinc supplementation is given, using oral zinc sulphate at 10 mg/kg preferably after a meal and in divided doses. For example, zinc methionine (Zinpro) may be given at a rate of 1 tablet per 10 kg daily; each is equivalent to 15 mg elemental zinc.

Should there be skin lesions requiring therapy, e.g. seborrhoea, antiseborrhoeals may be employed, e.g. seleen.

In most cases response to oral treatment is rapid and dramatic and other medication is not required.

Zinc deficiency in cats

This is a rare condition characterized by poor coat growth, alopecia and scaly skin. It responds to zinc supplementation (Kane *et al.*, 1981).

References

Degryse A-D., Fransen J., van Cutsem J. & Ooms L. (1987) Recurrent zinc responsive dermatosis in a Siberian Husky. *Journal of Small Animal Practice* **28**, 721–726.

Ihrke P.J. (1988) *BSAVA Congress Proceedings.*

Ihrke P.J. & Goldschmidt M.H. (1983) Vitamin A responsive dermatosis in the dog. *Journal of the American Veterinary Medical Association* **182**, 687.

Kane E., Morris J.G., Rogers Q.R., Ihrke P.J., & Cupps P.T. (1981) Zinc deficiency in the cat. *Journal of Nutrition* **111**, 488.

Kunkle G.H. (1980) Zinc responsive dermatosis in dogs. *Current Veterinary Therapy VII* (Ed. Kirk R.W.) pp. 472–476. W.B. Saunders, London.

Moynahan E.J. (1974) Acrodermatitis enteropathica: a lethal inherited human zinc deficiency disorder. *Lancet* **2**, 399.

Van den Broek A.H.M. & Thoday K.L. (1986) Skin disease in dogs associated with zinc deficiency. A report on 5 cases. *Journal of Small Animal Practice* **27**, 313–323.

Further reading

Fadok V. A. (1986) Nutritional therapy in veterinary dermatology. In *Current Veterinary Therapy XI. Small Animal Practice* (Ed. Kirk R.W.) pp. 591–596. W.B. Saunders, London.

11 / Physically and Chemically Induced Disease

Solar keratosis

Keratosis and chronic dermatosis occur in human skin when it is inadequately protected from prolonged exposure to sunlight. In humans, solar keratosis occurs in middle and old age. Hyperkeratosis and parakeratosis are prominent features in humans; squamous-cell carcinoma may develop in lesions of solar keratosis.

Hargis *et al.* (1977) reported lesions resembling solar keratosis on sparsely haired, lightly pigmented parts of the ventral body skin in 397 of 1680 beagle dogs in a colony; 34 dogs subsequently developed squamous cell carcinomata at these sites. Dogs in the colony were housed in a locality of prolonged sunshine in Colorado and regularly sunbathed for long periods on their backs. Hargis *et al.* (1977) considered that solar radiation was involved in the pathogenesis of the lesions. As reported elsewhere in this text, predilection sites for the development of squamous-cell carcinoma are those which are most exposed to sunlight — the tips of the ears and eyelids of lightly pigmented animals: white cats or cats with white ears are particularly at risk. The tips of the ears and their margins first show erythema, and a mild exfoliative dermatitis without pain; subsequently there is thickening, ulceration and encrustation with pain and excoriation. Continuing exposure to sunlight will, in some cases, result in frank neoplasia after several years.

Canine solar dermatitis, formerly called 'collie nose', is reported in the USA. Most cases are possibly a result of autoimmune disease, which is exacerbated by bright sunlight.

Caterpillar irritation

Members of the Lepidoptera (the moths and butterflies) may cause irritations to the skin or mucous membranes because they shed hair which irritate on penetration of the skin or because they are provided with defensive nettling hairs. A number of 'epidemics' in humans have been reported. An early one was in Boston, USA. White (1901) recognized that many cases of blistering eruptions were caused by the asp caterpillar of the brown tail moth, *Hylexia*. *Megalopyge opercularis* may also cause lesions in humans (McGovern, 1961). There have been a few reports of similar interactions in cats and dogs. The caterpillar of the brown tail moth, *Europroctis chrysorrhoea*, is protected by hollow setae which can cause irritation of the skin. There may be severe pruritus and erythema, particularly of the flank, with epiphora and ulceration of the tongue (Fig. 11.1). Cunningham and Mahon (1985) reported an episode in Portsmouth on the south coast of England during the summer months involving cats and dogs. Sticky tape pressed to the skin of the irritated area and then stripped may remove the implanted setae. Megestrol acetate 5 mg may then be given to control pruritus.

Several families of the Lepidoptera have species whose larvae possess stinging hairs and spines for self-defence. Probably many cases of urticating caterpillar dermatitis in cats and dogs go unreported. Harwood and James (1979) consider that the term 'erucism' should be used for the irritation caused by larvae, and 'lepidopterism' for that caused by adults. These authors reported severe stomatitis in dogs eating grasses contaminated with the setae of *Thaumetopoca pimivora*. Probably irritation is the result of physical reaction to setae and/or the presence of irritating chemicals.

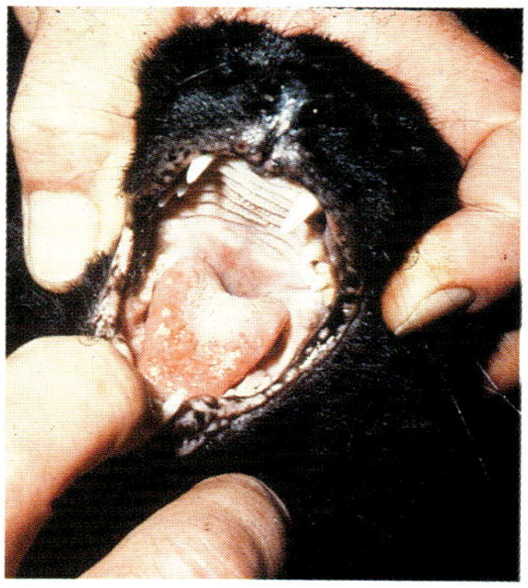

Fig. 11.1. Feline glossitis resulting from contact with irritant caterpillar setae. (Courtesy of S.M. Womar.)

Contact-irritant dermatitis

This is a dermatitis that develops rapidly after direct contact of the skin with an irritating substance. It does not involve an antibody–antigen reaction and is therefore to be distinguished from contact-allergic dermatitis (a cell-mediated immunity), which is characterized by the development of dermatitis after a latent period.

Irritants may be strong chemicals producing an immediate reaction, or solvents, detergents (Fig. 11.2) and soaps, which may produce irritation after several exposures. The skin of weak or anaesthetized animals may be severely inflamed by lengthy contact with urine.

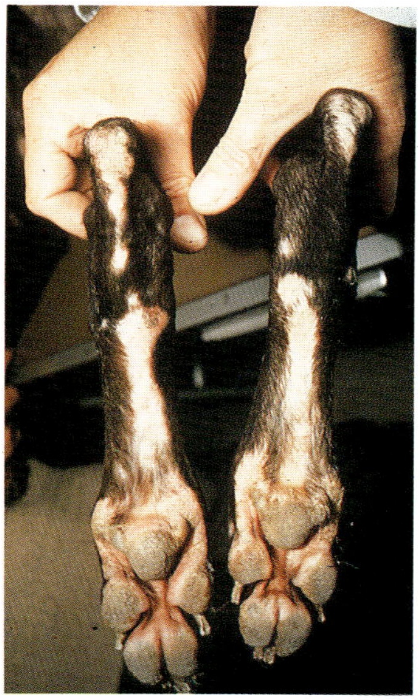

Fig. 11.2. Dermatitis of a greyhound, resulting from contact with hypochlorite used as a disinfectant.

CLINICAL SIGNS

The distribution of lesions is most usually on the hairless or relatively hairless parts of the body (Fig. 11.3); however, hairy parts of the body or the whole pelage may be affected if the reaction is to liquid or sprays. Reactions to plastic collars impregnated with a parasiticide to control flea infestation may be restricted to the area immediately beneath the collar or involve large areas of the neck and head.

The initial sign is erythema and there may be pruritus. The resulting licking and scratching may extend the primary

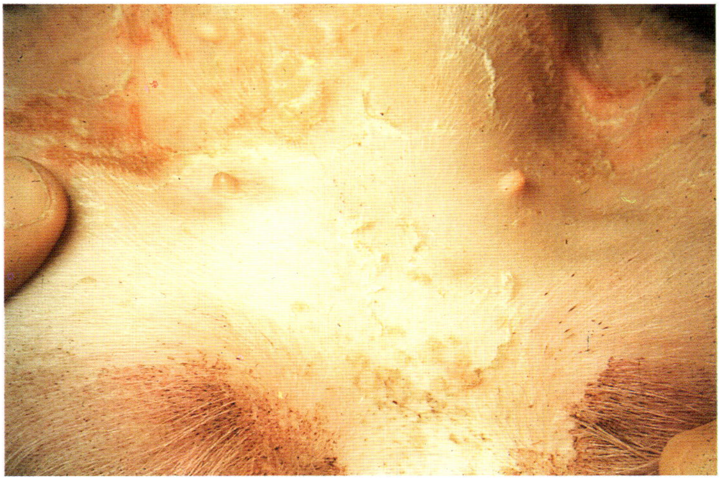

Fig. 11.3. Dermatitis of canine ventral trunk caused by contact with wart paint.

lesion or lesions to other parts of the body; thus, there may be erythema and ulceration of the lips and tongue. A mild irritant may not produce severe lesions; there may be healing with mild exfoliative dermatitis as the end point. With more corrosive chemicals there will be ulceration and severe erythema with secondary pyoderma developing.

The histopathology is not specific.

DIFFERENTIAL DIAGNOSIS

Contact-allergic dermatitis may be difficult to distinguish from contact-irritant dermatitis. In the former, frank ulceration is not seen, whilst the chronic case will show acanthosis and lichenification extending over a protracted period. Contact-irritant dermatitis is typically an exuberant dermatitis of sudden recent origin.

Atopic dermatitis presents with severe generalized pruritus with facial irritation.

DIAGNOSIS

Questioning the owner may reveal the recent use of paint stripper or other strong household chemicals in the pet's environment, whilst the distribution of the lesions themselves is helpful.

THERAPY

Further contact with the offending chemical, if known, must be avoided. Licking should be prevented by the use of an Elizabethan collar. The mouth should be examined to determine if there are associated buccal lesions, in which case antiseptic mouth-washes and soft feeding may be indicated. Severely inflamed lesions should be washed with saline or antiseptic and an emollient dressing (for example Siopel, ICI) applied. If there is severe inflammation betamethasone with neomycin may be applied.

Burns

Thermal damage may result from direct exposure to hot surfaces or scalding fluids or hair dryers. Anaesthetized or weak animals are particularly at risk if placed on heating pads for prolonged periods or if recovery lamps are placed too close to the skin (Fig. 11.4). Severe damage may result; this may not become obvious for several days, when there may be sloughing of the skin over large areas.

Thermal damage may be superficial, involving the epidermis only, or deep, with destruction of the epidermis, adnexae and dermis.

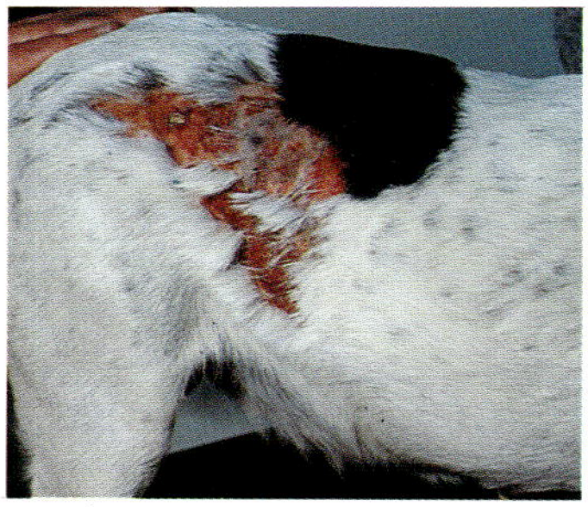

Fig. 11.4. Healing burns 2 weeks following surgery, caused by infrared lamp placed too near skin during recovery from anaesthesia.

CLINICAL SIGNS

The initial erythema of superficial burns and loss of sensation associated with deep burns may not be immediately apparent if the burns are not sufficiently extensive to produce systemic signs. Burns in cats and dogs are usually full-thickness burns, the pelage acting as an efficient insulator resulting in maximum damage. With superficial burns there is associated discomfort shown by attempts to lick or bite the affected area. Deep burns, unless extensive, may not be apparent for several days, the area being anaesthetized by destruction of the sensory nerve endings. Indeed the case may not be presented until the owner has noticed the affected skin becoming hard and leathery; often secondary infection is present with pus formation and the commencement of sloughing.

DIAGNOSIS

A history of recent thermal injury or exposure to heat during recovery is helpful. The appearance of full-thickness burns is characteristic. Superficial burns involving erythema and tenderness may present difficulties.

THERAPY

If the thermal damage is observed immediately, the affected area should be cooled with cold water, dried and close clipped, kept clean and licking prevented.

However, most burns are severe and not observed until extensive sloughing has commenced. The owner should be informed that burn healing, unless superficial or of a small area, is necessarily prolonged. The entire body surface should be closely examined for thermal damage and associated hair close clipped; anaesthetization may be necessary to enable this to be done. Extensive debridement may be necessary. The exposed surface should be daily washed with diluted povidone iodine and debrided as necessary. An Elizabethan collar should be worn to prevent licking. Myiasis is an attendant danger.

Frostbite

In temperate Europe environmental temperatures are rarely low enough to produce tissue damage in active, healthy animals. However, when frostbite does occur, the parts of the body affected are usually the extremities, although hairless areas, e.g. the scrotum, may also become frostbitten. When frozen, frostbitten areas are without sensation, the skin is blanched and cold. With thawing there is pain and functional erythema with swelling.

THERAPY

Gentle thawing is necessary by soaking in warm water. The frostbitten tissue is brittle and easily damaged so that careful handling is essential. When defrosted, an antiseptic emollient dressing should be applied after clipping surrounding hair. Healing may occur without necrosis. If there is necrosis the necrotic tissue should be surgically removed and routine therapy prescribed for surgical wounds.

Chemical depigmentation

A vitiligo-like depigmentation as a result of contact with chemical agents has been reported in humans, e.g. in tannery workers exposed to the monobenzylether of hydroquinone (MBEH), used as an antioxidant. MBEH depigmentation attributed to various rubber articles has been reported. Experimental evidence has been presented by Jimbowk *et al.* (1974); this involved melanocyte destruction in the skin of guinea pigs exposed to hydroquinone.

Chemical depigmentation occasionally occurs in dogs fed from rubber bowls, the contact area being white but without associated inflammatory changes (Fig. 11.5). The depigmentation is irreversible.

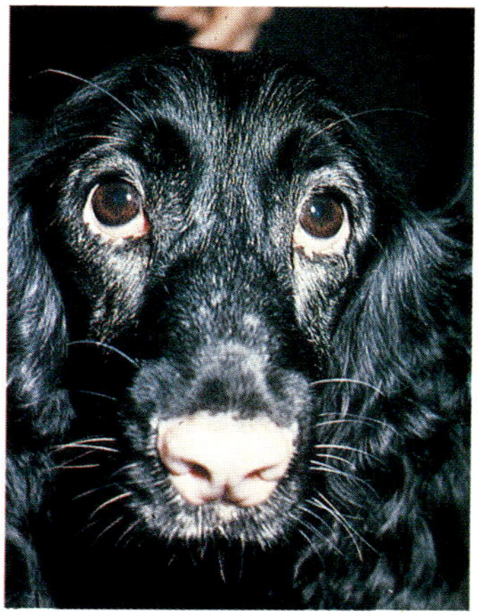

Fig. 11.5. Vitiligo of planum nasale due to contact with feeding bowl.

Thallium

This chemical was until comparatively recently widely used as a rodenticide. With acute toxicity, death occurs rapidly without the dermatological signs. With chronic toxicity there is a mild to severe exfoliative or ulcerative dermatitis.

References

Cunningham W.D. & Mahon F.J. (1985) Cats, dogs and caterpillars. *Veterinary Record* **117**, 71.

Hargis A.M., Thomassen R.W. & Phenister R.D. (1977). Chronic dermatosis and cutaneous squamous cell carcinoma in the Beagle dog. *Veterinary Pathology* **14**, 218–228.

Harwood R.F. & James M.T. (1979) *Entomology in Human and Animal Health*, 7th edn. Macmillan, London.

Jimbow K., Obata H. & Pathak M.K. (1974) Mechanisms of depigmentation by hydroquinone. *Journal of Investigational Dermatology* **62**, 436–449.

McGovern J.P. (1961) *Megalopyge opercularis*: observations of its life history, natural history of its sting in man. *Journal of the American Medical Association* **175**, 1155–1158.

White J.C. (1901) Dermatitis caused by caterpillar. *Boston Medicine and Surgery Journal* **144**, 599.

Appendix / Differential Diagnosis of Skin Disease

Skin disease	Pruritus	Alopecia	Pyoderma	Bulla
Skin-fold dermatitis	+		+	
Pruritic superficial folliculitis	+		+	
Pododermatitis	+	+	+	
Mycobacterial infection		+	+	
Dermatomycosis				
Dermatophytosis	±	+	±	
Leishmaniasis	+	+		
Ancylostomiasis				
Uncinariasis	+	+		
Pelodera dermatitis	+	+		
Schistosomiasis	+			+
Dracunculiasis	+		+ nodules	
Dirofilariasis	+		+	
Ticks				
spinous ear tick	+			
Ixodes	±			
Mites				
Dermanyssus	+	+		
Trombicula	+	+		
Otodectes cynotis	+	+		
Cheyletiella spp.	+	+		
Demodex	±	+	+	
Sarcoptes	++	+	+	
Notoedres	+	+		
Lice				
Linognathus setosus	+	+		
Felicola subrostratus	+	+		
Fleas	+	+		
Atopy	++	+		
Contact-allergic dermatitis	+	+		
Food hypersensitivity	+			
Drug eruption	+			
? Hormone hypersensitivity	+			
Intestinal parasite hypersensitivity	+			
Bacterial hypersensitivity	+			+
Pemphigus vulgaris				+
Pemphigus vegetans	±			
Pemphigus foliaceus	±			
Pemphigus erythematosus	±	+		+

Bullous pemphigoid	±			+
Systemic lupus erythematosus	±			
Discoid lupus	±			
Dermatitis herpetiformis	+			+
Toxic epidermal necrolysis	−			+
Vasculitis				
Linear IgA dermatitis	± or absent		+	
Hyperoestrogenism, female		+		
Sertoli-cell tumour, male		+		
Male hypogonadism		+		
Progesterone/progestagen		+		
Hyperadrenocorticism		+		
Pituitary dwarfism		+		
Adult growth hormone deficiency		+		
Feline endocrine alopecia		+		
Oestrogen responsive dermatosis, female		+		
Male feminizing syndrome		+		
Hypoandrogenism		+		
Diabetes mellitus		+	+	
Hypothyroidism		+	+	
Congenital/hereditary disease				
colour mutant alopecia		+	±	
feline alopecia universalis		+		
feline hypotrichosis		+		
canine congenital alopecia		+		
epidermolysis bullosa	±	+		
Alopecia areata		+		
Pinnal alopecia		+		
Seborrhoea	±	+	±	
Acne	+	+	+	
Feline psychogenic alopecia	+	+		
Solar dermatitis		+		
Contact-irritant dermatitis	+	+		
Frostbite				
Burns				
Thallium		+		
Protein deficiency		+		
Vitamin A deficiency				
Biotin deficiency				
Dalmatian bronzing syndrome	+	±	±	
'Acanthosis nigricans'		+		
Subcorneal pustular dermatosis	+	+		+
Feline miliary dermatitis	+	+		

Glossary

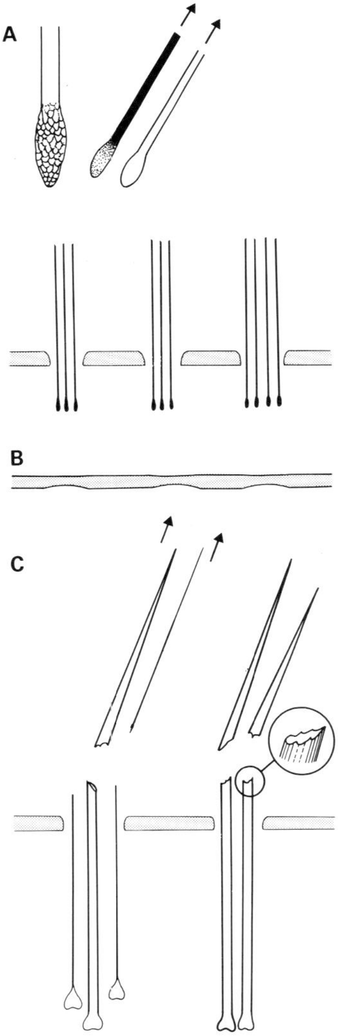

Alopecia.

Acantholysis Loss of cohesion between epidermal cells resulting in clefts, vesicles and bullae. Characteristically seen in autoimmune disease and other vesicular or pustular dermatoses.

Acanthosis Increase in thickness of the malpighian layer resulting in the formation of elongated rete pegs and consequent accentuation of the lines of cleavage of the skin. Commonly seen as a sequel to chronic skin damage.

Acne Secondarily infected hair follicles, often keratin plugged, resulting in papulopustular lesions commonly on the chin of the cat and short-haired dogs.

Adenoma A benign tumour of glandular tissue.

Allergy A state of changed reactivity, in an immunological sense. It may be protective or harmful.

Alopecia Hair loss. **A** Partial alopecia, e.g. hypothyroidism. Hair papillae inactive (telogen). **B** Complete alopecia, e.g. Cushing's disease, hypothyroidism. **C** Pruritic alopecia. Active (anagen) hair papillae. Primary and secondary hair loss, hair shafts ragged and broken.

Anagen The active growth phase of a hair.

Anaphylaxis An exaggerated immunological response to foreign protein.

Apocrine gland Sweat glands associated with each pilosebaceous complex, the secretion of which is produced by budding and disruption of the free portion of the secretory cells.

Arthrospore Spores formed from fungal hyphae.

Atopy A familial predisposition to an allergic state.

Autoimmunity The state of hypersensitivity in which the individual reacts against its own tissues. There may be high organ specificity, as in the pemphigus complex, or low organ specificity, as in systemic lupus erythematosus.

Bulla A large vesicle.

Calcinosis The deposition of amorphous calcium in the skin, e.g. calcinosis cutis in hyperadrenocorticism, or in the skin of the phalanges, foot pads or phrenum linguae — calcinosis circumscripta of unknown aetiology.

Carcinoma Malignant epithelial neoplasia, invasive of adjacent structures and causing metastases.

Catagen The intermediate stage in the hair growth cycle — between anagen and telogen.

Cerumen The lipid secretion produced by the glands of the ear canal.

Clear cell Specialized melanin-forming cells in the stratum germinativum — melanocytes.

Cleft A space caused by separation of the layers of the epidermis, as in the pemphigus complex, often giving rise to vesicles or bullae.

Collagen The substance of which the majority of the dermal fibres are composed.

Comedo, comedone A plug of keratin debris and sebum within the lumen and ostium of the hair follicle.

Crust Exudate from a lesion which has dried on the surface of the skin.

Cyst See under *Tumour*.

Demodicosis The disease caused by the multiplication of the mite *Demodex canis*.

Dermatophyte A fungus which lives upon the skin and other keratinized structures.

Dermatosis A disease of skin.

Desensitization A mechanism by which the immunological state of hypersensitivity is reduced or eliminated.

Diascopy Examination of a lesion through clear glass or plastic pressed down onto it. This will indicate whether the red colour of a lesion results from capillary dilatation or extravasation of blood.

Dyskeratosis Disordered keratinization as applied to keratinocytes.

Eczema A term used to indicate any exudative and erythematous skin disease which heals by scale and crust formation and is often followed by acanthosis and lichenification. (Often misused and misleading.)

Elastic fibres A complementary network of elastic fibrils around and between the collagen bundles.

Endocrine To do with the endocrine system or ductless glands.

Epidermal collarettes The peripheral desquamation at the edge of a lesion, as in annular lesions of bacterial dermatitis or bullous pemphigoid.

Epidermolysis Disruption of the dermo-epidermal junction to form vesicles.

Epithelioma Epithelial neoplasia.

Erosion A lesion of the skin insufficiently deep to scar on healing.

Erythema Reddening of the skin due to capillary dilatation and engorgement.

Excoriation Superficial physical damage to the skin.

Exfoliation Shedding of skin scales.

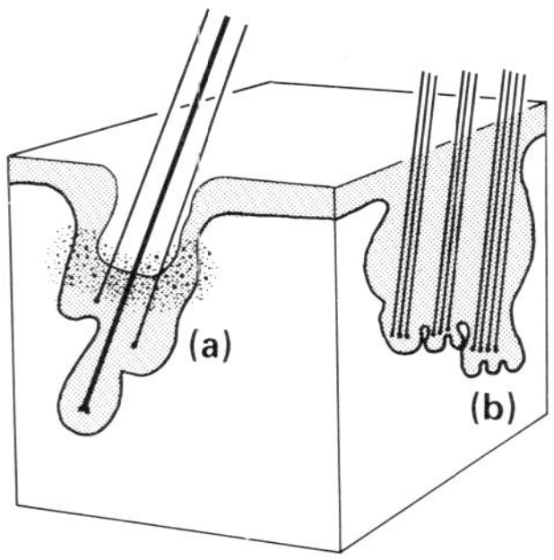

Folliculitis and furunculosis.

Exocytosis The migration of inflammatory cells from the dermis into the epidermis.

Fibroma A fibrous tumour, usually benign.

Fissure Discontinuity of the skin; a crack.

Follicular plug The accumulation of keratin debris within the lumen of an inactive hair follicle, as in endocrine alopecia.

Folliculitis (a) Inflammation of the hair follicle. The infiltrate may penetrate the pilary canal as in demodicosis.

Furunculosis (b) Rupture of hair follicles to form furuncles. There is inflammation of a large number of hair follicles with confluence and pus formation. Generalized demodicosis.

Glabrous skin The smooth skin of the less hairy or hairless areas of the body.

Granuloma Circumscribed subacute or chronic inflammation about a focus.

Hapten A substance conjugated with tissue protein, which is then antigenic.

Hydropic degeneration Vacuolization of basal cells with disintegration leading to destruction of the basement membrane and thus the dermo-epidermal junction.

Hyperhidrosis An increase in sweating.

Hyperkeratosis Increase in thickness of the stratum corneum. Unlike parakeratosis, nuclei are retained in the stratum corneum.

Hyperpigmentation Increase in melanin pigment in the stratum germinativum or upper dermis as in acanthosis nigricans.

Hypopigmentation Diminished pigmentation.

Hyposensitization See *Desensitization*.

Ichthyosis Disordered production of keratin, often congenital, giving rise to fish-scale-like hyperkeratosis.

Impetigo A superficial bacterial infection of the skin characterized by pustule formation and most commonly caused by pathogenic staphylococci.

Keratohyaline granules Granules in the stratum granulosum likely to be precursors of keratin.

Lanugo Down hair.

Lentigo A spot or freckle.

Lesion Any abnormality of tissue of pathological origin.

Lichenification An elevation of the skin resulting from irregular thickening of the epidermis. The surface markings are exaggerated and the surface is often scaly. Lichenification is usually extensive. It is seen, for example, in areas subjected to prolonged excoriation and in acanthosis nicricans. Diascopy does not cause blanching.

Lipoma A fatty tumour.

Macule A circumscribed area of altered skin colour without elevation or depression and not greater than 1 cm diameter. Causes:

1 Trauma — with extravasation of blood.

2 Hyperpigmentation or hypopigmentation due to altered melanocyte activity.

3 Local increased vascularity in erythema, petechiae, ecchymoses or haemangioma.

(1) and (3) can be distinguished by the pressure of a glass slide on the macule: blanching will occur at the site of increased vascularity.

Mastocytosis Increase in the number of mast cells.

Melanocyte A melanin-producing cell.

Melanophage A cell which engulfs and removes free melanin granules.

Merocrine Describing the process by which, through disruption of part of the secretory cell of apocrine glands, apocrine sweat is produced.

Metaplasia Alteration or change of one form of tissue into another.

Miliary Having the appearance of milia, small seeds.

Myiasis Parasitism by dipterous larvae.

Necrolysis Epidermal cell death, acute; as in acute epidermal necrolysis.

Necrosis Cell death.

Nikolsky sign Wrinkling or sliding of the epidermis by pressure where there is intra-epidermal or dermo-epidermal cleft formation, e.g. bullous pemphigoid.

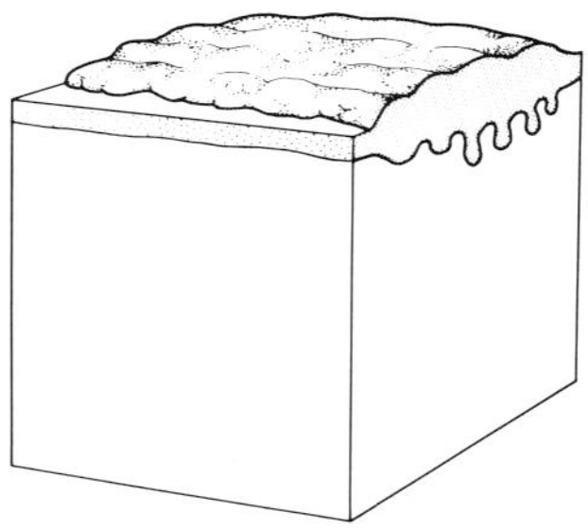

Nikolsky sign.

Nodule A small, circumscribed solid lesion of the skin, raised above the surface and extending into the dermis or deeper tissues of the skin.

Oedema Accumulation of fluid within the skin causing swelling due to an increase in thickness.

Panniculitis Inflammation of the fat layer of the skin.

Papilloma A pendunculated projection of the epidermis consisting of neoplastic epidermal cells. May be multiple.

Papillomatosis Irregularity of the surface of the skin due to upward proliferation of dermal papillae, e.g. in chronic lichenification due to self trauma.

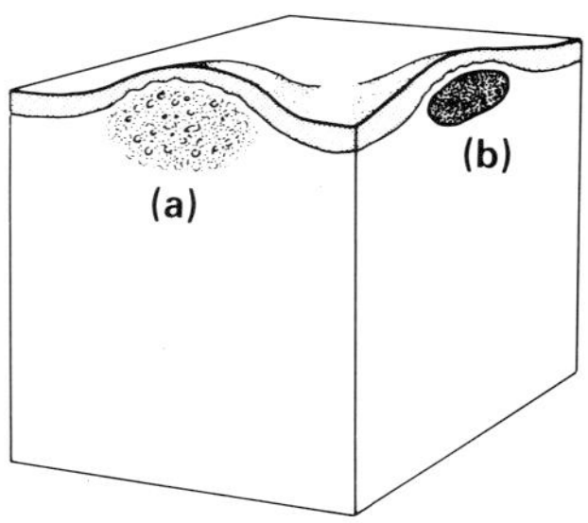

Papule.

Papule A small (less than 1 cm diameter), solid elevation of the skin caused by aggregations in the dermis displacing the epidermis. Aggregations may be (a) cellular or (b) metabolic infiltrates.

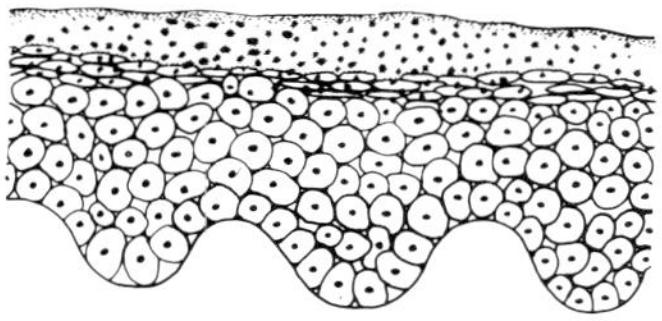

Parakeratosis.

Parakeratosis Abnormal or imperfect keratinization of epidermal cells characterized by retention of nuclei in the stratum corneum and follicle wall, e.g. in zinc-deficiency dermatosis or adjacent to inflammatory skin lesions.

Paronychia Inflammation of the nail bed.

Patch A circumscribed area of discoloration of the skin that is larger than a macule.

Pemphigus A blistering disease; the cause is considered to be autoimmune acantholysis.

Petechiae Small haemorrhages penetrating the skin.

Pilosebaceous complex The structures of the hair follicles together with their adjacent sebaceous glands.

Plaque A flat-topped, steep-sided elevation of the skin.

Polymorphic Having a variety of forms.

Prickle cells Cells of the epidermis showing the presence of desmosomes (prickles), as of the malpighian layer.

Pruritus Itching.

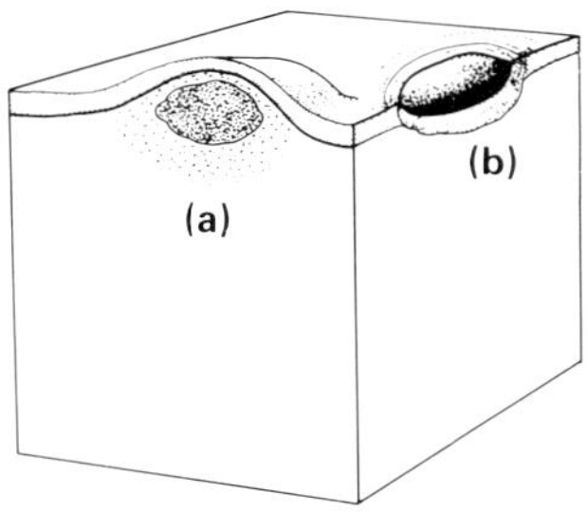

Pustule.

Pustule A small (less than 1 cm diameter), elevated, pus-filled skin lesion (a). These rupture to heal with a collarate perimeter typical of staphylococcal hypersensitivity (b).

Pyoderma A purulent skin disease.

Sarcoma A malignant mesodermal tumour.

Scab An accumulation of exudate, cell debris and blood clot covering a wound. See *Crust*.

Scale Accumulations of desquamating epidermal cells.

Scar A mass of dense fibrous tissue at the site of previous dermal damage.

Seborrhoea An increase in scale formation with or without concurrent increase in sebum production.

Sebum The lipid secretion of the sebaceous glands.

Spongiosis Intercellular oedema, as between keratinocytes, causing stretching of the desmosomes.

Squame A scale, e.g. desquamating, cornified cells.

Subcutis The layers immediately beneath the skin.

Telogen The resting phase of the hair follicle in the hair growth cycle.

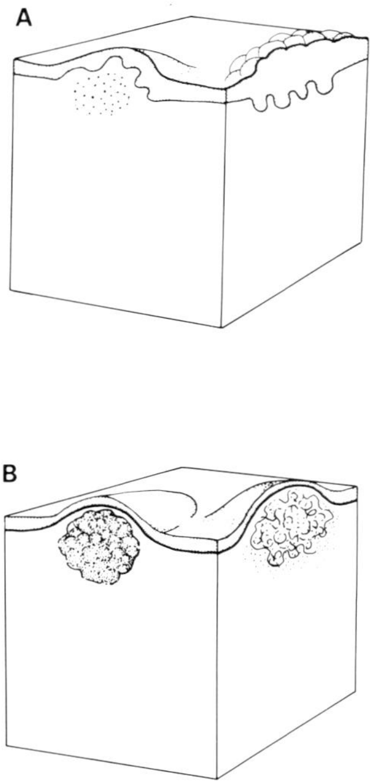

Tumours.

Tumour A skin swelling, not always neoplastic.

A *Papule*. A small, solid elevation, less than 1 cm diameter, raised above surrounding skin. This may be warty (verrucose).

B *Nodule*. A small, solid elevation, less than 1 cm diameter,

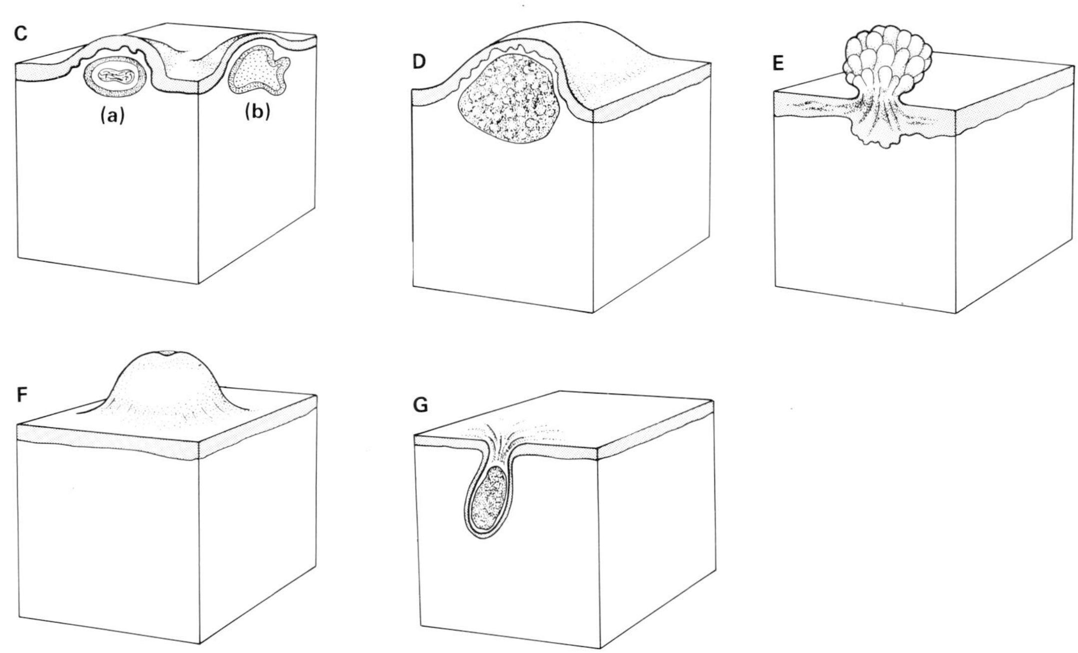

Tumours.

extending into the dermis more than a papule. May be ulcerated.

C *Cyst*. Although not neoplastic, the cyst is included because of its superficial resemblance to a tumour. It is a small, fluid-filled sac in the dermis. Cysts may be *epidermal* in origin (a) when they are lined with stratified squamous epithelium and produce whorled keratin or *pilar* or *sebaceous* (b) when no mature granular layer is present and keratin is not produced.

D *Sessile*. The sessile tumour has a broad base. If encapsulated and freely mobile it is probably non-malignant. May be ulcerated if in an area subjected to pressure.

E *Verrucose*. These are warty tumours which may be malignant or benign. Viral papillomata of young dogs are characteristically verrucose and malignant because of their viral aetiology.

F *Umbilicate*. Sessile tumours with a central dimple.

G *Pedunculate*. These are usually benign tumours with a definite constricted 'neck'.

Ulcer Loss of integrity of the epidermis to expose the moist dermis and underlying structures which quickly become

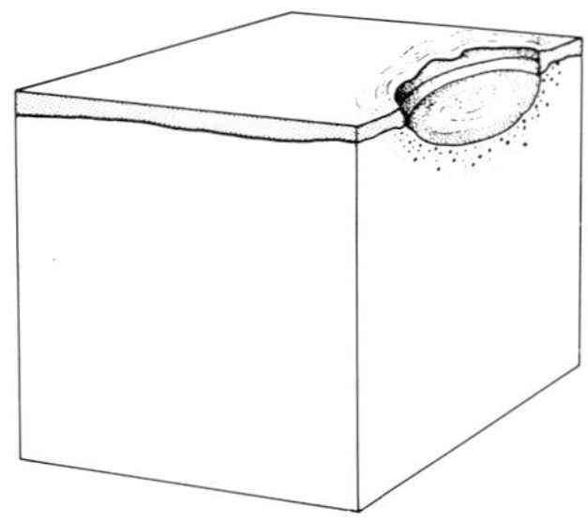

Ulcer.

secondarily infected. They often heal indolently. Ulcers may result from pressure, self-excoriation or chemical damage.

Urticaria A skin condition characterized by the formation of oedematous plaques or wheals.

Vasculitis Inflammatory vascular changes usually associated with hypersensitivity reactions and recognized by thickening and endothelial swelling accompanied by infiltration of the walls of the vessels by neutrophils, eosinophils and erythrocytes.

Verrucose Wart-like.

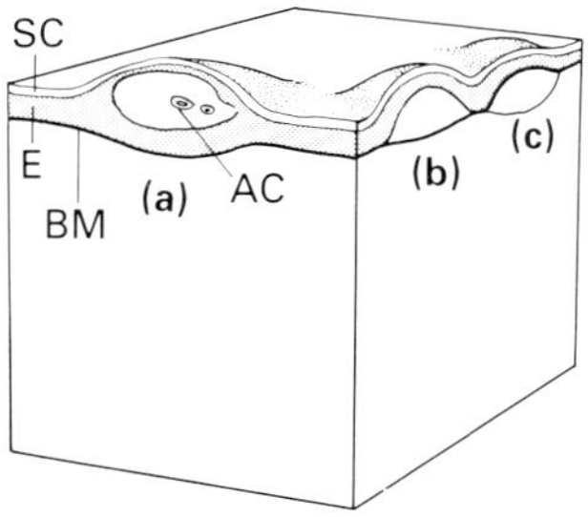

Vesicle.

Vesicle Spherical elevation containing clear fluid. They are small, easily ruptured and may form either subcorneally (SC), intra-epidermally, at the dermo-epidermal junction or subepidermally. (a) Cavity containing fluid within the epidermis (E) formed as a result of an autoimmune reaction. Free epidermal cells may be seen. (b) An autoimmune reaction may occur at the basement membrane (BM) level. (c) Vesicles may be the result of allergic and other reactions in the dermis, with the formation of serous fluid, e.g. contact allergy, irritant plant or animal hairs.

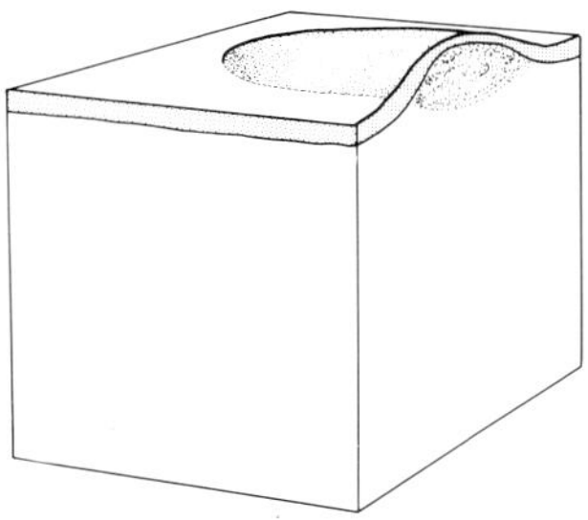

Wheal.

Vibrissae Long, coarse tactile hairs. Whiskers found mainly around the muzzle.

Vitiligo Acquired patchy loss of pigment.

Wheal A circumscribed area of dermal oedema. They may result from trauma or insect bites, for example. Pressure on the wheal by a glass slide produces blanching diascopy and some flattening. See *Urticaria*.

Index

Box - 1+1+1+1+1+1+1+1+1+1+1+1

Books - 10+10+10+10+10+10+10+10+10+10+12+10

=122

N-15015